Case Studies in Vascular Medicine

Case Studies in Vascular Medicine

Editor: Sebastian Edwards

AMERICAN
MEDICAL PUBLISHERS
www.americanmedicalpublishers.com

AMERICAN
MEDICAL PUBLISHERS
www.americanmedicalpublishers.com

Cataloging-in-Publication Data

Case studies in vascular medicine / edited by Sebastian Edwards.
p. cm.
Includes bibliographical references and index.
ISBN 979-8-88740-619-0
1. Blood-vessels--Diseases. 2. Peripheral vascular diseases. 3. Cardiology.
I. Edwards, Sebastian.
RC691 .V38 2023
616.13--dc23

American Medical Publishers,
41 Flatbush Avenue,
1st Floor, New York,
NY 11217, USA

ISBN 979-8-88740-619-0 (Hardback)

Contents

Preface

In my initial years as a student, I used to run to the library at every possible instance to grab a book and learn something new. Books were my primary source of knowledge and I would not have come such a long way without all that I learnt from them. Thus, when I was approached to edit this book; I became understandably nostalgic. It was an absolute honor to be considered worthy of guiding the current generation as well as those to come. I put all my knowledge and hard work into making this book most beneficial for its readers.

Vascular medicine is an area of medical science that involves the diagnosis and management of diseases affecting the blood vessels, including arteries, veins, and lymphatic vessels. The blood vessels play a crucial role in the transport of oxygen, nutrients, and waste products within the body. Vascular diseases can disrupt this important function, leading to a range of health issues. Some of the common vascular conditions are peripheral artery disease (PAD), deep vein thrombosis (DVT), varicose veins, venous insufficiency, and aneurysms. Vascular medicine utilizes various diagnostic tools, such as ultrasound, computed tomography (CT) and magnetic resonance imaging (MRI), to assess the structure and function of blood vessels. This book unfolds the innovative aspects of vascular medicine which will be crucial for the progress of this field in the future. Those in search of information to further their knowledge will be greatly assisted by it.

I wish to thank my publisher for supporting me at every step. I would also like to thank all the authors who have contributed their researches in this book. I hope this book will be a valuable contribution to the progress of the field.

Editor

1

Angiographic Embolization with Histoacryl in Combination with Direct Injection of Bone Cement of an Intraosseous Venous Malformation of the Mandible: Report of a Case with 22-Year Follow-Up

Antoine Berberi,[1] Georges Aoun,[2] Georges Aad,[2] Saad Khairallah,[3] and Ghassan Abi Chedid[4]

[1]*Department of Oral and Maxillofacial Surgery, Faculty of Dental Medicine, Lebanese University, Lebanon*
[2]*Department of Oral Medicine and Maxillofacial Radiology, Faculty of Dental Medicine, Lebanese University, Lebanon*
[3]*Department of Pathology, Faculty of Medicine, Lebanese University and Director Institute National de Pathology, Lebanon*
[4]*Department of Radiology, Sacre-Coeur Hospital, Baada Lebanon and Head Department of Medical Imaging, Lebanese German University, Beirut, Lebanon*

Correspondence should be addressed to Antoine Berberi; aberberi@ul.edu.lb

Academic Editor: Hiroyuki Nakajima

Vascular malformations of the maxillofacial region are unusual, and they occur more rarely in bone than in soft tissue. Mandibular intraosseous vascular lesions represent 0.5-1.0% of all bone tumors, and they are classified as venous malformation, lymphatic malformation, arterial malformation, arteriovenous malformations, and arteriovenous fistulae. Venous malformation is the most common vascular malformation, accounting for 44-64% of all vascular malformations, and is considered a low-flow malformation. Endovascular therapy as selective angiographic embolization is considered as the first-choice treatment associated or not with emboli injections with a success rate of 70%, and this evades mutilating surgery and related sequelae. We report a case of mandibular venous malformation on a 45-year-old female complaining of unilateral swelling of the left body of the mandible with facial deformation. The computed tomography scan images and the T1-weighted MR images showed a lesion that expresses an expansible lesion in the spongy bone of the left of the mandible with a buccal cortical rupture. Signal voids were not identified, suggesting a low-flow vascular lesion. The T2-weighted images exposed hypersignals; accordingly, a vascular lesion was suspected. The treatment was done under locoregional analgesia; after selective angiography, direct histoacryl injection was completed, followed by bone cement injection. The patient was followed yearly since1998. Radiological images of 10-year follow-up MRI showed a stabilization of the lesion without any new extensions. The panoramic radiograph after 22 years showed a bone formation inside the body of the mandible. The long follow-up period and the absence of any complications are favorable for the adopted treatment plan.

1. Introduction

Vascular lesions were considered as hemangiomas before the1980s, and it was in 1982 that Mulliken and Glowacki proposed a classification for vascular anomalies based on pathological features [1]. Afterwards, the International Society for the Study of Vascular Anomalies (ISSVA) updated the old classification and splits vascular anomalies into two categories: vasoproliferative neoplasms (VN) and vascular malformations (VM) [2].

VMs include capillary malformation (CM), venous malformation (VM) (intraosseous vascular malformation), lymphatic malformation (LM), arterial malformation (AM), arteriovenous malformations (AVM), and arteriovenous fistulae (AVF) [2].

In addition, VMs can be divided based on the degree of blood flow: "slow flow" (CM, VM, or LM), "fast flow" (AM, AVM, or AVF), and combined vascular malformations [3].

VMs are the most common vascular malformation, accounting for 44-64% of all vascular malformations, and are considered as low-flow malformations [4].

Management of VMs is very complex and needs a multidisciplinary team for successful results [5]. At present, super-selective angiographic embolization is considered as the first-choice treatment [6, 7], in association with injectable embolic [8–10].

We describe a case of intraosseous multilocular VM of the mandible where a conservative treatment was applied with a follow-up period of 22 years.

2. Case Report

A 45-year-old female was oriented to our department complaining of unilateral swelling of the left body of the mandible with facial deformation.

Clinical exam revealed a well-delimited hard swelling at the left of the mandible (body and angle) with submandibular adenopathy. Intraorally, a hard tumefaction that fills the buccal posterior area of the mandible was noticed. Mobility scale 3 of the second premolar was observed, and no paresthesia was noted (Figures 1(a) and 1(b)).

History reveals that the swelling started three years ago without any pain, and the left mandibular first and second molars were extracted as they were mobile without any complications or hemorrhage.

A 2D-panoramic radiograph showed then a well-defined multilocular radiolucency, spreading from the left mandibular mental nerve region anteriorly to the ramus posteriorly; small loculations and fine trabeculae were noted inside the lesion (Figure 2(a)).

Blood test analysis was performed, and the results were in the range of normality (bleeding time: 2 min; blood platelet count: 322 K/μL).

The differential diagnosis varies between ameloblastoma, odontogenic myxoma, giant-cell granuloma, fibrous dysplasia, aneurysmal cyst, and vascular malformations.

After concertation with the patient and her family, the mobile second premolar was extracted and a biopsy of the lesion was taken through the alveolar socket. No hemorrhage was noted, but for safety, a Gelfoam® sponge was placed in the alveolar socket, stabilized with resorbable sutures, and covered with cyanoacrylate tissue glue.

The histological findings of the biopsy (×10 with hematoxylin and eosin coloration) showed a single layer of endothelial cells lining the dilated vascular spaces with mild inflammatory polymorphous leucocytic infiltrates in the surrounding tissue with thin-walled and dilated vascular spaces of variable diameter (Figures 2(b) and 2(c)).

Following the clinical, radiological, and histological results, a CT scan and MRI were requested to determine the soft and hard tissue extensions of the lesions.

2.1. CT Scan and MRI Examinations. The CT scan images presented an expansible multilocular lesion with a distinct periosteum reaction on the buccal cortical bone. No loculations were detected, and the axial images displayed a trabeculated lesion in the body of the left mandible (Figure 2(d)).

MRI images with 1.5 T using routine T1- and T2-weighted spin-echo sequences showed the existence of a lesion of the entire left part of the body of the mandible and extending to the ramus without reaching the condyle.

The T1-weighted MR images showed a lesion with hyposignals that express an expansible lesion in the spongy bone of the left of the mandible with a buccal cortical rupture. Signal voids were not identified, suggesting a low-flow vascular lesion (Figure 2(e)).

The T2-weighted images exposed hypersignals; accordingly, a vascular lesion was suspected. Axial cuts displayed high signal intensity and an expansible lesion in the bone marrow of the left hemimandible, with a buccal bone discontinuity and extension towards the soft parts of the vestibular edge of the mandible, producing a subcutaneous tumefaction. Inner loculations were present in the axial cuts suggesting multilocularity (Figure 2(f)).

Clinical, radiological, and histological findings leaded to a conservative treatment, based on embolization and bone cement injections. The treatment plan was suggested and discussed with the patient and her family who signed a consent form.

2.2. Angiography/Embolization/Bone Cement Injection. Angiography, through a transfemoral approach, was achieved under local anesthesia in the hospital, and selective arteriography of the left external carotid artery was performed.

Digital subtraction angiograms clearly displayed the facial and its branches, inferior alveolar, and left lingual arteries (Figure 3(a)).

After this and under locoregional analgesia of the left mandible, direct histoacryl injection was completed with a low speed under fluoroscopy monitoring, in the angiographic suite through a percutaneous puncture performed with a 22-gauge puncture needle.

The volume of the histoacryl used varied around 4 to 5 ml (diluted 25% with lipiodol) (Figures 3(b) and 3(c)).

Then, bone cement with gentamicin (CMW3™) mixed with lipiodol was injected through the same 22-gauge puncture needle, first in the posterior part of the lesion (Figure 3(d)), followed by the anterior part (Figure 3(e)).

The percutaneous injections revealed abnormal venous lakes or pouch which depicts the venous lesion.

No complications were noted in the postoperative period, and the patient was discharged the same day. The patient was followed yearly from 1998 till 2020 (Figures 4(a)–4(d)).

The swelling was maintained with the same volume, and the only difficulties were losing her mandibular teeth.

Radiological images of 10-year follow-up MRI showed a stabilization of the lesion without any new extensions (Figures 5(a) and 5(b)).

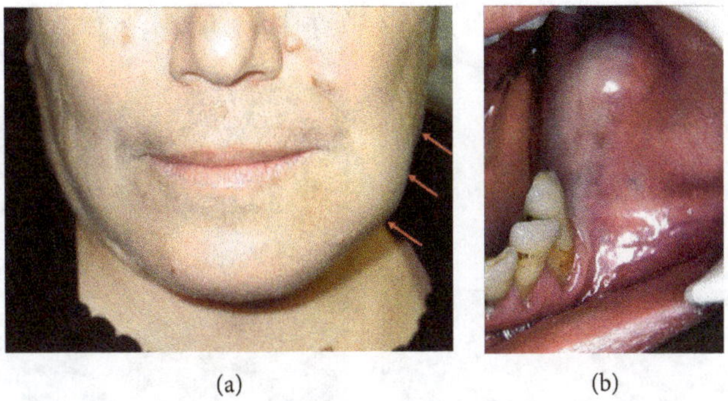

Figure 1: (a) Facial deformation in regard with the left mandible. (b) Tumefaction filling the buccal posterior area of the mandible.

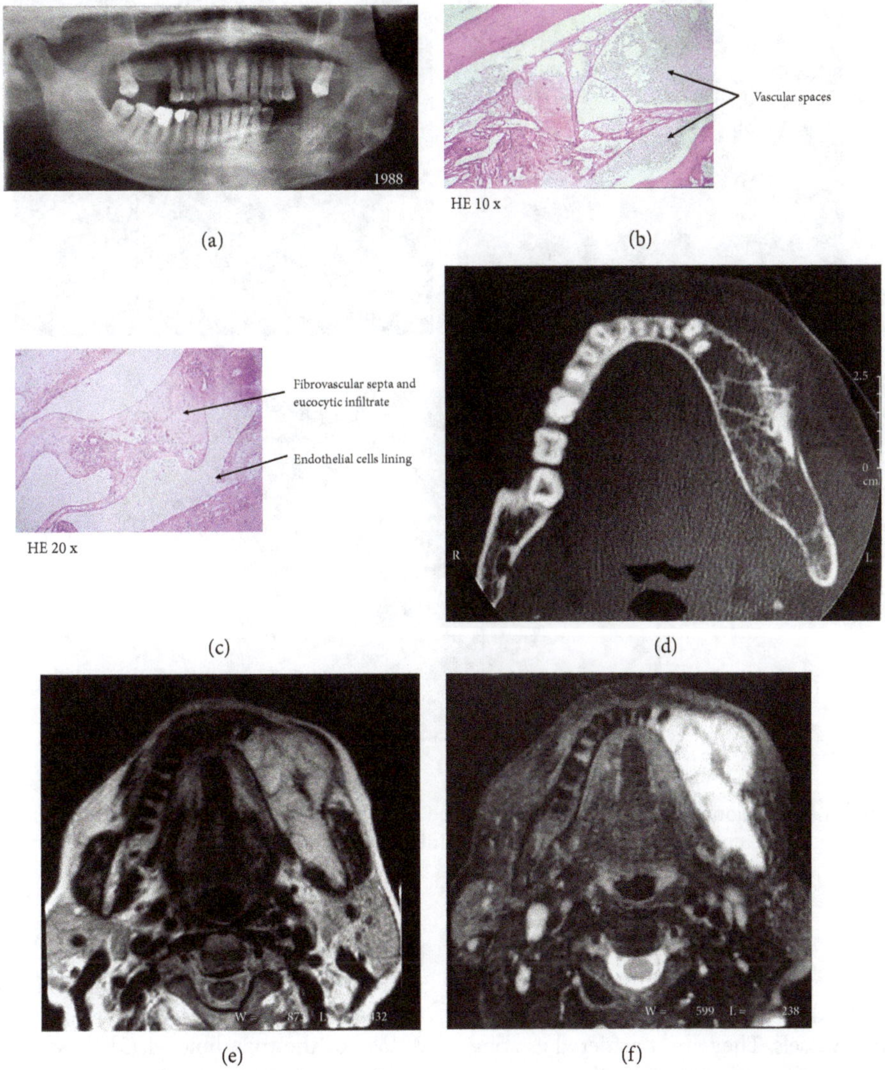

Figure 2: (a) Panoramic radiograph showing a well-defined multilocular radiolucency extending from the mental nerve region to the ramus. (b) Thin-walled and dilated vascular spaces of variable diameter (HE ×10). (c) Regular endothelial lining of the vascular spaces with mild inflammatory polymorphous leucocytic infiltrates in the surrounding tissue (HE ×20). (d) An axial CT image showing an expansible multilocular radiolucency lesion with periosteal reaction on the buccal cortex. (e) An axial T2WI MR image revealing a hyposignal intensity expansible low-intensity lesion in the marrow of the left hemimandible with cortical rupture and soft tissue extension. (f) An axial T2 WI FSE image presented a hypersignal and expansible lesion with internal loculations suggesting a multilocular lesion.

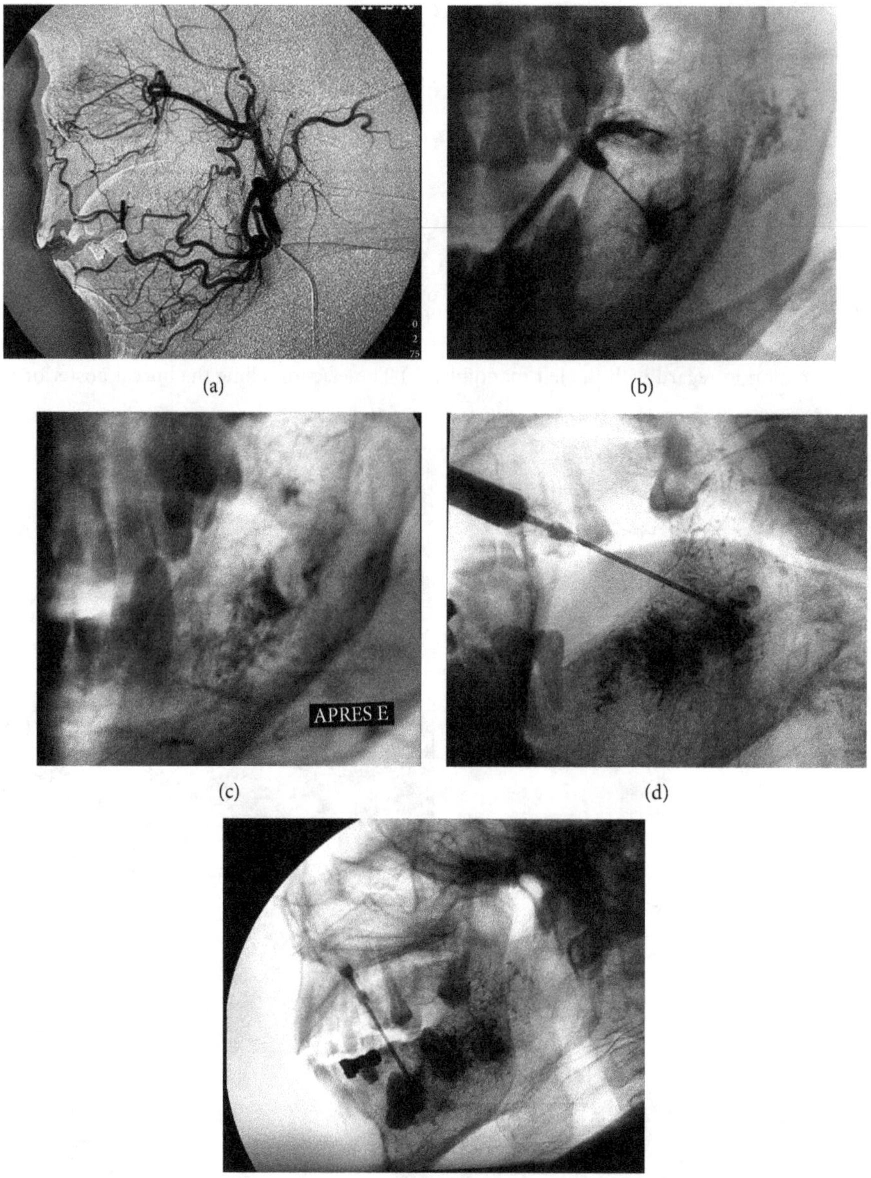

Figure 3: (a) Lateral digital subtraction angiography image displayed the inferior alveolar and lingual arteries. (b) Direct intraosseous histoacryl injection. (c) Image after ending of histoacryl injection. Intraosseous injection of CMW3™ (d) in the posterior part of the lesion and (e) in the anterior part.

3. Discussion

VMs are characterized by the irregular proliferation of endothelial cells of the blood vessels. They are considered as congenital inaccuracies of vascular morphogenesis that result in fragile endothelial cell proliferation inside the network of blood vessels [2].

VMs appear more frequently in soft tissue than in bone. In the mandible, they are very rare and represent only 0.2–1.0% of all intraosseous tumors, and the most common symptoms are pain, swelling, and tooth mobilities [5, 11]. Previous studies suggested that VMs appear more commonly in females than in males (ratio 3/1) [4]. Zlotogorski et al. reported that the molar region and angle of the mandible are affected in 69%, and the lesions were multilocular in 66% and unilocular in 33%, and 1% demonstrated a sunray radiographic shape [12].

Surgery is considered as the last treatment choice for AVMs of the mandible [4, 5]. Resection with block of the affected area in the mandible or maxilla has been proposed, and rehabilitation with autogenous or alloplastic bone materials has been recommended [13].

Endovascular therapy has been proposed for the treatment of the mandibular VMs with a success rate of 70%, and this evades mutilating surgery and related sequelae [4, 5]. Additionally, embolization can maintain functional anatomy and morphology [5].

Injection of emboli is suggested in a direct intraosseous technique; embolization should be achieved before to reduce

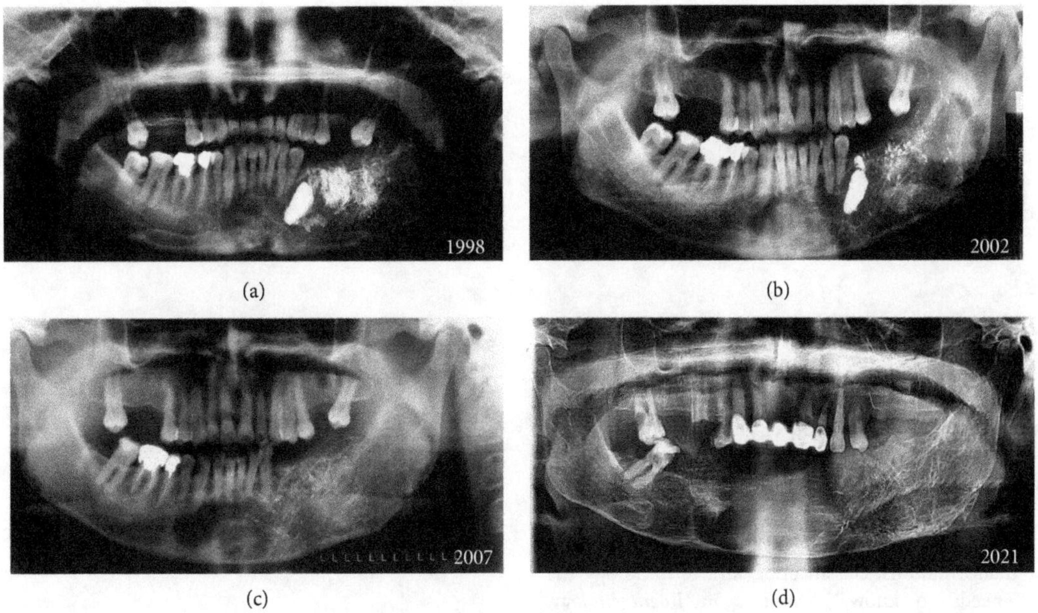

Figure 4: (a) The same day panoramic radiograph. (b) 4-year panoramic radiograph. (c) 9-year panoramic radiograph. (d) 22-year panoramic radiograph; note the calcification inside the lesion.

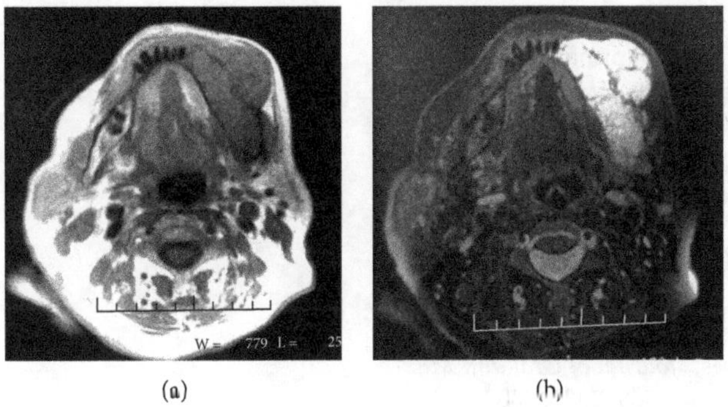

Figure 5: 10-year MRI images: (a) after an axial T1WI MR image showing the stabilization of the old lesion; (b) an axial T2WI image presented the same hypersignals and expansible lesion.

the blood flow and to admit more precise accumulation of bone cement inside the lesion [7].

The biomaterials used as injectable embolic for the treatment of vascular lesions are intended to become occlusive by provoking thrombosis or directly obstructing the lesion when hardening of the embolic appears [14].

Different biomaterials have been used such as polymethylmethacrylate, n-butyl-2-cyanoacrylate, cellulose acetate polymer, fibrin glue, and bone cement [10].

In general, intraosseous VMs display hyposignals on T1WI and hypersignals on T2WI [15]. Slow-flow VMs are categorized by a varied intermediate signal without flow, voids on T1WI, and hypersignals on T2WI [15]. On T2WI, the lesions show well-defined borders and high contrast with the surroundings, with the lesion appearing as multispatial or multicystic [15].

The present case displayed homogenous hyposignals on T1WI and hypersignals on T2WI. The absence of signal voids advocates that we are facing a vascular malformation classified as a slow-flow lesion.

The MR images showed that the lesion was multilocular with bone cortical discontinuity with extension to the soft tissue.

The conservative treatment adopted a superselective angiographic embolization with the direct injection of histoacryl mixed with lipiodol and followed with the injection of bone cement in the two parts of the lesion. The first step reduces blood flow, and the second step is aimed at inducing thrombosis and at directly blocking the lesion.

The MR images 10 years later revealed stabilization of the size and extensions of the lesion. The panoramic radiograph after 22 years showed a bone formation inside the body of the mandible. The long follow-up period and the absence of any complications are favorable for the adopted treatment plan.

4. Conclusion

VMs need a very close multidisciplinary collaboration involving interventional radiology, otorhinolaryngology, oral/maxillofacial surgery, and plastic surgery in the arrangement and application of an appropriate treatment plan for these lesions.

Consent

Patient signed the consent.

References

[1] J. B. Mulliken and J. Glowacki, "Hemangiomas and vascular malformations in infants and children," *Plastic and Reconstructive Surgery*, vol. 69, no. 3, pp. 412–420, 1982.

[2] M. Wassef, M. Borsik, P. Cerceau et al., "Classification des tumeurs et malformations vasculaires. Apport de la classification ISSVA 2014/2018," *Annales de Pathologie*, vol. 41, no. 1, pp. 58–70, 2021.

[3] L. H. Lowe, T. C. Marchant, D. C. Rivard, and A. J. Scherbel, "Vascular malformations: classification and terminology the radiologist needs to know," *Seminars in Roentgenology*, vol. 47, no. 2, pp. 106–117, 2012.

[4] S. Behravesh, W. Yakes, N. Gupta et al., "Venous malformations: clinical diagnosis and treatment," *Cardiovascular Diagnosis and Therapy*, vol. 6, no. 6, pp. 557–569, 2016.

[5] J. W. Zheng, H. M. Mai, L. Zhang et al., "Guidelines for the treatment of head and neck venous malformations," *International Journal of Clinical and Experimental Medicine*, vol. 6, no. 5, pp. 377–389, 2013.

[6] X. D. Fan, L. X. Su, J. W. Zheng, L. Z. Zheng, and Z. Y. Zhang, "Ethanol embolization of arteriovenous malformations of the mandible," *AJNR. American Journal of Neuroradiology*, vol. 30, no. 6, pp. 1178–1183, 2009.

[7] D. Liu, X. Ma, F. Zhao, and J. Zhang, "Intraosseous embolotherapy of central arteriovenous malformations in the jaw: long-term experience with 8 cases," *Journal of Oral and Maxillofacial Surgery*, vol. 67, no. 11, pp. 2380–2387, 2009.

[8] V. Gluncic, R. R. Reid, F. M. Baroody, L. J. Gottlieb, and S. A. Ansari, "Hemostasis and obliteration of mandibular arteriovenous malformation through direct hydroxyapatite cement injection into the molar cavity," *Journal of NeuroInterventional Surgery*, vol. 3, no. 1, pp. 92–94, 2011.

[9] K. Öztürk, S. Göde, G. Gürsan, G. Turhal, C. Çınar, and H. Bozkaya, "Obliteration of a large mandibular arteriovenous malformation with polymethyl methacrylate bone cement," *Turkish Archives of Otorhinolaryngology*, vol. 53, no. 2, pp. 80–83, 2015.

[10] O. Jordan, E. Doelker, and D. A. Rüfenacht, "Biomaterials used in injectable implants (liquid embolics) for percutaneous filling of vascular spaces," *Cardiovascular and Interventional Radiology*, vol. 28, no. 5, pp. 561–569, 2005.

[11] S. Okura, C. Igarashi, S. Wakae-Morita et al., "A case of venous malformation of the mandible," *Oral Radiology*, vol. 35, no. 2, pp. 194–197, 2019.

[12] A. Zlotogorski, A. Buchner, I. Kaffe, and D. Schwartz-Arad, "Radiological features of central haemangioma of the jaws," *Dento Maxillo Facial Radiology*, vol. 34, no. 5, pp. 292–296, 2005.

[13] S. Akita, K. Akino, K. Tanaka, K. Anraku, H. Yano, and A. Hirano, "Therapeutic choice for craniofacial venous malformations," *The Journal of Craniofacial Surgery*, vol. 17, no. 4, pp. 729–735, 2006.

[14] A. Laurent and L. Moine, "Les nouveaux biomatériaux de l'embolisation," *Medical Science (Paris)*, vol. 33, no. 1, pp. 25–31, 2017.

[15] N. Kakimoto, K. Tanimoto, H. Nishiyama, S. Murakami, S. Furukawa, and S. Kreiborg, "CT and MR imaging features of oral and maxillofacial hemangioma and vascular malformation," *European Journal of Radiology*, vol. 55, no. 1, pp. 108–112, 2005.

2

Renal Artery Thrombectomy Causing Functional and Symptomatic Recovery after 50-Hour Delay in Reperfusion of Acute Main Renal Artery Thrombosis

Kevin Singh Kang[1] and John Steven Wilson[2]

[1]*Department of Cardiology, University of Pittsburgh Medical Center Hamot, Erie, PA 16550, USA*
[2]*Department of Cardiology, Meadville Medical Center, Meadville, PA, USA*

Correspondence should be addressed to Kevin Singh Kang; kevinsinghkang@gmail.com

Academic Editor: Hiroyuki Nakajima

Acute renal artery thrombosis is rare and even rarer in the thrombus occluding the main renal artery and compromising the entire kidney. We report on a 46-year-old female smoker with no past medical history and no hypercoagulability who developed sudden severe left flank pain, hematuria, acute renal failure, and severe hypertension. A CT angiogram showed totally occluded renal artery at the ostium with a thrombus and severely hypoperfused left kidney with multiple infarcts. Initial course of treatment was with intravenous heparin but with no improvement after 50 hours since symptom onset; angiography was done. This revealed totally occluded renal artery at ostium with no vessels or kidney blush seen. After aspiration thrombectomy, blush was seen in kidney parenchyma along with flow in the arcuate renal arteries although with some distal embolic events. The ostial lesion was treated with a drug eluting stent with excellent result angiographically. However, 8 months later, severe restenosis occurred. This time, the patient did not flank pain or renal failure but had progressive hypertension. The patient was treated this time with rheolytic thrombectomy followed by intravascular ultrasound-guided drug-eluting stenting. The patient has been followed for a year and a half since and recent CT scan revealed widely patent renal arteries bilaterally with normal kidney function, BP, and good perfusion to the left kidney with only tiny areas of infarct. Ultrasound of the kidneys also showed the size of the left kidney as within normal range now, and she has good distal flow velocities in the branch renal arteries. Our case report shows that even delayed reperfusion of complete renal artery occlusion with jeopardized arterial flow to the entire kidney could result in restoration of function to most of the kidney.

1. Introduction

Acute renal artery occlusion is rare when involving the entire kidney due to total occlusion of the main renal artery and rarer when due to in situ thrombosis and not embolic event [1]. However, this was noted in our patient as reported here. As expected, acute renal artery occlusion would result in diffuse ischemia and risk of total kidney loss [1, 2]. As noted, embolic events from atrial fibrillation, cardiomyopathy, or valvular heart disease are far more common than in situ thrombosis [1, 3]. In our patient, there were no cardiovascular risk factors of embolic events as confirmed after a two-year follow-up, and clinically and angiographically, in situ thrombus was the most likely scenario. Additionally, the angiographic criteria based on coronary literature were suggestive of plaque rupture and thrombosis [4]. The irregular and ulcerated angiographic appearance in ostial and proximal renal artery suggested in situ thrombosis related to underlying atherosclerotic plaque [4]. The smoking history was the contributor to the plaque rupture appearance and in situ renal artery occlusion.

The diagnosis of acute main renal occlusion is difficult clinically and must be considered in patients presenting with acute renal failure, flank pain, hematuria, high LDH, and new or worsening hypertension even though fever and nausea may be seen also [5, 6]. Often, the complication may

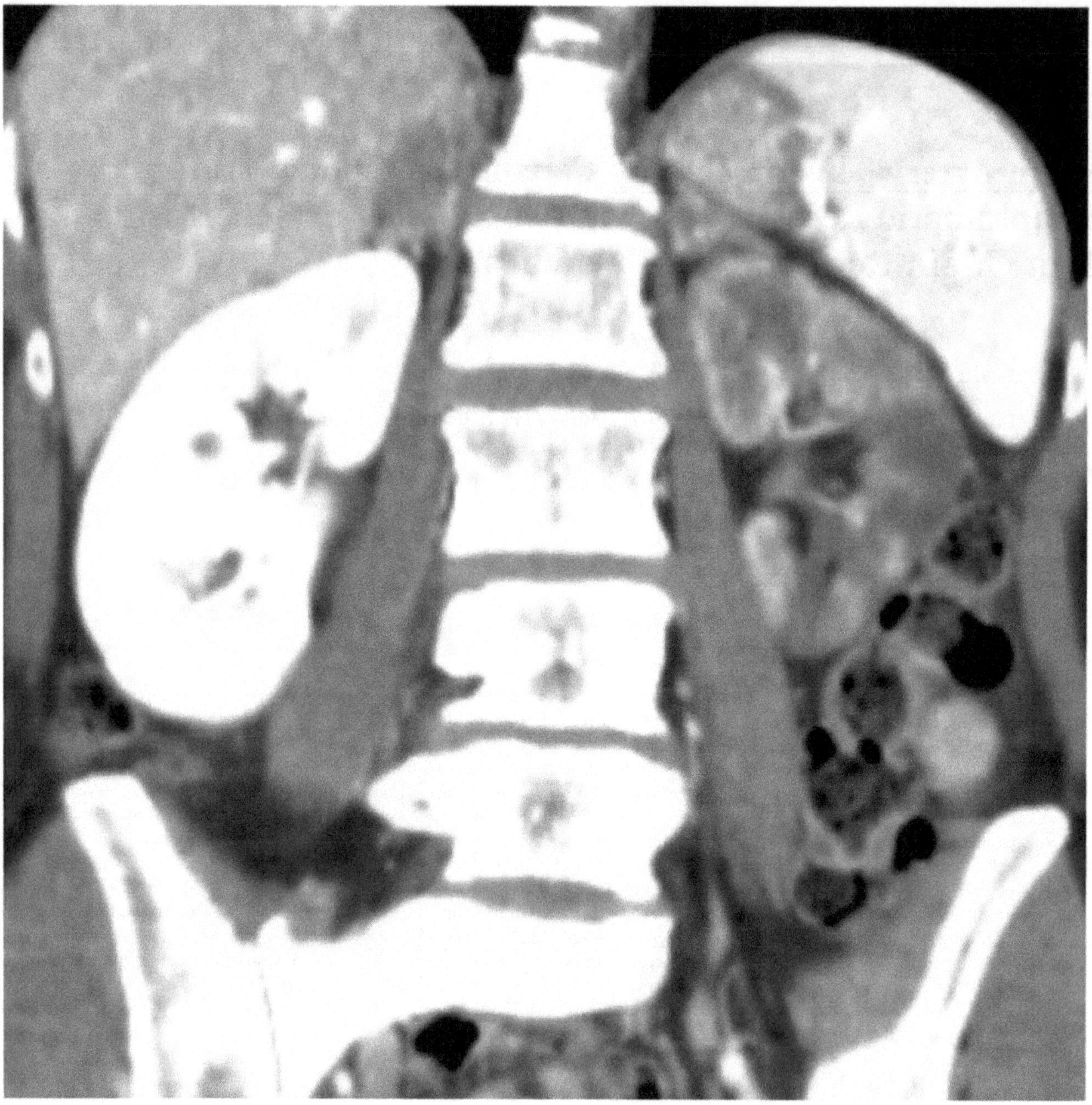

Figure 1: CT angiogram showing normal findings on the right side but the left kidney is severely hypoperfused with probably multiple renal infarcts.

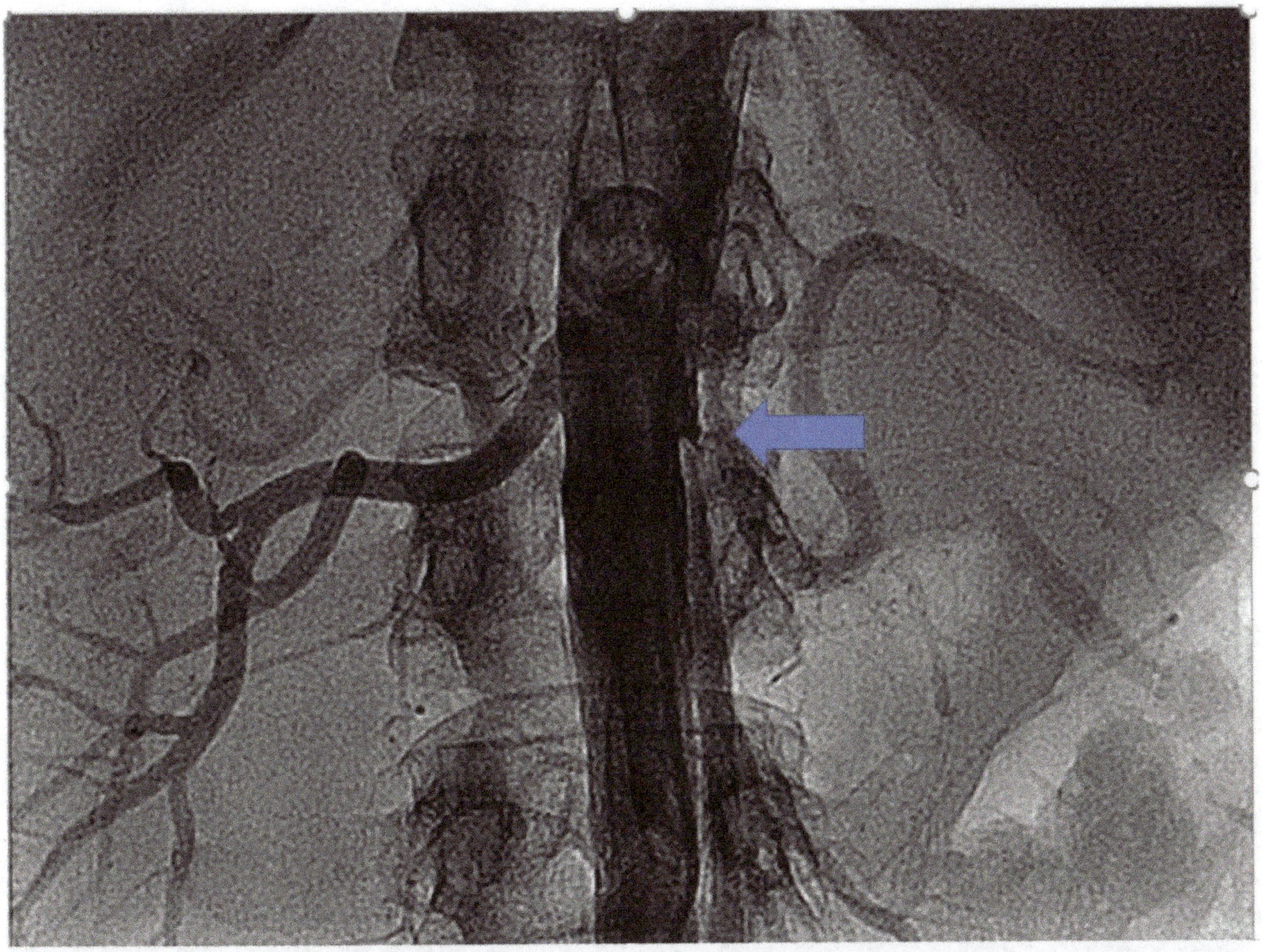

FIGURE 2: Abdominal aortic angiography revealing normal right-sided findings. In contrast, the left renal artery is totally occluded at the ostium (blue arrow) with angiographic appearance of a thrombus at the ostium with contrast staining.

arise after renal or aortic endovascular interventions due to dissection [1, 2, 6]. It is clear that if there is acute occlusion of main renal artery, early reperfusion would preserve kidney function but the benefits of late revascularization are unclear [1, 7]. There is also limited information on long-term outcomes for BP and renal function recovery after reperfusion of acute main renal artery thrombosis [1, 7].

Treatment of renal artery thrombosis is initially with anticoagulation, and the benefits are questionable [7]. The more invasive treatments after failure of anticoagulation to improve the patients signs, symptoms, and renal function are anecdotal from small retrospective series or case reports [7]. Often catheter directed thrombolysis is endorsed for the treatment of thrombotic occlusion of the main renal artery but this has been tested mostly in embolic forms of occlusion and not associated with complete restoration of renal function [1]. Since angiography would be mandated for this treatment, and our patient's angiographic as well as clinical characteristics suggested in situ thrombosis, we elected aspiration and rheolytic thrombectomy techniques. There are no data to suggest superiority of catheter directed thrombolysis over thrombectomy techniques [7, 8].

2. Case Report

We report on a 46-year-old female smoker with no past medical history and no hypercoagulability who developed sudden severe left flank pain, hematuria, acute renal failure, and severe hypertension. The symptoms had been going on for about a day prior to presentation. The patient was hypertensive, and the laboratory values showed hematuria and reduced renal function. A CT angiogram showed totally occluded renal artery at the ostium with a thrombus and severely hypoperfused left kidney suggestive of large infarcts in the left kidney (Figure 1). Initial course of treatment was anticoagulation with intravenous heparin but with no improvement over next 24 hours totaling about 48 hours prior to her onset of symptoms without kidney reperfusion. At that point, she was transferred to our hospital. Angiography was done with 6-French sheath in right common femoral artery and 6-French pigtail catheter in the abdominal aorta at the level of renal arteries; this revealed totally occluded renal artery at ostium with no visualization of distal renal arterial tree (Figure 2). There was also no renal blush noted suggestive of renal perfusion from renal artery

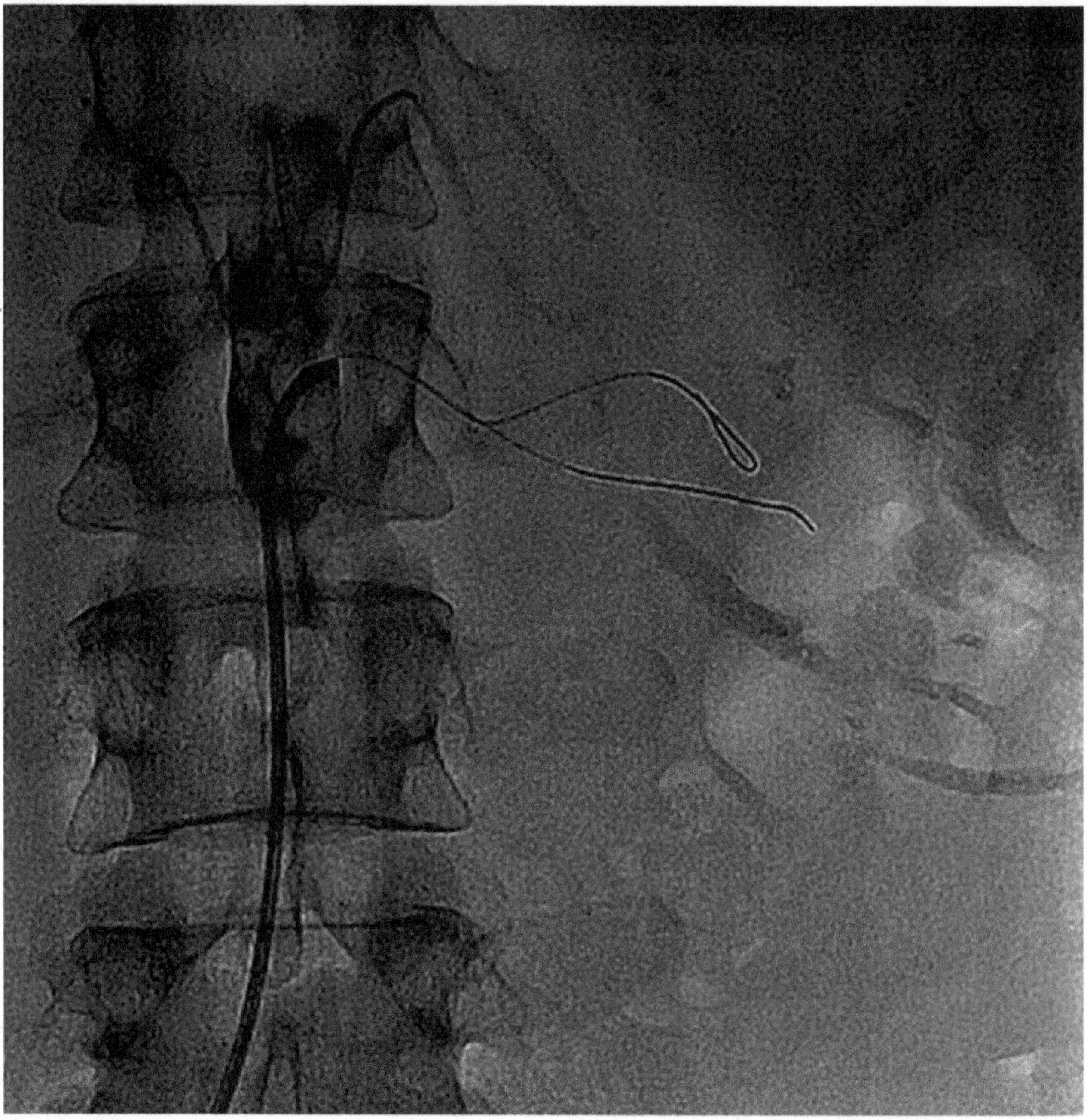

FIGURE 3: 0.014-inch wire across the occlusion still showing no renal blush and no distal arterial vasculature. Second wire placed in the renal artery due to difficulty in advancing the thrombectomy catheter into multiple distal renal artery branches to restore perfusion to multiple renal lobes.

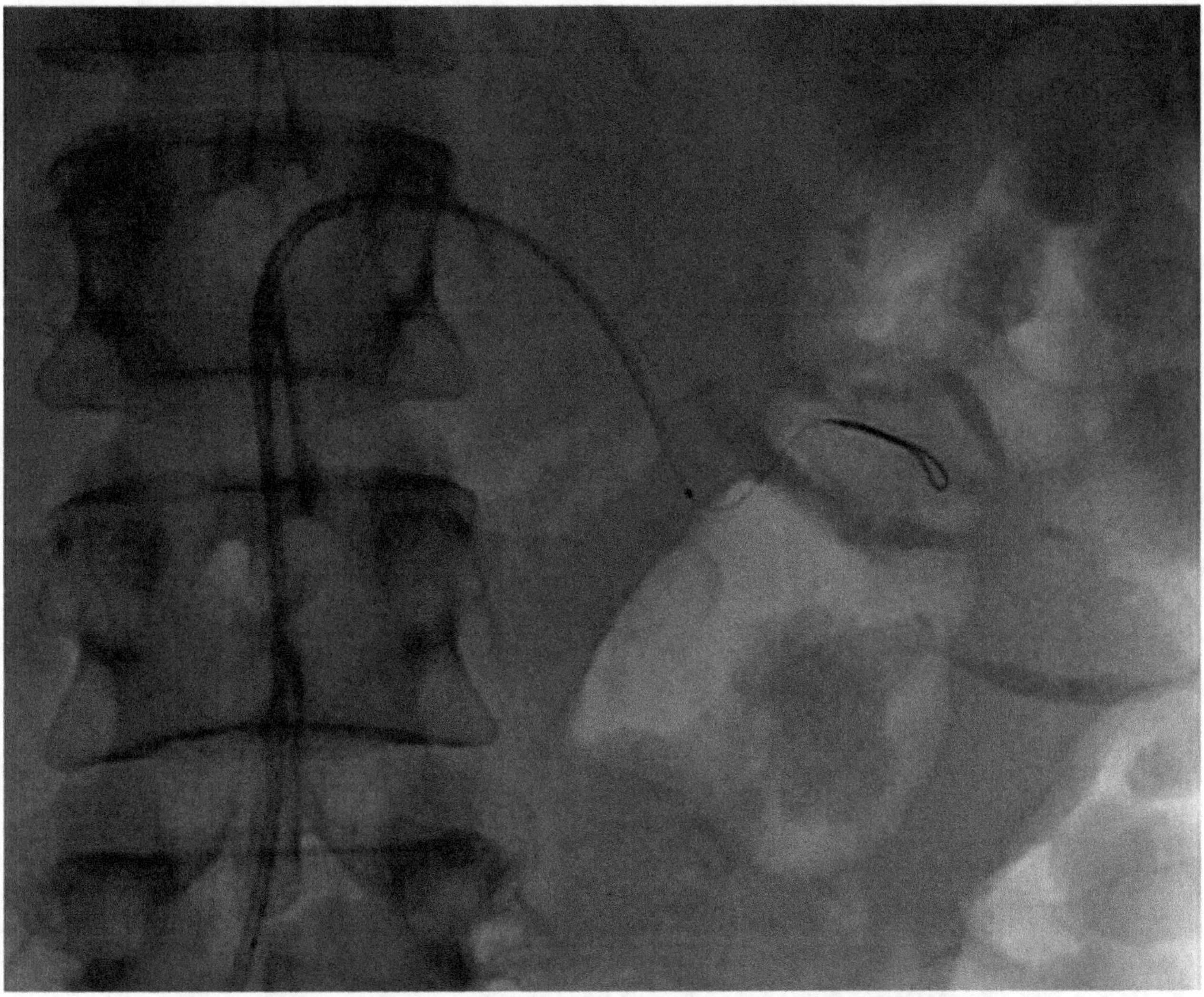

FIGURE 4: Aspiration thrombectomy catheter taken down multiple interlobar arteries.

contrast injections (Figure 3). Selective engagement of left renal artery was done with 6-French internal mammary guiding catheter, and the main renal artery total occlusion at the ostium was crossed with two 0.014-inch nonhydrophilic tipped wires and left in two different lobular branches to allow aspiration thrombectomy of multiple branches (Figure 4). The renal artery thrombus was then treated by aspiration thrombectomy with 6-French-sized Medtronic Xport aspiration catheter with removal of visible clots outside the body (Figure 4). This led to restoration of flow to the kidney, and the ostial lesion looked irregular and had an angiographic appearance of plaque rupture rather than an embolic site which would have resulted in a smooth angiographic appearance (Figure 5). Finally, blush was seen in kidney parenchyma along with flow in the arcuate renal arteries despite a distal embolic event to lobular artery noted by distal vessel cut off (Figure 6). The ostial lesion was treated with a drug eluting stent with excellent result angiographically (Figure 7). The symptoms of severe left flank pain and nausea that were present up to the initiation of procedure resolved completely by the next morning. Blood pressure (BP) was better and within normal range the next day, and the patient was noted to improve renal function. Glomerular filtration rate that was 59 (units are ml/min/ $1.73\,m^2$) on the morning of the procedure improved to 93, the next morning. A month later, CT angiogram showed much better left kidney perfusion, and the kidney was normal in size (Figure 8).

However, 8 months later, severe restenosis occurred. This time, the patient did not flank pain or renal failure but had progressive hypertension. Ultrasound of the kidney suggested severe left renal instent restenosis, and angiography was done again with the same technique showing severe instent restenosis with mil contrast staining and possible thrombus in the stent (Figure 9). The patient was treated this time with rheolytic thrombectomy using 6-French angiojet device inside the stent (Figure 10). Intravascular ultrasound (IVUS) showed severe instent intimal proliferation (Figure 11). Repeat drug eluting coronary stent was placed with widely patent left renal arterial system angiographically

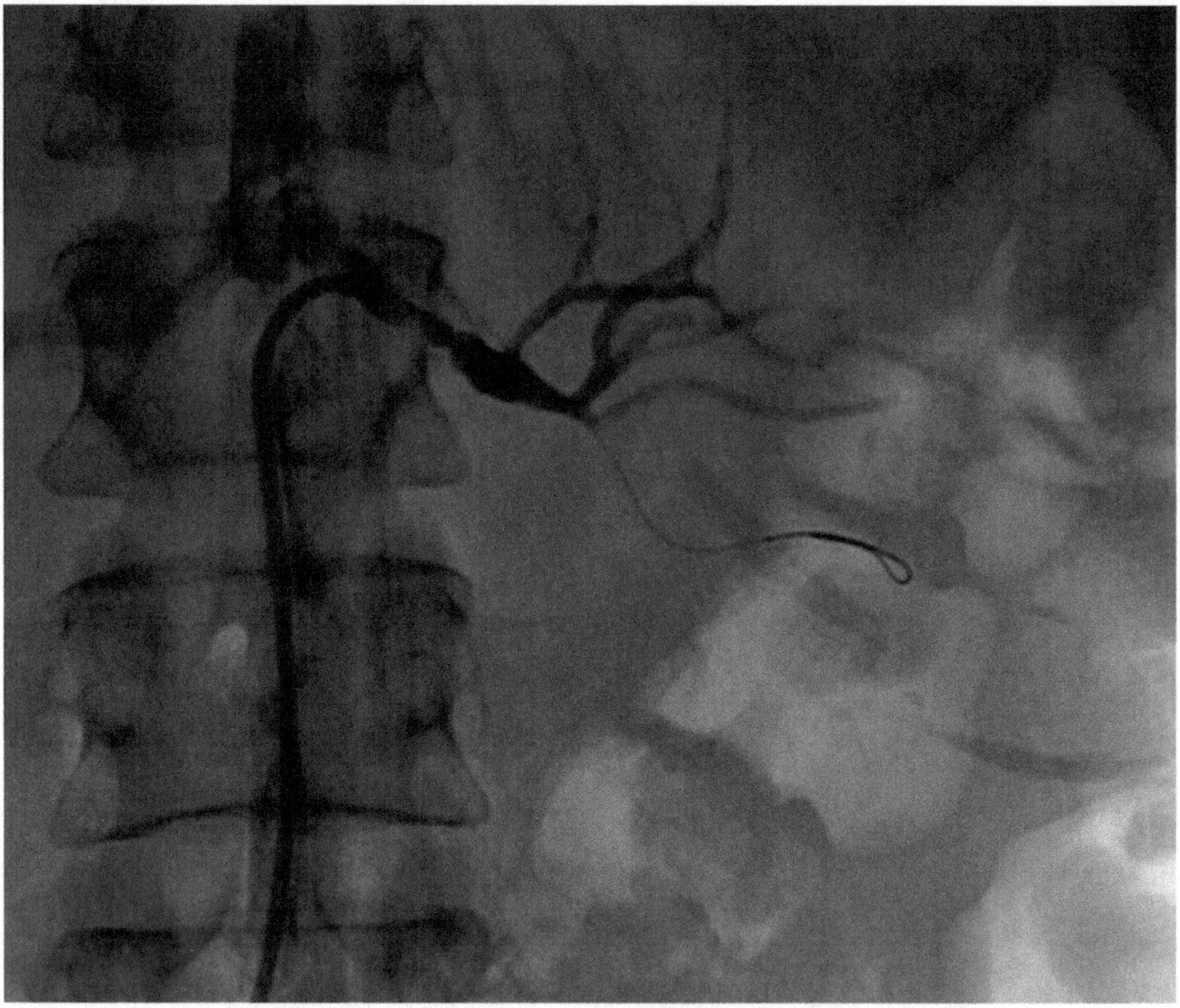

Figure 5: After aspiration thrombectomy, underlying irregular angiographic appearance looks like a plaque rupture at the ostial left renal artery suggesting in situ thrombosis rather than embolism.

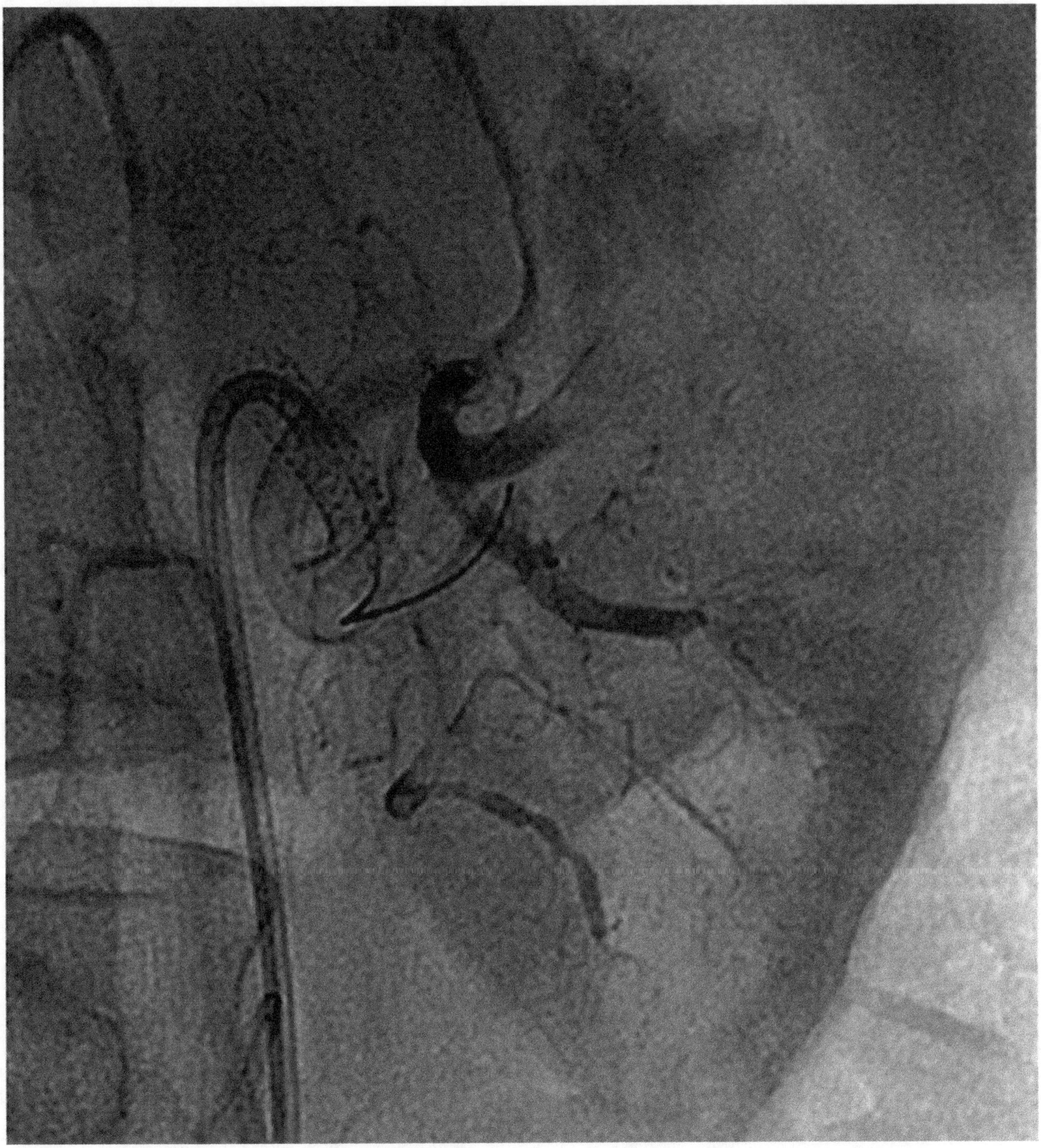

Figure 6: After stenting of the ostium, renal blush is noted.

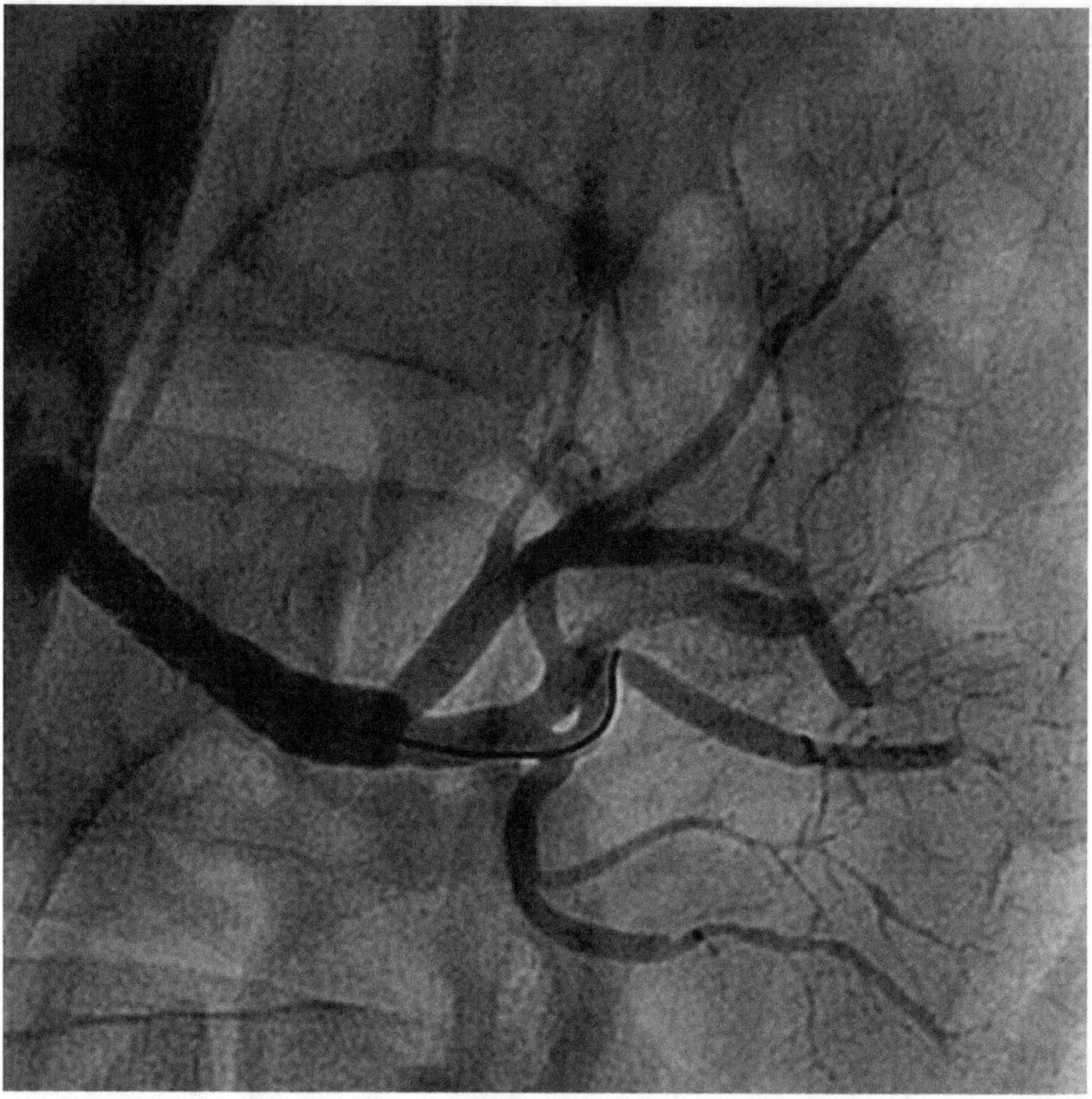

FIGURE 7: The poststent angiography reveals much better renal perfusion with patent renal lobular and arcuate arteries, but distal vessels still look in spasm and with some distal embolization.

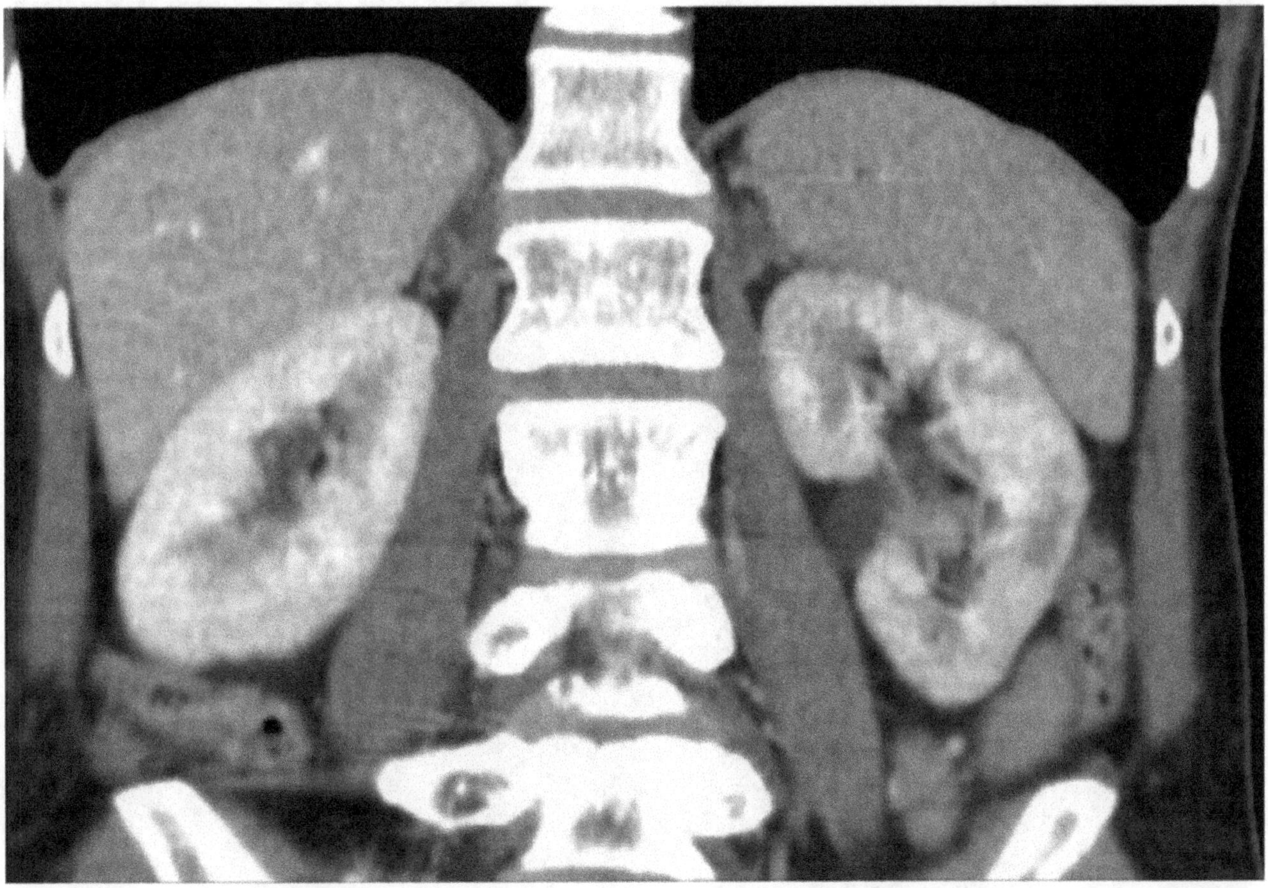

FIGURE 8: CT angiogram a month later now shows much better renal perfusion with minimal infarcts on the left side, compared to Figure 1.

(Figure 12). This was followed by repeat intravascular ultrasound showing widely patent stent lumen (Figure 13).

Follow-up CT angiogram had revealed much better perfusion to the left kidney with only a tiny area of infarct. Incidentally a nuclear cardiac stress test that was done with technetium pyrophosphate showed normal perfusion to both kidneys as well. An ultrasound of the kidneys 1 year postinitial presentation had also showed the size of left kidney as within normal range and good distal flow velocities in the branch renal arteries (Figure 14).

The patient has been followed for more than 2 years since her initial event and the recent CT scan revealed widely patent renal arteries bilaterally. On a recent outpatient visit, 49 months after initial presentation, she was asymptomatic with normal creatinine and glomerular filtration rate and with a normal BP on the same antihypertensives that had failed to control her BP in the past.

3. Discussion

Acute renal artery thrombosis causing acute renal infarction is a rare clinical syndrome and more often is related to embolic than in situ thrombus [1, 2]. Patients often have risk factors like diabetes, hypertension, spontaneous dissection, fibromuscular dysplasia, or hypercoagulability or may be post an endovascular procedure. Atrial fibrillation is a frequent association causing embolic renal arterial occlusion. Our patient had no prior medical history except for nicotine abuse, and clinical and angiographic findings favored a plaque rupture and in situ thrombosis and hence was treated with thrombectomy and drug eluting stenting [3, 4]. The diagnosis of acute renal artery thrombosis or acute renal infarct is rare and often missed due to rarity of the syndrome [3]. The patient presents often like an acute abdomen with severe abdominal pain and may be confused to have a renal stone like our patient was initially suspected to have nephrolithiasis [5, 6]. There may be acute renal failure and hypertension as in our patient especially if the entire kidney is at risk of infarct and is hypoperfused [1, 7]. There is hematuria, and LDH is high due to renal infarct [1, 5, 6]. Our patient incidentally had all these findings.

The urgency of intervention is not clear at this stage, but the previous case reports have suggested that up to 30 hours of delay in reperfusion of an occluded renal artery may result in salvage of renal function [6, 7].

Diagnosis is often delayed due to rarity of the presentation, but diagnosis can be confirmed by CT angiography (CTA), gadolinium-enhanced MRA, or renal angiography [7]. In our patient, she had a CTA that showed renal artery thrombosis of the main left renal artery at its ostium and severe hypoperfusion of the entire left kidney with initial CTA multiple infarcts in the left kidney.

Goals of therapy are symptom relief, improvement in renal function, and BP control. Most of the available

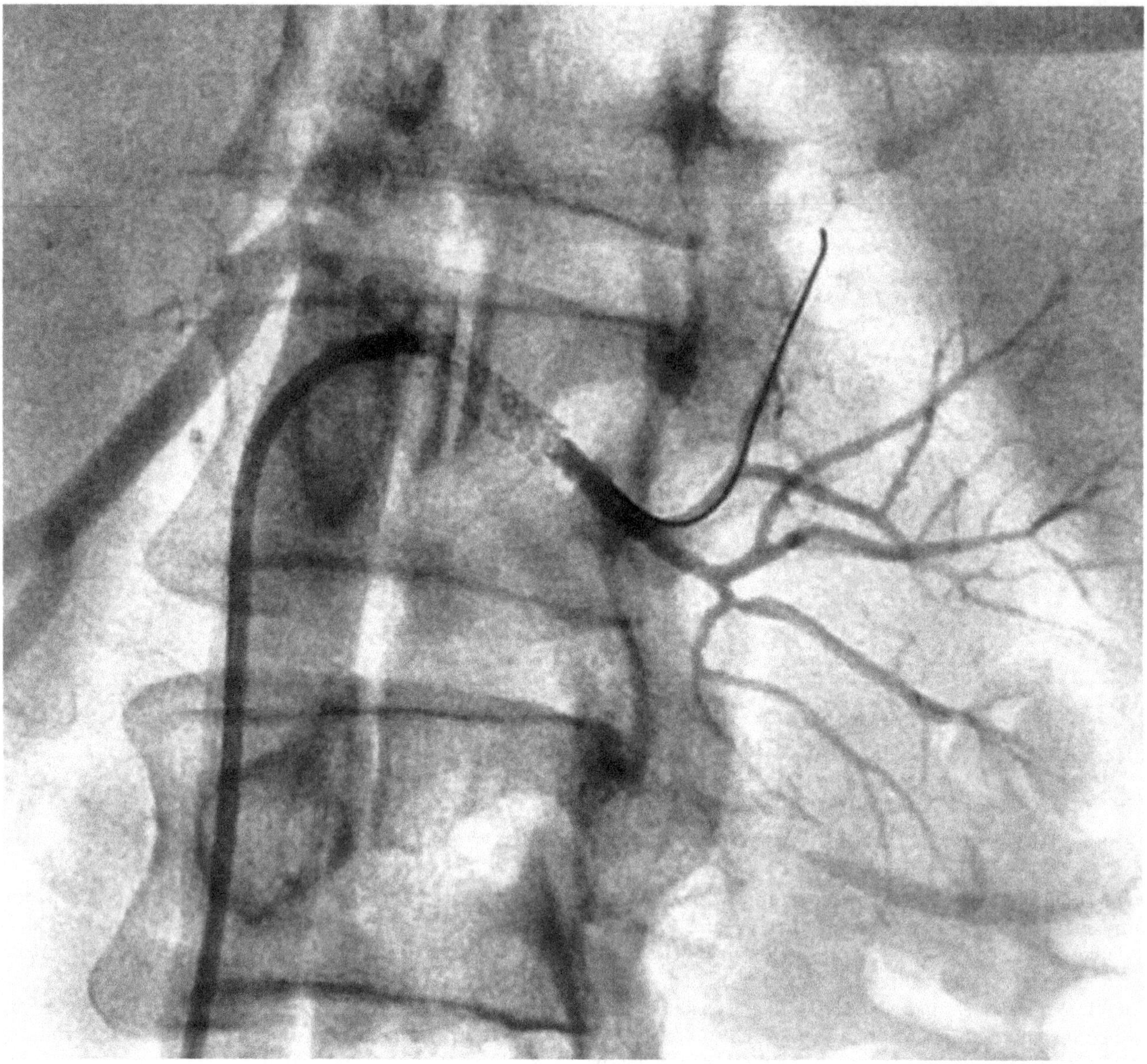

Figure 9: 8 months after atherectomy and stenting, angiography shows that the patient has severe instent restenosis with potential thrombus formation as well.

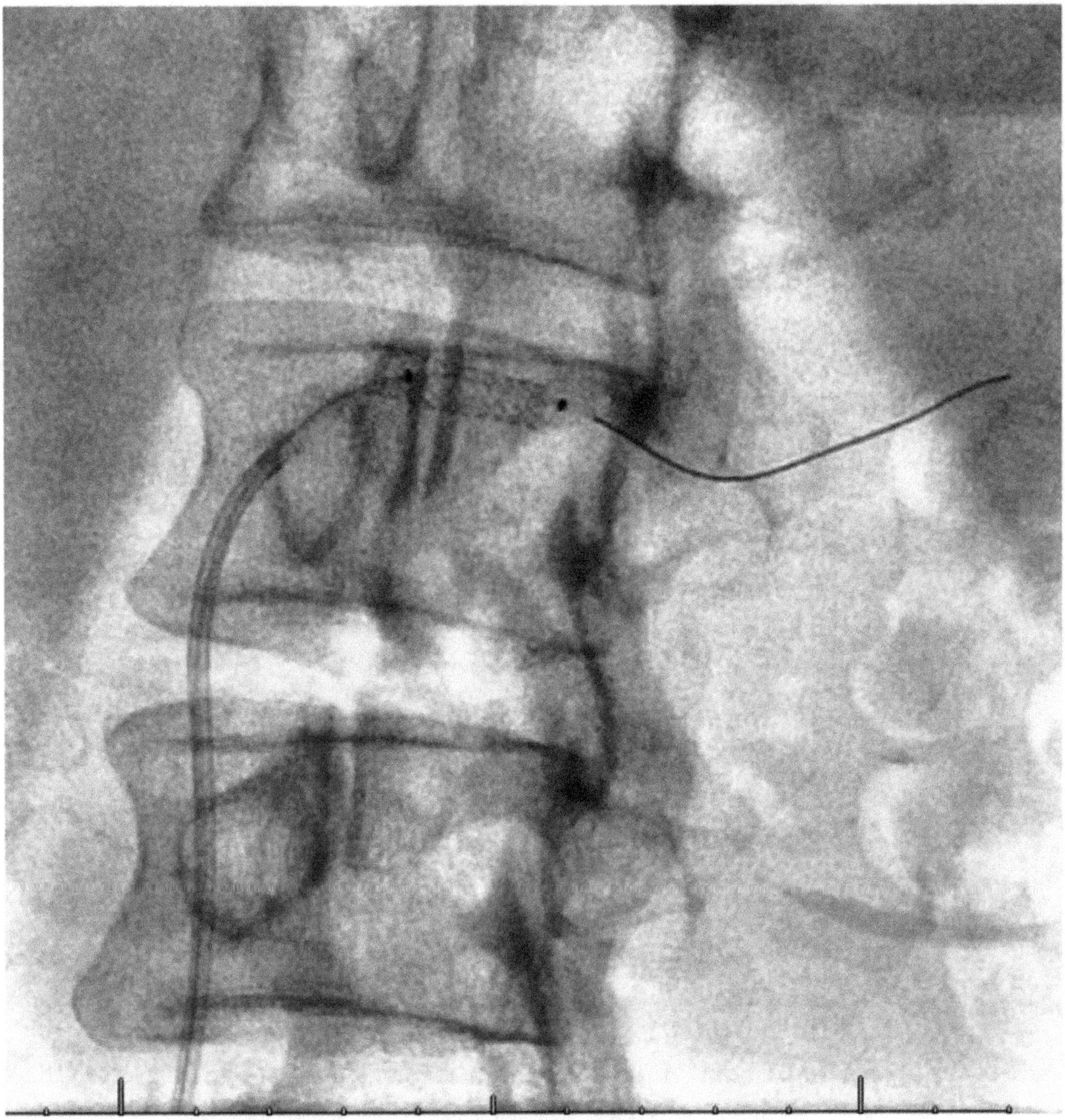

FIGURE 10: The angiojet thrombectomy was done inside the stent.

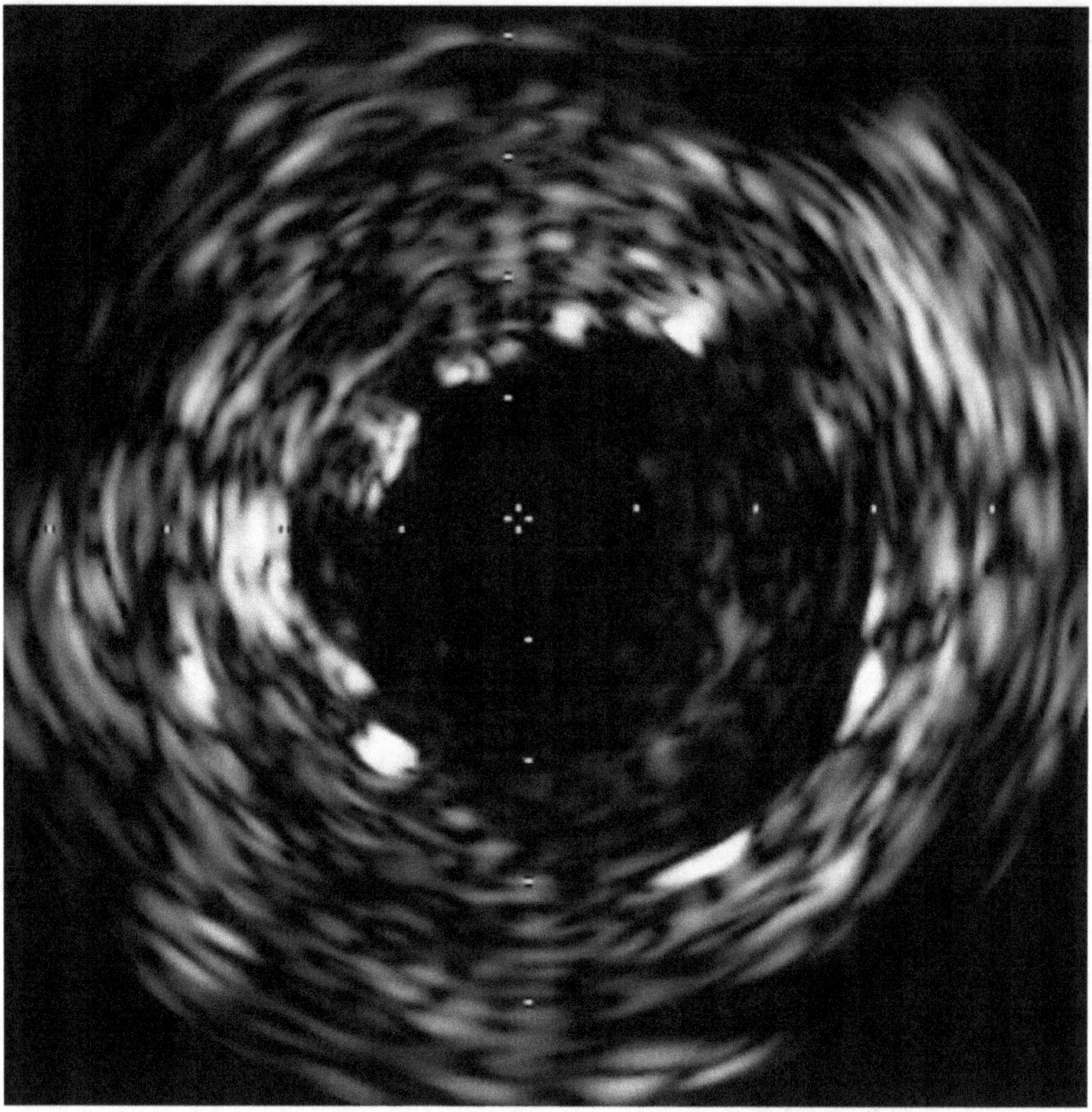

Figure 11: The patient has IVUS view of severe instent restenosis after anjiojet thrombectomy.

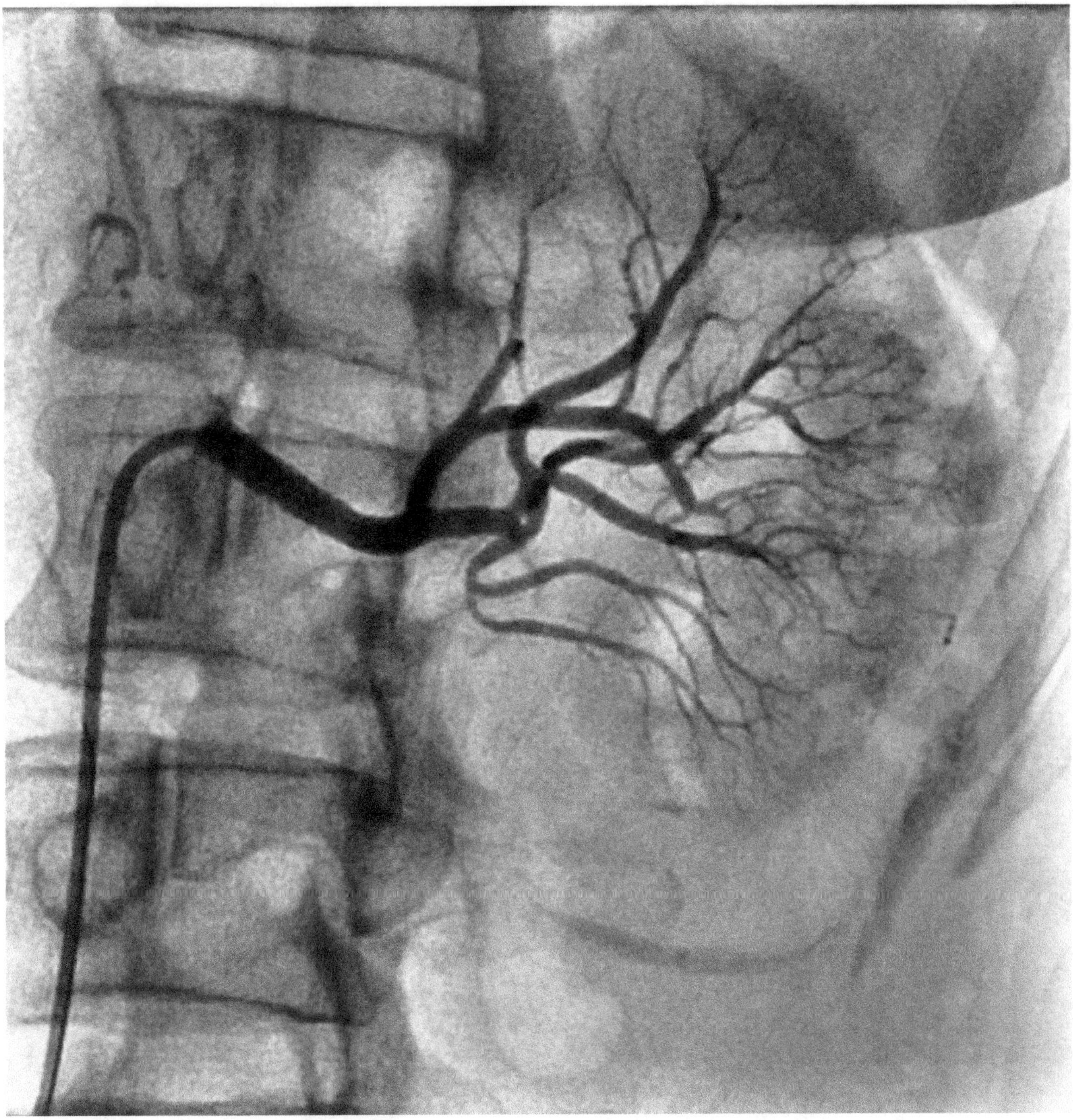

Figure 12: Postrestenting of the renal artery now shows excellent left kidney blush and patent lobular, arcuate and distal kidney vessels with less spasm, and no embolic cut offs, compared to Figure 7.

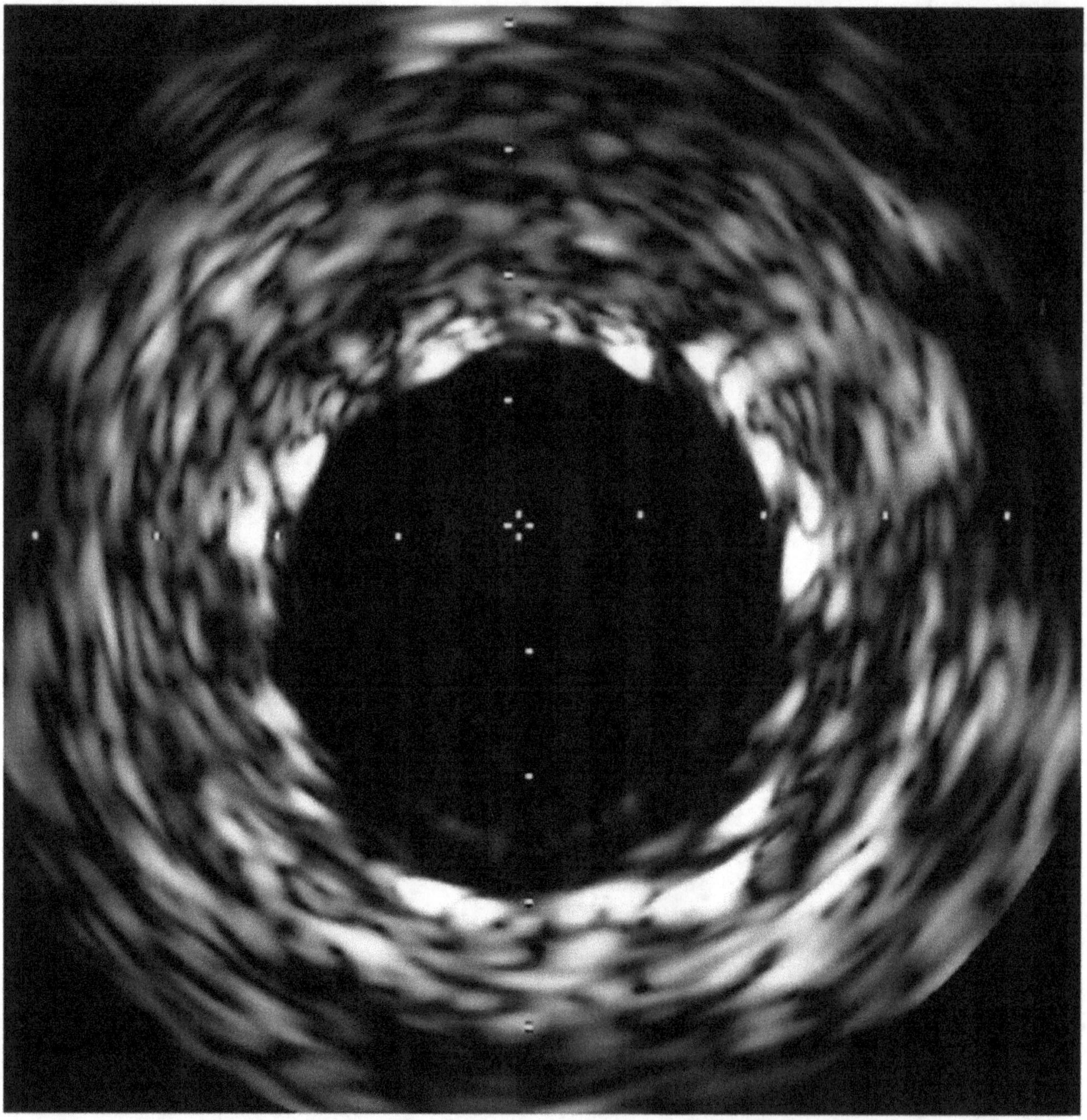

Figure 13: IVUS shows poststent, lumen diameter of over 4 mm with excellent stent expansion.

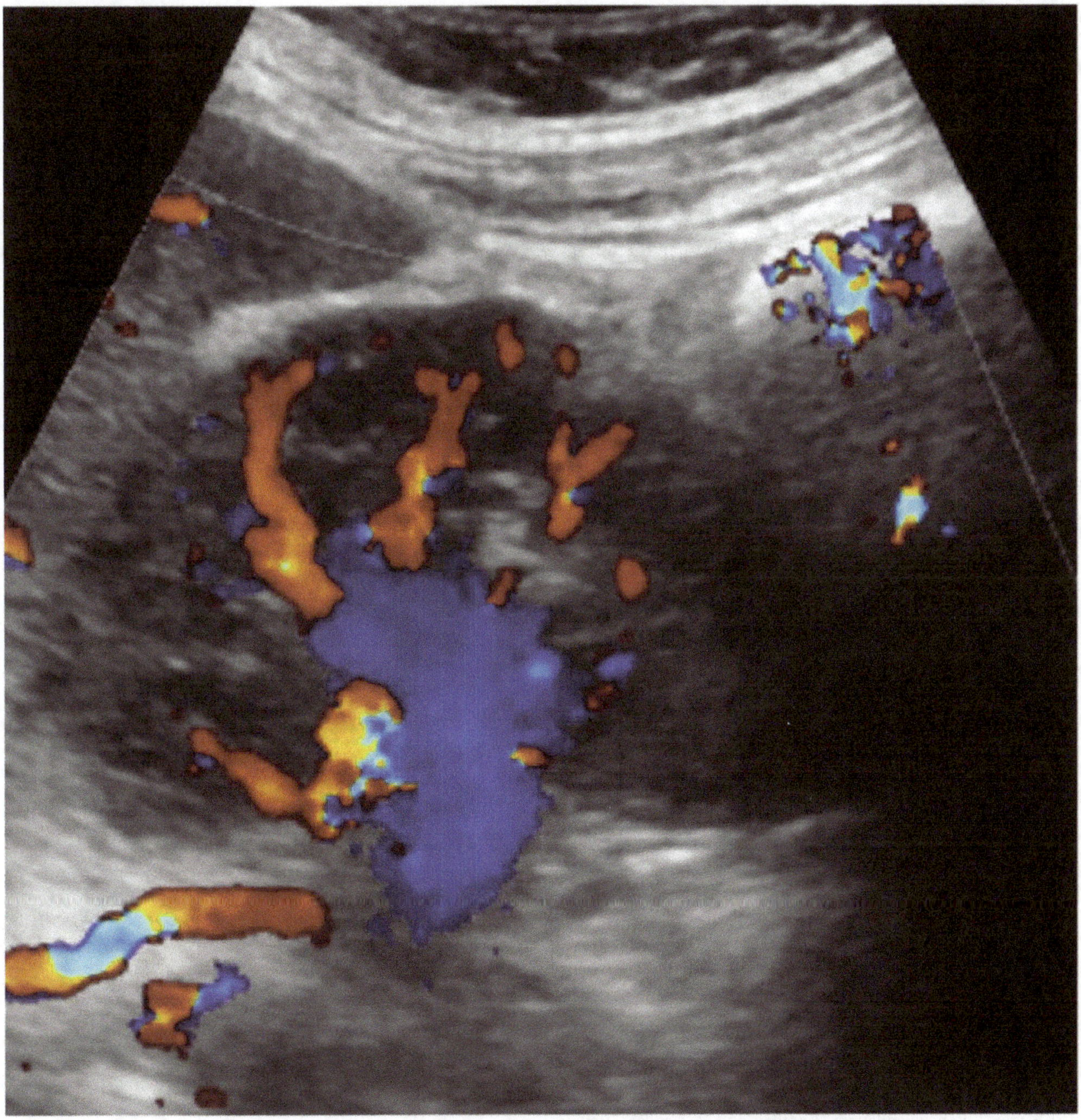

FIGURE 14: US color Doppler shows patent color flow in distal vessels.

treatments are based on small series or case reports [1, 7]. The initial treatment of acute renal artery thrombosis is anticoagulation but in our patient, anticoagulation with intravenous heparin did not lead to any clinical benefit and resulted in continued symptoms [7]. Systemic thrombolytic therapy has low success and high complication risk in renal arterial thrombosis, and surgical and endovascular options are preferred [7–9]. Surgical treatment includes thrombectomy and aortorenal bypass, but given the high morbidity and mortality of open surgical options, endovascular therapy is preferred [7].

Percutaneous options for in situ or embolic renal artery thromboembolism include intra-arterial thrombolytic and various thrombectomy techniques along with angioplasty and stenting [1, 2, 7]. Thrombectomy techniques, when available, may be preferred given the higher bleeding complications with thrombolytic therapy [7]. Renal artery angioplasty and stenting for thrombosis has been done in case reports [7].

In conclusion, our case report is unusual for using both rheolytic and aspiration thrombectomy as well as stenting and then repeat stenting. It is also unusual for very late reperfusion leading to improvement in symptoms, renal function, and then, improved kidney perfusion on CTA.

References

[1] D. Silverberg, T. Menes, U. Rimon et al., "Acute renal artery occlusion: presentation, treatment and outcome," *Journal of Vascular Surgery*, vol. 64, pp. 1026–1032, 2016.

[2] N. Ganju, S. Sondhi, and A. Kandoria, "Acute renal artery embolisation: role of local catheter-based intra-arterial thrombolysis," *BML Case Reports*, vol. 2018, 2018.

[3] H. J. Lim, J. H. Hwang, J. H. Kim, S. Park, K. H. Lee, and S. H. Park, "Spontaneous renal artery thrombosis: a rare cause of acute flank pain," *Radiology Case Reports*, vol. 16, no. 1, pp. 9–12, 2021.

[4] H. S. Al-Sergani, P. J. Fitzpatrick, and S. Waxman, "Angiographic and ultrasonic evidence of plaque rupture causing myocardial infarction," *Circulation*, vol. 98, no. 13, p. 1348, 1998.

[5] Z. Korzets, E. Plotkin, J. Bernheim, and R. Zissin, "The clinical spectrum of acute renal infarction," *Israel Medical Association*, vol. J4, pp. 781–784, 2002.

[6] T. Cinar, I. Rencuzogullari, Y. Karabag, and M. Cagdas, "Renal arterial atherothrombosis due to catheter-induced dissection: Necessity of urgent intervention in a patient with a solitary functioning kidney," *Heart & Lung*, vol. 48, no. 1, pp. 69–71, 2019.

[7] T. W. Tan, W. T. Bohannon, M. A. Mattos, K. J. Hodgson, and A. Farber, "Percutaneous mechanical thrombectomy and pharmacologic thrombolysis for renal artery embolism: case report and review of endovascular treatment," *International Journal of Angiology*, vol. 20, no. 2, pp. 111–116, 2011.

[8] U. G. Rossi, G. A. Rollandi, R. Dallatana, and M. Cariati, "Mechanical aspiration thrombectomy in the treatment of acute intrastent renal artery thrombosis," *Cardiovascular Revascularization Medicine*, vol. 20, no. 4, pp. 344–346, 2019.

[9] K. Ouriel, C. H. Andrus, J. J. Ricotta, J. A. DeWeese, and R. M. Green, "Acute renal artery occlusion: when is revascularization justified?," *Journal of Vascular Surgery*, vol. 5, no. 2, pp. 348–355, 1987.

3

85-Year-Old Postsurgical Complex Patient Successfully Managed Remotely at the Novel Mayo Clinic's Hospital at Home

Margaret R. Paulson,[1] Ricardo A. Torres-Guzman,[2] Francisco R. Avila,[2] Karla Maita,[2] John P. Garcia,[2] Abdullah Eldaly,[2] Luiza Palmieri-Serrano,[2] Antonio J. Forte,[2] Jonathan C. Thompson,[3] and Michael J. Maniaci[4]

[1]*Division of Hospital Internal Medicine, Mayo Clinic Health Systems, Eau Claire, 2321 Stout Road, Menomonie, Wisconsin 54751, USA*
[2]*Division of Plastic Surgery, Mayo Clinic, 4500 San Pablo Road, Jacksonville, Florida 32224, USA*
[3]*Division of Orthopedics, Mayo Clinic Health Systems, 1400 Bellinger Stree, Eau Claire, Wisconsin 54703, USA*
[4]*Division of Hospital Internal Medicine, Mayo Clinic, 4500 San Pablo Road, Jacksonville, Florida 32224, USA*

Correspondence should be addressed to Michael J. Maniaci; maniaci.michael@mayo.edu

Academic Editor: Nilda Espinola-Zavaleta

An 85-year-old male presented to the podiatry clinic following a 1st to 5th left toe amputation as a complication of severe peripheral arterial disease and nonhealing wound despite endovascular intervention with an angiogram. At the visit, cellulitis with gangrene of the surgical site was noted. The patient was admitted to the brick and mortar (BAM) hospital and taken to surgery for a transmetatarsal amputation of the left limb. In the immediate postoperative period, the incisional margins appeared dusky creating concern for flap viability. The medical team recommended a vascular bypass versus a below-knee amputation. However, given the age, comorbidities, and nutritional status, the family refused further surgical intervention. As such, Mayo Clinic's home hospital program, Advanced Care at Home (ACH), was consulted for continued nonsurgical acute management at home. The patient was transferred to ACH and transported home three days after BAM admission to continue IV antibiotic therapy and wound care. Discharge from ACH occurred 11 days after admission to the BAM hospital. This case highlights the importance of developing health care alternatives to traditional hospitalization and demonstrates that ACH can manage highly complex, elder postoperative patients from the comfort of their homes.

1. Introduction

Increased hospital occupancy around the U.S. during the coronavirus pandemic meant that many surgical services required adaptions to traditional models of care for surgical patients requiring hospitalization. Elderly hospitalization is becoming more common in surgical departments. To date, almost two out of five surgical procedures are performed on patients over 65 years old [1]. Advanced Care at Home (ACH) is a unique hospital-at-home program for delivering acute and postacute care. This offering seeks to provide high-acuity care in the home setting while also aiming to reduce healthcare expenditures as well as decrease readmissions and healthcare-associated infections [2–7]. We report a case of a complex surgical patient managed at their home in northwest Wisconsin through the ACH centralized command center in Florida.

2. Case Presentation

An 85-year-old retired truck driver was seen by his family medicine physician after a recent hospitalization for atrial fibrillation with a rapid ventricular response. He had a past medical history of atrial fibrillation on anticoagulation, congestive heart failure, coronary artery disease status postcoronary artery bypass surgery, hypertension, aortic valve replacement, chronic kidney disease stage 3, obstructive sleep apnea, and peripheral vascular disease. Four months prior to his visit, he had undergone stenting of the right common iliac artery, angioplasty and stenting of the right superficial femoral artery, and angioplasty of the right tibioperoneal trunk and popliteal artery and ultimately required a right transmetatarsal amputation for osteomyelitis.

In the months leading up to his clinical visit, he started to develop digital gangrene in his left foot affecting the second and third digits. He had undergone an angiogram one month prior that showed severe stenosis of the left distal external and proximal common femoral arteries. Due to these findings, an atherectomy and drug-eluting balloon angioplasty were performed on the left distal iliac and common femoral arteries at that time. After that procedure, he was seen in follow-up in the podiatric clinic, where palpable pedal pulses were appreciated.

Now at his clinical visit his family medicine physician discovered worsening erythema in the left foot in the setting of persistent digital gangrene classified by the Society for Vascular Surgery Lower Extremity Threatened Limb: Wound, Ischemia, and foot Infection (SVS WIfI) as a W2I-fI1. Acute cellulitis of the left foot was diagnosed, and oral antibiotic management with cephalexin was initiated.

Two days after initiating management with cephalexin, the patient was assessed by his podiatrist who discovered full-thickness gangrene extending down to the base of the digit and onto the dorsal and plantar forefoot adjacent to the 2nd and 3rd digits (W3I-fI2). Due to the extension of the gangrene, a 1st through 5th toe amputation was deemed necessary and conducted at the brick and mortar (BAM) hospital at Mayo Clinic Health Systems at Eau Claire, Wisconsin, USA.

Four days postoperatively, the patient was seen in the podiatric clinic for routine follow-up. Upon physical exam, diffuse incisional dehiscence with progressive gangrenous changes was noted. The patient was admitted back to BAM hospital for IV antibiotics, vascular intervention, and definitive surgical management. Anesthesiology noted during its pre-operative risk assessment a Duke Activity Status index of 3.97 METs, a Gupta cardiac risk of myocardial infarction or cardiac arrest intraoperative or 30 days postoperative of 0.9%, a STOP-Bang Total Score of 5 (high risk for obstructive sleep apnea) and an ASA Physical Status Classification System of 4. During this hospitalization, the patient was also noted to both meet the ASPEN criteria of malnutrition as well as to have bacteremia with *Bacteroides fragilis*. Broad-spectrum antibiotics were first initiated and then subsequently downgraded to cefepime and metronidazole.

A transmetatarsal amputation was performed the day after readmission to BAM hospital. Marginal bleeding was appreciated intraoperatively with duskiness of the plantar flap and incisional margins, raising concern for insufficient vascular status to support healing of the amputation site (see Figure 1). Vascular Surgery was consulted for further discussion of revascularization options. An open femoral-popliteal vascular bypass was recommended versus the secondary option of a below-knee amputation. After considering the options presented in an informed consent discussion, the patient and family wished to pursue neither option and ultimately opted for palliative measures.

The medical team considered it appropriate to request a consultation by the ACH team to ensure that he was a potential candidate to continue acute management at home. The ACH team evaluated the patient at the bedside to determine eligibility based on insurance, demographic, social, and clinical criteria to be admitted into the program. The patient was transferred from the Medical Surgical floor to his home hospital three days after the transmetatarsal amputation. The technological kit consisting of a tablet device for video communication and data collection, a one way telephone to the centralized command center, and a personal emergency response system was given and tested. The patient and family received daily virtual rounds with the medical team coordinated by the single telemedicine command center located in Jacksonville, Florida, USA. Additionally, the patient had twice daily visits by a paramedic and nurse to evaluate peripheral pulses using a portable Doppler, change the dressings, take pictures for the command center, and administer the IV antibiotics (see Figure 2).

After the patient transferred to ACH, pain, erythema (W3I-fI2), and confusion increased progressively (see Figure 1). The patient, family, and healthcare team engaged in ongoing discussions about goals of care. Five days after transfer to the ACH program, the patient and the family decided to pursue hospice care. Seven days after admission, shared decision-making with the patient, family, and medical team, led to discharge from the ACH program and a smooth transition to hospice services.

3. Discussion

The traditional practice of medicine involves in-person consultation and examination. However, the current COVID-19 pandemic has obligated that many surgery services adapt quickly and implement telemedicine in their services by the degree of complexity of the patient and telehealth resources available at the different surgery service hospitals [8–10]. Telehealth has granted providers the ability to evaluate, diagnose, treat, and provide follow-up to surgical patients, particularly in places where resources and subspecialists are insufficient. Moreover, telemedicine has been accepted by the public views as an acceptable substitute for in-person visits [9, 11], especially during the COVID-19, pandemic as shown in a recent publication by Sorensen et al. [9] where a 43-question survey was performed assessing respondents' attitudes toward telehealth for initial consultations with surgeons, both in the context of COVID-19 and during non-COVID-19 circumstances. The results showed that out of 1.827 responses, 86% of responders reported being satisfied (either extremely or somewhat) with telehealth encounters. The percentage of preference for virtual visits declined with the surgical procedure's complexity, even during the pandemic [9].

The ACH program was implemented at Mayo Clinic in July 2020. Patients in Florida and Wisconsin are admitted into the ACH program and monitored by a single telemedicine command center through telehealth. The command center conducts virtual rounds on the patient and delivers in-home care through a smart supply chain. The patient

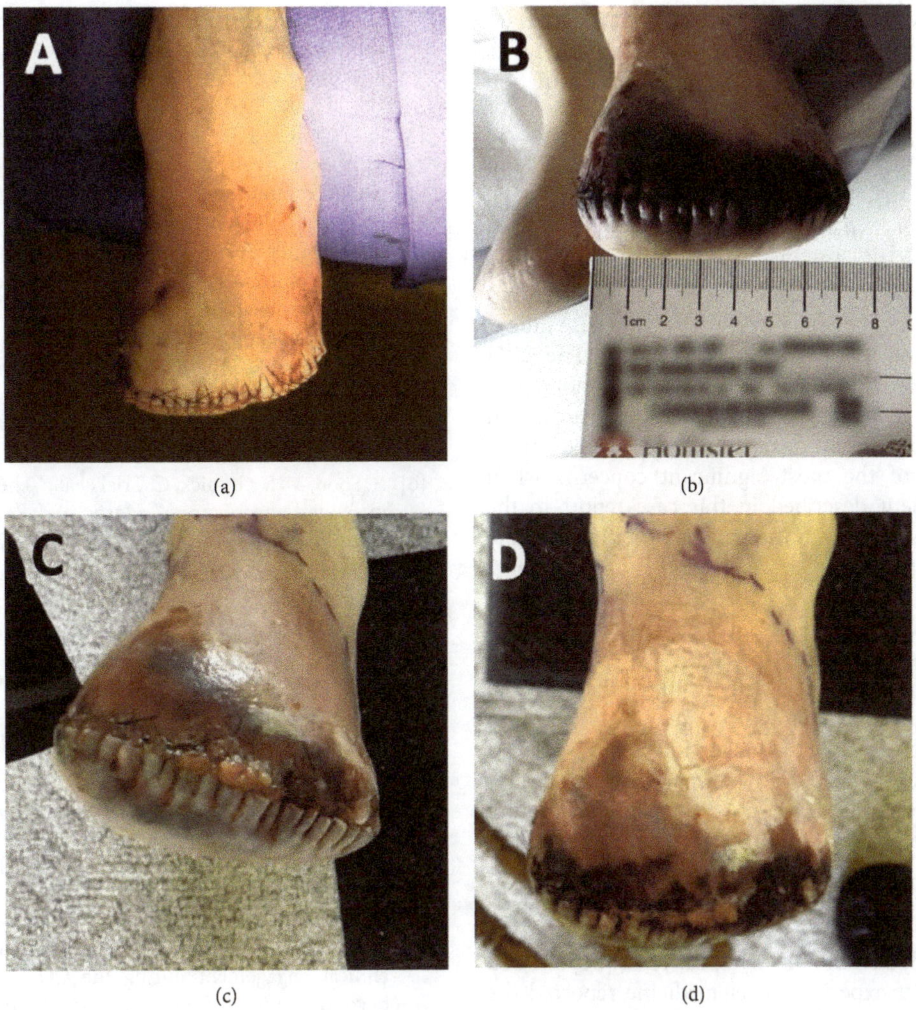

Figure 1: Follow-up pictures of the patient. (a) Intraoperative photograph of the transmetatarsal amputation. (b) ACH follow-up day three after transmetatarsal amputation. (c) The picture was taken on day 2 of the ACH program. (d) The image was taken on day 3 of the ACH program.

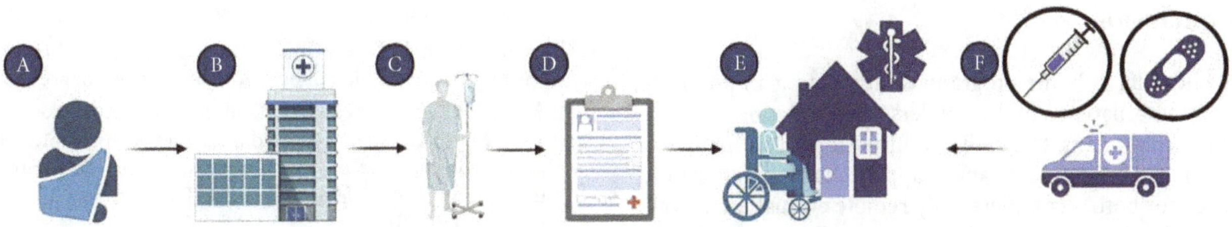

Figure 2: Patient transit flow chart. (a) The patient is sent to the ED after a clinic visit, where skin changes of the left foot were noticed. (b) The patient is hospitalized and evaluated by the podiatrist at Mayo Clinic Health Systems, Eau Claire, Wisconsin. (c) The patient is recommended to undergo the surgical procedure. (d) The family denies further procedures. The medical team consults the ACH team. The patient meets the criteria to be admitted to the program. (e) The patient is transported home, where the technological kit is given. (f) The command center located in Jacksonville, Florida, evaluated the patient daily. Additionally, a medical team visited the patient's home to administer antibiotics, perform a vascular assessment with a Doppler, and change the dressing of the wounds.

reported he had both daily virtual rounds by the Internal Medicine and Orthopedics hospital teams and in-home administered antibiotics, wound care, laboratory studies, and physical therapy. Furthermore, the ACH program differs from other hospital-at-home programs since it combines the two classifications of telemedicine in one. For instance, the two major classifications that characterize telemedicine are synchronous and asynchronous [12, 13]. Synchronous telemedicine or real-time telemedicine encompasses the use of telecommunication in real-time to simplify provider-patient interaction. On the other hand, asynchronous telemedicine uses data or images to transmit them electronically to be reviewed later. The ACH program allows providers and patients to interact using both types, synchronous and asynchronous, depending on the situation required.

A hospitalization is a threatening event for patients 65 years and older. The complexity of diseases and other health conditions make older patients prone to adverse hospital outcomes, including institutionalization, mortality, and functional decline [14, 15]. The mortality rate in these patients is approximately 20%; meanwhile, 30% of the survivors decrease their level of daily living activities (DLA) functioning three months after hospital discharge [16]. The ACH program seeks to provide high-acuity care in the home setting while also reducing healthcare expenditures and decreasing readmissions and healthcare-associated infections [2–7]. One of the most significant concerns when admitting the patient described in this case report to the ACH program was that given the patient's multiple comorbidities, his transition from the brick and mortar hospital to home would be hazardous. Nevertheless, not only the transition was successful, but 30-day readmission after hospital discharge was prevented [1].

Telemedicine in the surgical field exhibited the potential to increase productivity, follow-up rates, and access to healthcare by lessening travel-associated limitations [8, 17] and reducing costs [8, 18–20]. However, some of the limitations reported include the risk of misdiagnoses, information protection, technological literacy, and failure to identify abuse victims [8]. Additionally, the lack of in-person physical examination creates the need for a reliable virtual examination, especially in acute and complex conditions [8]. An online survey conducted in 2019 by Spear et al. [21] showed that out of 781 that experienced telemedicine reported the lack of hands-on care, intimacy, and technical difficulties as the main disadvantages [21]. There is a need to demonstrate that remote physical examination is reliable to follow-up complex postoperative patients as reported.

4. Conclusion

While hospital at home programs continue to gain popularity with both patients and providers, the limitations of successfully conducting telemedicine in postoperative patients, such as the equipment and supply chain organization required for both a complete daily remote evaluation as well as delivering high-acuity in-home care, still exist. However, the present case study highlights the ability of the Mayo Clinic's virtual hybrid hospital at home program to manage a complex postoperative patient with relative ease using telemedicine combined with coordinated in-person resources.

Acknowledgments

Figure 2 was created using https://BioRender.com.

References

[1] A. Zurlo and G. Zuliani, "Management of care transition and hospital discharge," *Aging Clinical and Experimental Research*, vol. 30, no. 3, pp. 263–270, 2018.

[2] R. G. Bentvelsen, E. Holten, N. H. Chavannes, and K. E. Veldkamp, "eHealth for the prevention of healthcare-associated infections: a scoping review," *The Journal of Hospital Infection*, vol. 113, pp. 96–103, 2021.

[3] R. L. Gunter, S. Fernandes-Taylor, S. Rahman et al., "Feasibility of an image-based mobile health protocol for postoperative wound monitoring," *Journal of the American College of Surgeons*, vol. 226, no. 3, pp. 277–286, 2018.

[4] R. L. Gunter, S. Chouinard, S. Fernandes-Taylor et al., "Current use of telemedicine for post-discharge surgical care: a systematic review," *Journal of the American College of Surgeons*, vol. 222, no. 5, pp. 915–927, 2016.

[5] E. M. Bogen, K. M. Augestad, H. R. Patel, and R. O. Lindsetmo, "Telementoring in education of laparoscopic surgeons: an emerging technology," *World J Gastrointest Endosc.*, vol. 6, no. 5, pp. 148–155, 2014.

[6] A. Sood, M. S. Granick, C. Trial et al., "The role of telemedicine in wound care, France," *Plastic and Reconstructive Surgery*, vol. 138, 3 Supplement, pp. 248s–256s, 2016.

[7] E. Y. Huang, S. Knight, C. R. Guetter et al., "Telemedicine and telementoring in the surgical specialties: a narrative review," *American Journal of Surgery*, vol. 218, no. 4, pp. 760–766, 2019.

[8] P. Moisan, B. Barimani, and J. Antoniou, "Orthopedic surgery and telemedicine in times of COVID-19 and beyond: a review," *Current Reviews in Musculoskeletal Medicine*, vol. 14, no. 2, pp. 155–159, 2021.

[9] M. J. Sorensen, S. Bessen, J. Danford, C. Fleischer, and S. L. Wong, "Telemedicine for surgical consultations - pandemic response or here to stay?: a report of public perceptions," *Annals of Surgery*, vol. 272, no. 3, pp. e174–e180, 2020.

[10] C. M. Contreras, G. A. Metzger, J. D. Beane, P. H. Dedhia, A. Ejaz, and T. M. Pawlik, "Telemedicine: patient-provider clinical engagement during the COVID-19 pandemic and beyond," *Journal of Gastrointestinal Surgery*, vol. 24, no. 7, pp. 1692–1697, 2020.

[11] V. Sathiyakumar, J. C. Apfeld, W. T. Obremskey, R. V. Thakore, and M. K. Sethi, "Prospective randomized controlled trial using telemedicine for follow-ups in an orthopedic trauma population," *Journal of Orthopaedic Trauma*, vol. 29, no. 3, pp. e139–e145, 2015.

[12] N. S. Lanham, K. J. Bockelman, and B. J. McCriskin, "Telemedicine and orthopaedic surgery," *JBJS reviews*, vol. 8, no. 7, 2020.

[13] A. Buvik, E. Bugge, G. Knutsen, A. Småbrekke, and T. Wilsgaard, "Patient reported outcomes with remote orthopaedic consultations by telemedicine: a randomised controlled trial," *Journal of Telemedicine and Telecare*, vol. 25, no. 8, pp. 451–459, 2019.

[14] G. R. Baker, P. G. Norton, V. Flintoft et al., "The Canadian Adverse Events Study: the incidence of adverse events among hospital patients in Canada," *CMAJ*, vol. 170, no. 11, pp. 1678–1686, 2004.

[15] A. J. Forster, H. J. Murff, J. F. Peterson, T. K. Gandhi, and D. W. Bates, "The incidence and severity of adverse events affecting patients after discharge from the hospital," *Annals of Internal Medicine*, vol. 138, no. 3, pp. 161–167, 2003.

[16] B. M. Buurman, J. L. Parlevliet, B. A. van Deelen, R. J. de Haan, and S. E. de Rooij, "A randomised clinical trial on a comprehensive geriatric assessment and intensive home follow-up after hospital discharge: the Transitional Care Bridge," *BMC Health Services Research*, vol. 10, no. 1, p. 296, 2010.

[17] W. F. DeNino, T. Osler, E. G. Evans, and P. M. Forgione, "Travel distance as factor in follow-up visit compliance in postlaparoscopic adjustable gastric banding population," *Surgery for Obesity and Related Diseases*, vol. 6, no. 6, pp. 597–600, 2010.

[18] L. A. Aponte-Tinao, G. L. Farfalli, J. I. Albergo et al., "Face to face appointment vs. telemedicine in first time appointment orthopedic oncology patients: a cost analysis," *Studies in Health Technology and Informatics*, vol. 264, pp. 512–515, 2019.

[19] K. Harno, E. Arajärvi, T. Paavola, C. Carlson, and P. Viikinkoski, "Clinical effectiveness and cost analysis of patient referral by videoconferencing in orthopaedics," *Journal of Telemedicine and Telecare*, vol. 7, no. 4, pp. 219–225, 2001.

[20] P. Wallace, A. Haines, R. Harrison et al., "Joint teleconsultations (virtual outreach) versus standard outpatient appointments for patients referred by their general practitioner for a specialist opinion: a randomised trial," *Lancet*, vol. 359, no. 9322, pp. 1961–1968, 2002.

[21] K. L. Spear, P. Auinger, R. Simone, E. R. Dorsey, and J. Francis, "Patient views on telemedicine for Parkinson disease," *Journal of Parkinson's Disease*, vol. 9, no. 2, pp. 401–404, 2019.

4

Lingual Raynaud's Phenomenon after Surgical and Radiotherapeutic Intervention for Oral Squamous Cell Carcinoma

Nicholas J. Murphy,[1] Loay S. Kabbani,[2] Alexander D. Shepard,[2] and Farzan Siddiqui[3]

[1]Wayne State University School of Medicine, 540 E. Canfield Ave. Detroit, MI 48201, USA
[2]Department of Surgery, Henry Ford Hospital, 2799 W Grand Blvd Detroit, MI 48202, USA
[3]Department of Radiation Oncology, Henry Ford Hospital, 2799 W Grand Blvd Detroit, MI 48202, USA

Correspondence should be addressed to Farzan Siddiqui; fsiddiq2@hfhs.org

Academic Editor: Muzaffer Sindel

Raynaud's phenomenon of the tongue after radiation therapy with or without chemotherapy is an exceedingly rare complication. Symptoms are similar to Raynaud's disease of other sites and involve pallor and discomfort on exposure to cold temperatures that resolve with rewarming. Presentation occurs approximately 18-24 months after radiotherapy on average and can usually be managed effectively with lifestyle modification and pharmacotherapy. Here, we present a case of lingual Raynaud's following surgery and adjuvant radiation therapy in a patient with squamous cell carcinoma of the oral cavity.

1. Introduction

Raynaud's phenomenon (RP) is a vasospastic process that typically affects the digits of the hands, causing painful discoloration on exposure to cold temperatures or strong emotions [1]. It is estimated that 3-5% of the general population is affected by RP with a predilection for females and those in more northerly regions [1]. Classically, it presents in three phases beginning with pallor, which represents the initial vasoconstrictive ischemic phase. After a prolonged period of ischemia, the second phase of a cyanotic blue color results from the presence of desaturated blood in the affected part. With recovery, there is a final hyperemic phase of vasodilation which produces a red color. This classic color progression from white to blue to red is only infrequently present. Episodes of vasospasm usually last from minutes to one hour but can last multiple hours [1].

The precise mechanism for RP has not yet been elucidated but current thinking points to a combination of probable neural and vascular factors. The neural pathway involves sympathetic nervous system stimulation by cold temperatures or stress. The resulting release of norepinephrine activates vascular smooth muscle alpha adrenoreceptors leading to vasoconstriction. However, local factors can override this neural response as seen in patients with local anesthesia of sympathetic nerves or postsympathectomy who can still experience episodes of RP [1]. Another postulated mechanism for RP is production of reactive oxygen species (ROS) by mitochondria in response to cold temperatures [1]. Signaling through the Rho/Rho-kinase pathway leads to translocation and subsequent activation of α2C-adrenoreceptors causing vasoconstriction [1].

Small artery occlusive disease (e.g., vasculitis) is more commonly implicated in secondary RP, which is associated with collagen vascular diseases such as systemic sclerosis [1]. Some of the vascular causes include endothelial cell damage, disparate vasoactive substance production, intravascular narrowing, and increasing vasoconstriction [1]. Once exposed to cold, these factors increase the body's natural vasoconstrictive response leading to the classical pale skin of affected areas [1, 2].

Development of management strategies has been hampered by the complex etiology of RP and a poor understanding of its exact mechanisms. Many therapies have been tried with varying degrees of success. They are broadly divided into nonpharmacologic and pharmacological interventions.

Treatment is stratified based on severity, beginning with nonpharmacological approaches for mild symptoms. These include lifestyle modification to avoid triggers such as keeping the affected areas warm with clothing and avoiding exposure to cold temperatures [1]. Smoking cessation is always advised, if applicable [1]. For more severe symptoms, vasodilator therapy is added, typically beginning with dihydropyridine calcium channel blockers—nifedipine being the most studied and drug of choice [1]. Other potential agents include alpha-1 adrenoreceptor antagonists (prazosin), angiotensin-converting enzyme inhibitors, nitric oxide, prostaglandin analogs, phosphodiesterase inhibitors, selective serotonin reuptake inhibitors, antioxidants, botulinum toxin A, endothelin receptor antagonists, and Rho inhibitors [1]. Alternative approaches include herbal remedies such as Ginkgo biloba extract and rosemary oil, acupuncture, transcutaneous nerve stimulation, and sympathectomy among others [1].

Although the primary regions affected by RP are the digits of the hands and feet, rarely affected regions include the nose, ears, lips, and nipples. Raynaud's of the tongue is exceedingly rare and to date is only described in a handful of case reports.

2. Case

A 63-year-old postmenopausal female with a history of hypertension, hyperlipidemia, and former 25 pack-year tobacco use presented with squamous cell carcinoma of the oral cavity pathological stage IVA (pT1N2bM0). She had undergone wide local excision of an alveolar ridge lesion with, left neck dissection of levels I-IV, and reconstruction with a right radial forearm free flap; the margins were negative, and there was no extranodal extension. She subsequently completed postoperative radiation therapy to a dose of 60 Gy in 30 fractions using intensity-modulated radiation therapy (IMRT) to the areas shown in Figures 1(a) and 1(b). At follow-up, 19 months after radiation, she continued to suffer from xerostomia and diminished taste sensation but showed no evidence of disease based on clinical and radiologic examination. Approximately two years after completion of radiation, in the month of October, she began to notice intermittent lingual pallor. She reported that the tip and anterior 1/4 of her tongue predominately on the left side began to tingle and turn white, lasting 10-15 minutes and occurring two to three times per day as shown in Figure 2. This change occurred mostly with exposure to cold ambient temperatures and resolved with rewarming. Interestingly, it did not occur with drinking cold beverages. There were no motor, sensory, balance, or hearing changes or similar symptoms in the digits of the hands or feet. She had no history of Raynaud's disease, cerebrovascular accident, transient ischemic attack, or other neurologic disease. Physical examination revealed no visible abnormality of the tongue and flexible laryngoscopy was unremarkable. A computed tomography angiogram of the head and neck done to investigate possible vascular causes showed no significant extracranial arterial occlusive disease or aneurysm. She was referred to vascular surgery for further evaluation, and laboratory studies were ordered, showing an ESR 4 mm/Hr, CRP 0.2 mg/dL, PT 12.9 sec, PTT 25 sec, INR 0.97, DRVVT 35 sec, and lupus anticoagulant negative. Her presentation was noted to be most consistent with Raynaud's phenomenon of the tongue, and a trial of nifedipine extended release 30 mg daily was started. During follow-up several weeks later, she reported significant improvement in the frequency and severity of symptoms and was tolerating treatment, though attacks continued to occur intermittently when outdoors in cold temperatures.

3. Discussion

Raynaud's phenomenon of the tongue is exceedingly uncommon and often occurs in the setting of primary Raynaud's disease of the digits. There have been at least 22 cases of lingual involvement reported in the literature, usually associated with systemic sclerosis, Sjögren's syndrome, or other connective tissue disorders [3–8]. Of the lingual Raynaud's cases found in the literature, four were identified without preexisting connective tissue disease all occurring after the use of radiotherapy for head and neck squamous cell carcinomas [2, 9–11]. In three cases, there was no history of Raynaud's disease affecting the digits and in all cases, radiotherapy had occurred between 18 and 54 months prior to the onset of symptoms. One of the patients was noted to have a smoking history while the other three were either nonsmokers or not specified. Nicotine is noted to be a risk factor for Raynaud's disease and was potentially a contributing factor in our patient [1].

Interestingly, 2/4 cases involved male patients, while typical RP tends to affect females more than males. One risk factor for RP is the hormone estrogen, which potentiates vasoconstriction occurring via alpha adrenoreceptors [1]. Further evidence for this factor comes from estrogen therapy increasing the risk of RP in postmenopausal women [1]. Our patient was not on estrogen therapy. Raynaud's phenomenon can result from either increased vasoconstriction or impaired vasodilation or a combination of the two in small arteries. Underlying arterial occlusive disease can be a major contributing factor. Arteries narrowed by such a process have a lower "critical closing pressure," and normal cold-induced vasoconstriction can lead to temporary vessel closure. Radiation leads to a progressive obliterative endarteritis of small vessels which makes them prone to such changes and may be a contributing factor to the rare occurrence of RP [2]. Additionally, radiation damage to the endothelium disrupts normal chemical mediators of vasorelaxation. The result is exaggerated vasoconstriction, both in intensity and duration, to normal adrenergic-mediated stimuli (e.g., cold or stress) and impaired vasodilation leading to the classic symptoms of RP [2]. Surgery is also likely a contributing factor from scarring leading to compression of small arterial beds [11].

Non-RT-associated cases in this group of lingual Raynaud's patients tended to occur in younger people and females, often

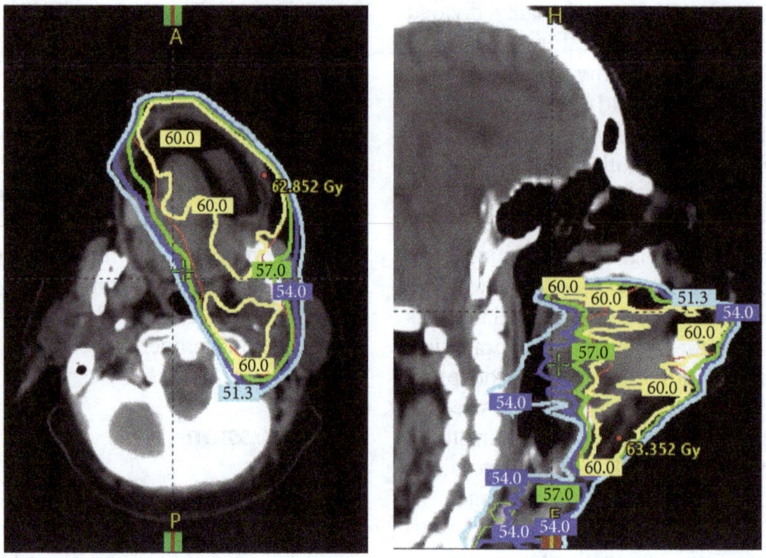

(a) (b)

FIGURE 1: (a, b) Dose lines of radiotherapy treatment showing irradiated regions of the oral cavity.

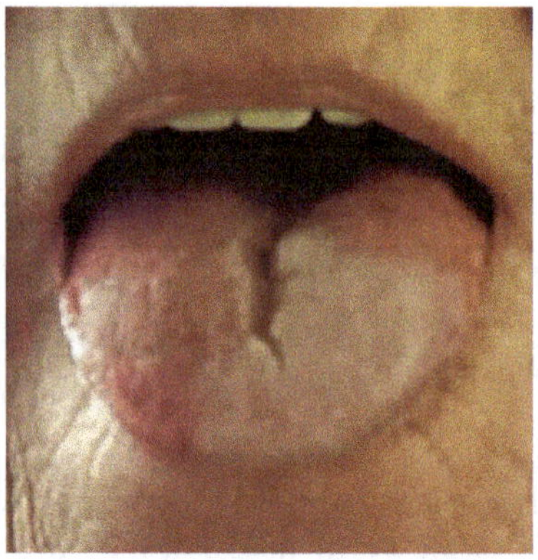

FIGURE 2: Picture of the oral tongue demonstrating left-sided tongue pallor.

with a previously diagnosed systemic sclerosis with digital Raynaud's symptoms [3–8].

Treatment of our patient using calcium channel blockers was apparently effective, though other options ranging from lifestyle changes of avoiding colder temperatures up to recurrent botulinum toxin injections seemed acceptable [2, 9–11]. Three of the other cases demonstrated stable disease with nonpharmacologic management, leading to ongoing intermittent pain attacks that were reported as self-limiting and tolerable [2, 9, 10]. One patient was treated with fifty units of botulinum toxin injected along the sternocleidomastoid muscle, which provided complete resolution of the patient's discoloration, paresthesia, and dysphagia for 3 months until symptoms gradually returned [11]. Repeat injections reportedly had similar effect to the first [11]. Overall, the treatment paradigm for lingual Raynaud's after RT seems to mirror the general consensus for primary Raynaud's disease. Severity of symptoms and patient preference for intervention should be the main considerations until further data in this specific patient population become available.

4. Conclusion

In summary, lingual Raynaud's phenomenon is a rare complication of radiation therapy to the oral cavity. Although the exact mechanism is currently unknown, the etiology is likely related to radiation-induced small artery damage resulting in an exaggerated vasoconstrictive response to normal adrenergic stimulation. Treatments can be effective in mitigating symptoms and include lifestyle changes and pharmacologic intervention.

Disclosure

This study is performed as part of employment with Henry Ford Health System.

References

[1] I. Nawaz, Y. Nawaz, E. Nawaz, M. R. Manan, and A. Mahmood, "Raynaud's phenomenon: reviewing the pathophysiology and management strategies," *Cureus*, vol. 14, no. 1, article e21681, 2022.

[2] C. B. Westbury, K. J. Harrington, P. Rhys-Evans et al., "Raynaud's phenomenon after radical radiotherapy for tumours of the head and neck," *Postgraduate Medical Journal*, vol. 79, no. 929, pp. 176-177, 2003.

[3] B. Lioger and E. Diot, "Raynaud's phenomenon of the tongue: uncommon presentation of a classical sign," *QJM: An International Journal of Medicine*, vol. 106, no. 6, pp. 583-584, 2013.

[4] S. Chatterjee, "Raynaud phenomenon causing lingual pallor and dysarthria," *Canadian Medical Association Journal*, vol. 188, no. 15, pp. E396–E396, 2016.

[5] V. Grémain, L. Richard, V. Langlois, and I. Marie, "Raynaud's phenomenon of the tongue," *Joint, Bone, Spine*, vol. 84, no. 2, article 231, 2017.

[6] J. Cohen, M. Lia Palomba, and L. Morris, "Raynaud's phenomenon of the tongue," *The Journal of Rheumatology*, vol. 40, no. 3, article 1093, 2013.

[7] E. Casey and N. Lawton, "Progressive systemic sclerosis presenting with Raynaud's phenomenon in the tongue and sensory trigeminal neuropathy," *Rheumatology*, vol. 11, no. 3, pp. 131–133, 1971.

[8] M. Perry, S. Surtee, and Z. Nawaz, "Raynaud's of the *tongue*," *Internal Medicine*, vol. 4, no. 8, 2017.

[9] A. Mittal and A. Mittal, "Raynaud's of the tongue following chemoradiation for squamous cell carcinoma of the oropharynx," *Molecular and Clinical Oncology*, vol. 6, pp. 187-188, 2017.

[10] A. F. Ghiam and J. Cho, "Lingual Raynaud phenomenon," *Canadian Medical Association Journal*, vol. 187, no. 15, pp. 1160–1160, 2015.

[11] S. Boukovalas, A. C. Mays, and J. C. Selber, "Botulinum toxin injection for lower face and oral cavity Raynaud phenomenon after mandibulectomy, free fibula reconstruction, and radiation therapy," *Annals of Plastic Surgery.*, vol. 82, no. 1, pp. 53-54, 2019.

5

Ruptured Superficial Femoral Artery Anastomotic Pseudoaneurysm after 30 Years

D. Baldwin,[1] H. Mashbari,[1,2] K. L. Chow,[1] and M. Sarhan[3]

[1]*Department of General Surgery, University of Illinois at Chicago, Chicago, IL, USA*
[2]*Department of General Surgery, Jazan University, Saudi Arabia*
[3]*Department of Surgery, Division of Vascular Surgery, Advocate Christ Medical Center, Oak Lawn, IL, USA*

Correspondence should be addressed to D. Baldwin; dustinbaldwin21@gmail.com

Academic Editor: Nikolaos Papanas

Introduction. Anastomotic pseudoaneurysms are a complication of vascular reconstructive surgery with the majority in the femoral region. Although rare, ruptured femoral anastomotic pseudoaneurysms have high mortality and require emergency surgery. *Case Presentation.* A 60-year-old male with a history of a left leg crush injury was treated with a superficial femoral artery interposition vein graft 30 years ago. He presented nowadays with a three-day history of severe pain in his left thigh. CT angiography demonstrated a ruptured anastomotic pseudoaneurysm with contrast extravasation into an intramuscular hematoma. He had significant scarring from his previous surgeries which made the leg hostile for an open repair. Therefore, percutaneous access selectively cannulated the left iliofemoral vasculature. An angiogram showed a distal superficial femoral artery pseudoaneurysm. Subsequently, two 10mmx15cm Viabahn covered stents (Gore & Associates, Flagstaff, AZ) were placed bridging healthy superficial femoral artery. A completion angiogram demonstrated no extravasation into the pseudoaneurysm. The patient recovered and was discharged home two days postoperatively. *Conclusion.* Ruptured femoral anastomotic pseudoaneurysms are traditionally repaired with open pseudoaneurysm excision and arterial reconstruction, although endovascular repair has been reported. Furthermore, most femoral anastomotic pseudoaneurysms form less than 10 years after initial operation. We present a unique case of ruptured superficial femoral artery pseudoaneurysm, 30 years after the initial operation. Endovascular stents offer effective treatment for ruptured anastomotic pseudoaneurysms.

1. Introduction

Pseudoaneurysms are localized arterial disruptions that communicate with an artery through a defect in the arterial wall. They are different from true aneurysms as they do not contain all three layers of the vessel wall. Pseudoaneurysms are commonly associated with penetrating trauma, iatrogenic injury during cardiac, endovascular, or radiological intervention, or arterial-graft anastomotic disruption. Other less common causes of pseudoaneurysm formation include bacterial, mycobacterial, or amoebic infection, inflammatory processes such as pancreatitis, or arterial degeneration from Marfans syndrome or fibromuscular dysplasia.

Complications from pseudoaneurysms include thrombosis, distal embolization, and potential free rupture. Rupture of anastomotic pseudoaneurysms results in high morbidity and mortality ranges from 20 to 46.6% [1, 2]. Patients need emergency surgery to prevent loss of life or limb. Traditional treatment involves open surgery with pseudoaneurysm excision and arterial reconstruction. However, the emergence of endovascular therapy has permitted another option for interventionalists in treating pseudoaneurysms. Endovascular techniques are limited with regard to availability and access but are invaluable in scarred or difficult to reach locations. To illustrate this, we present a unique case of ruptured superficial femoral artery pseudoaneurysm presenting 30 years after a reverse saphenous vein interposition graft repair in a hostile

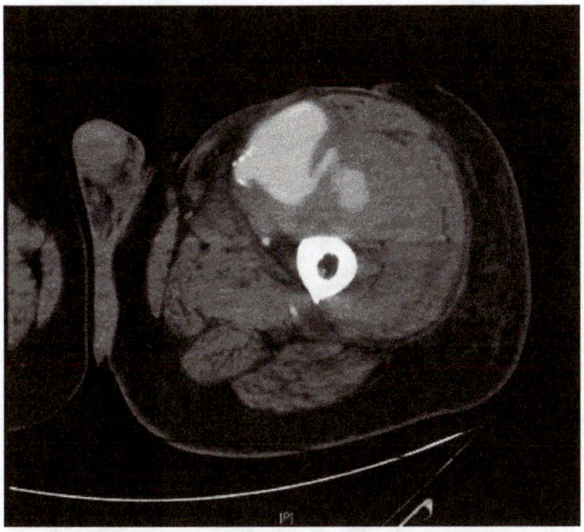

FIGURE 1: CTA of left lower extremity, axial images showing the anastomosis pseudoaneurysm with active extravasation.

surgical field. The 30-year timeframe in which the femoral pseudoaneurysm ruptured and the inability to perform an open repair offered unique challenges.

2. Case Presentation

A 60-year-old obese male with a history of smoking, hypertension, diabetes, and chronic kidney disease had a previous left leg crush injury requiring a superficial femoral artery reverse saphenous vein interposition graft repair 30 years ago. Postoperatively, he suffered from chronic lymphedema and developed a left superficial femoral artery anastomotic pseudoaneurysm which was followed with serial imaging. Two months prior to presentation, ultrasound imaging showed the pseudoaneurysm had grown significantly to 6.8 x 5.7 x 5.0 cm, yet he refused surgery.

Upon presentation, the patient endorsed a three-day history of progressive, severe pain and swelling in his left thigh causing him to present to the emergency room. He presented with mild tachycardia, but other vital signs were within normal limits. CT angiography demonstrated a ruptured anastomotic pseudoaneurysm with contrast extravasation into an intramuscular hematoma measuring 12.4 x10.6 x 28.2 cm (Figures 1 and 2). On examination, he had significant scarring of the left groin from his previous surgeries and skin grafting which precluded open vascular repair (Figure 3). As such, we elected to perform an endovascular repair to avoid the hostile surgical field.

Ultrasound guided percutaneous access was obtained via the right common femoral artery. A catheter was inserted and the left iliofemoral system was selectively cannulated using a guidewire and omniflush. A left lower extremity angiogram was obtained showing a pseudoaneurysm coming from the distal superficial femoral artery (Figure 4). At this point, a stiff wire along with an 11 French sheath was positioned at the normal superficial femoral artery just proximal to the pseudoaneurysm. Then two 10mm x 15cm Viabahn covered

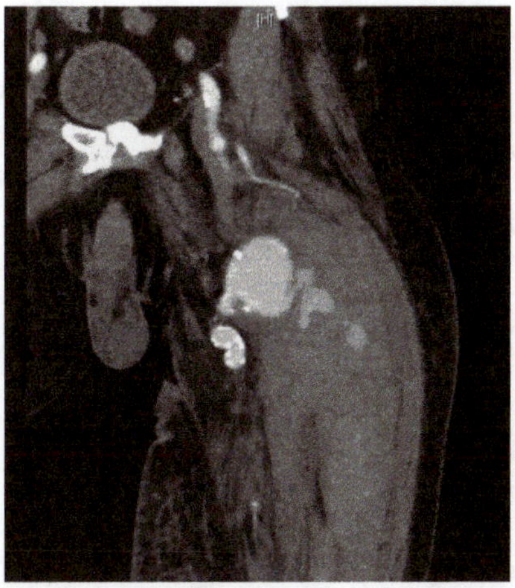

FIGURE 2: CTA of left lower extremity, coronal images showing the anastomosis pseudoaneurysm with active extravasation.

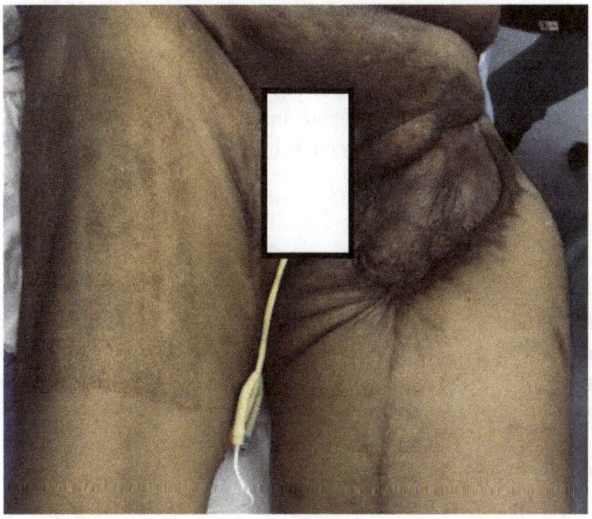

FIGURE 3: Left thigh of the patient on physical exam.

stents (Gore & Associates, Flagstaff, AZ) were placed with 8 cm of stent overlap bridging healthy superficial femoral artery proximally and distally. The stented segment was around 20 cm long. After 10mm balloon dilation of the stents, a completion angiogram demonstrated no extravasation to the pseudoaneurysm (Figure 5). We then made a small counter incision in the left groin to allow hematoma evacuation. The hematoma was not sent for culture. The patient had an uneventful recovery and was discharged home two days postoperatively. He required no postoperative anticoagulation. Although the patient had minimal follow-up, to our knowledge the stents remain patent.

3. Discussion

Current studies theorize anastomotic pseudoaneurysms form due to turbulent blood flow which progressively weakens the arterial wall promoting the development of anastomotic leaks [3]. The most common location for anastomotic

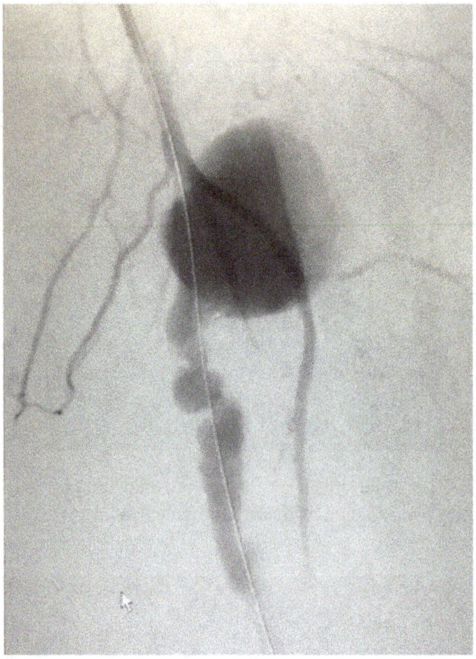

FIGURE 4: Intraoperative angiogram showing the left superficial femoral artery pseudoaneurysm with wire in place.

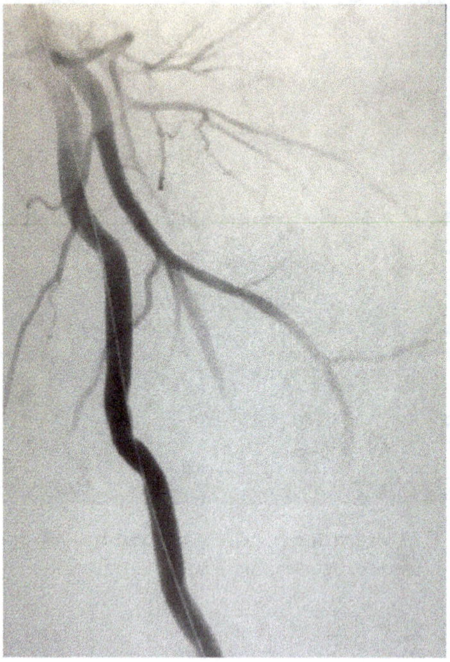

FIGURE 5: Intraoperative angiogram showing complete resolution the left superficial femoral artery pseudoaneurysm after stents placement.

pseudoaneurysms is the common femoral artery to bypass graft junction, which occurs in 0.8–2.2% of revascularization procedures [3]. In evaluating pseudoaneurysms, cultures of the graft and vessel wall are essential to exclude infection as an etiologic factor in the development of the anastomotic aneurysm [4]. Patients with known pseudoaneurysms are followed with serial ultrasounds and should be repaired if symptomatic.

Treatment of pseudoaneurysms depends on size, location, and feasibility. Arterial catheterization pseudoaneurysms less than 2cm can be observed, with most spontaneous resolving [5]. For larger or symptomatic pseudoaneurysms, nonoperative techniques include ultrasound-guided compression, thrombin injection, and coil embolization. However, these techniques are rarely used for anastomotic pseudoaneurysms. These are best treated with open surgery or endovascular repair [4, 5].

Skourtis et al. reported a case series of 49 patients with anastomotic pseudoaneurysms [2]. Most (85.7%) occurred at the femoral anastomosis site and emergency surgery for ruptured pseudoaneurysms was associated with 46.6% mortality [2]. In their case series, all patients were operated on with open surgery. Due to high mortality, free rupture of femoral anastomotic pseudoaneurysms is the most dreaded complication. Several papers have described ruptured femoral pseudoaneurysms mainly from infectious etiologies [1, 6, 7]. Klonaris et al. reported 6 patients with ruptured femoral artery anastomotic pseudoaneurysms secondary to infection. All patients were treated with emergency percutaneous covered stent deployment with surgical debridement in the following days to remove the infected pseudoaneurysm [1]. With the stent grafts covering the neck of the pseudoaneurysm, proximal and distal control were not needed, which limited the amount of open dissection. Patients were then placed on 6 weeks of intravenous antibiotics. At median follow-up of 14 months, there had been no indication of recurrent infection or pseudoaneurysm [1]. Until recently, open surgical repair had been the sole management option of such entities, despite its well-known limitations including scar tissue, distorted anatomy, and difficulty obtaining vascular control. This study highlights the expanding possibilities for endovascular covered stents.

Along with covered stents, there are several options for endovascular repair. Embolism with coils or liquid embolic agents, gelfoam, or vascular plugs have all been successfully used [8]. These options work well for most pseudoaneurysms, even in infected fields. Moulakakis et al. conducted a systematic review looking at infected pseudoaneurysms of the iliofemoral region treated with covered stent grafts. The most commonly used covered stents were Viabahn (22.9 %), Jostent (17.1 %), Fluency (14.3 %), and Wallgraft (14.3 %). Even in the infected field, stent patency was 94.3% at 16 months' follow-up with stent infection rate only at 3.4% [9].

In our patient, there was no evidence of infection leading to the pseudoaneurysm rupture. The most likely etiology was degeneration of the reverse saphenous vein bypass conduit. The incidence of femoral anastomotic aneurysms occurs less frequently with saphenous vein grafts than synthetic vascular grafts, a reflection of more complete healing of autogenous tissue [4]. Marković et al. examined 87 patients with pseudoaneurysms following bypass surgery. The causes were primarily arterial degeneration (66%) and infection

(25%). These patients presented mainly with ruptured pseudoaneurysm, thrombosis, chronic limb ischemia, or acute limb ischemia. Most patients presented between 2 and 5 years after the initial operation and were treated with open repair. Furthermore, only 12.6% of patients presented after 10 years [10].

The timeframe for development of anastomotic pseudoaneurysms varies based on study but is reported between 5 and 9.2 years after primary operation [7, 10]. Skourtis et al. in their case series of 49 patients with anastomotic pseudoaneurysms reported that mean time of pseudoaneurysm developed to be 6.8 years [2]. In a larger study by Levi et al. with 76 patients who had femoral anastomotic pseudoaneurysms, the interval between the primary operation and the operation for the femoral pseudoaneurysm was 9.2 years, with a range from 1 month to 26 years [7]. To our knowledge, we present the first noninfected anastomotic femoral pseudoaneurysm rupture after 30 years.

Such late presentations of anastomotic pseudoaneurysms from venous conduits are rare. It is unclear if this is due to durable anastomotic integrity or due to the unfortunate reality that many vascular patients do not survive for 30 years with their bypass. The etiology of long-term failure is still unclear but a combination of progression of the host's underlying disease, increased graft intimal hyperplasia, and the development of atherosclerosis-like lesions within the vein graft appears to be the principal cause [11]. However, as evidenced by this case report, there may be an upper limit to anastomotic integrity even amongst well established and long-standing anastomoses. This case report may serve clinicians as evidence for vascular anastomosis surveillance even up to 30 years.

4. Conclusion

Ruptured femoral anastomotic pseudoaneurysms are rare but have high mortality. Traditional repair involves open pseudoaneurysm excision and arterial reconstruction, although endovascular repair has been reported. Furthermore, most femoral anastomotic pseudoaneurysms form between 5 and 9.2 years after initial operation. To our knowledge, we present the first noninfected anastomotic femoral pseudoaneurysm rupture after 30 years successfully treated with covered endovascular stents. The late presentation of rupture adds to the literature and may serve clinicians as evidence for vascular anastomosis surveillance even up to 30 years.

Consent

All participants have agreed and consented to be included in this case report. The images, figures, or patient data used are included in this consent.

References

[1] C. Klonaris, A. Katsargyris, I. Vasileiou, F. Markatis, C. D. Liapis, and E. Bastounis, "Hybrid repair of ruptured infected anastomotic femoral pseudoaneurysms: Emergent stent-graft implantation and secondary surgical debridement," *Journal of Vascular Surgery*, vol. 49, no. 4, pp. 938–945, 2009.

[2] G. Skourtis, I. Bountouris, G. Papacharalambous et al., "Anastomotic pseudoaneurysms: our experience with 49 cases," *Annals of Vascular Surgery*, vol. 20, no. 5, pp. 582–589, 2006.

[3] H. Naouli, H. Jiber, and A. Bouarhroum, "False aneurysm of perforating branch of the deep femoral artery—Report of two cases," *International Journal of Surgery Case Reports*, vol. 14, pp. 36–39, 2015.

[4] Greenfield's Surgery: Scientific Principles and Practice, 5e. Chapter 101. Lower Extremity Aneurysms.

[5] I. Kronzon, "Diagnosis and treatment of iatrogenic femoral artery pseudoaneurysm: A review," *Journal of the American Society of Echocardiography*, vol. 10, no. 3, pp. 236–245, 1997.

[6] C. D. Karkos, I. T. Giagtzidis, T. E. Kalogirou, P. Christoforou, and K. O. Papazoglou, "Endovascular management of ruptured anastomotic pseudoaneurysm at the distal end of a prosthetic femoro-popliteal bypass: A 'quick and easy fix'," *Hippokratia*, vol. 19, no. 2, pp. 179–181, 2015.

[7] N. Levi and T. V. Schroeder, "Anastomotic femoral aneurysms: Increase in interval between primary operation and aneurysm formation," *European Journal of Vascular and Endovascular Surgery*, vol. 11, no. 2, pp. 207–209, 1996.

[8] P. Entezami, J. Dalfino, M. W. O'Brien, and A. Paul, "Endovascular embolisation of an iatrogenic superficial temporal artery pseudoaneurysm using liquid embolic," *BMJ Case Reports*, vol. 12, no. 1, Article ID e227742, 2019.

[9] K. G. Moulakakis, V. G. Alexiou, G. S. Sfyroeras et al., "Endovascular management of infected iliofemoral pseudoaneurysms – a systematic review," *Vasa*, vol. 46, no. 1, pp. 5–9, 2017.

[10] D. M. Marković, L. B. Davidović, D. M. Kostić et al., "Anastomotic pseudoaneurysms," *Srpski Arhiv za Celokupno Lekarstvo*, vol. 134, no. 3-4, pp. 114–121, 2006.

[11] M. G. Davies and P. O. Hagen, "Pathophysiology of vein graft failure: a review," *European Journal of Vascular and Endovascular Surgery*, vol. 42, no. 1, pp. S19–S29, 2011.

6

Combined use of Excimer Laser and High-Speed Rotational Atherectomy to Overcome a Severely Calcified Lesion in Endovascular Therapy

Keisuke Nakabayashi, Shinya Hata, Nobuhito Kaneko, Akihiro Matsui, Kazuhiko Tanaka, Hiroshi Ando, and Minoru Shimizu

Kasukabe Chuo General Hospital, Heart Center, Saitama, Japan

Correspondence should be addressed to Keisuke Nakabayashi; keisuke2018@gmail.com

Academic Editor: Atila Iyisoy

Although endovascular therapy (EVT) is commonly used in treatment of peripheral artery disease (PAD), severely calcified lesions pose a challenge, in spite of the technical advancement. In this report, we discuss the case of a 74-year-old male with coronary artery disease and end-stage renal disease who presented at our institution with bilateral intermittent claudication. Angiography showed chronic total occlusion (CTO) of the right superficial femoral arteries (SFA). Because the bilateral external iliac arteries demonstrated moderate stenosis, we performed endovascular therapy on the right SFA-CTO using a contralateral approach. With the antegrade wire progressing into the subintimal space, direct distal-SFA puncture was performed and wire externalization was established. However, no devices (minimal balloon, microcatheter, or Crosser system) were able to pass the lesion in antegrade or retrograde manner, even though the child catheter support or needle cracking technique from outside/inside was applied. Therefore, we used a combination of an excimer laser and high-speed rotational atherectomy to overcome the severely calcified lesion. First, the excimer laser catheter (Turbo Elite 0.9 mm) ablated the entry to the CTO; however, it did not pass through completely. Thereafter, the thin microcatheter (Caravel) succeeded in crossing the CTO in an antegrade manner using the BAlloon Deployment using FORcible Manner (BADFORM) technique. After wire-exchange to the Rota-wire, rotational atherectomy (RotaLink Plus 1.5 mm) passed through the CTO. Subsequently, we could dilate the CTO lesion with a conventional balloon followed by bare metal stent deployment. The right ankle-brachial index of the patient improved from being unmeasurable to 0.79, and the intermittent claudication disappeared. This combination therapy, described as the "RASER" technique in coronary section, is accepted for reimbursement. However, these devices in EVT section are considered off-label use in Japan. Therefore, we have to refrain from frequent use of this strategy; however, this method provides an option for severely calcified lesions.

1. Introduction

Endovascular therapy (EVT) has developed over the past decade because of advancement in techniques and devices [1, 2]. Therefore, the clinical indication of EVT for peripheral artery disease (PAD) becomes widely spread. However, severely calcified lesions still remain challenging. To overcome this situation, some techniques and devices have been developed. Excimer laser atherectomy (ELA) is a unique procedure [3] that modifies the morphology of the surface-plaque as well as the hard tissues underneath the calcification to facilitate easy device crossing, balloon dilatation, and subsequent stenting. High-speed rotational atherectomy (RA) with Rotablador (Boston Scientific, Natick, MA, USA) is also an important device that modifies and debulks the calcified lesion in the coronary section [4]. These two options complete each other by utilizing their characteristics.

Here, we report the case in which combination therapy using ELA and RA successfully treated chronic total occlusion (CTO) of the superficial femoral artery (SFA) with severe calcification.

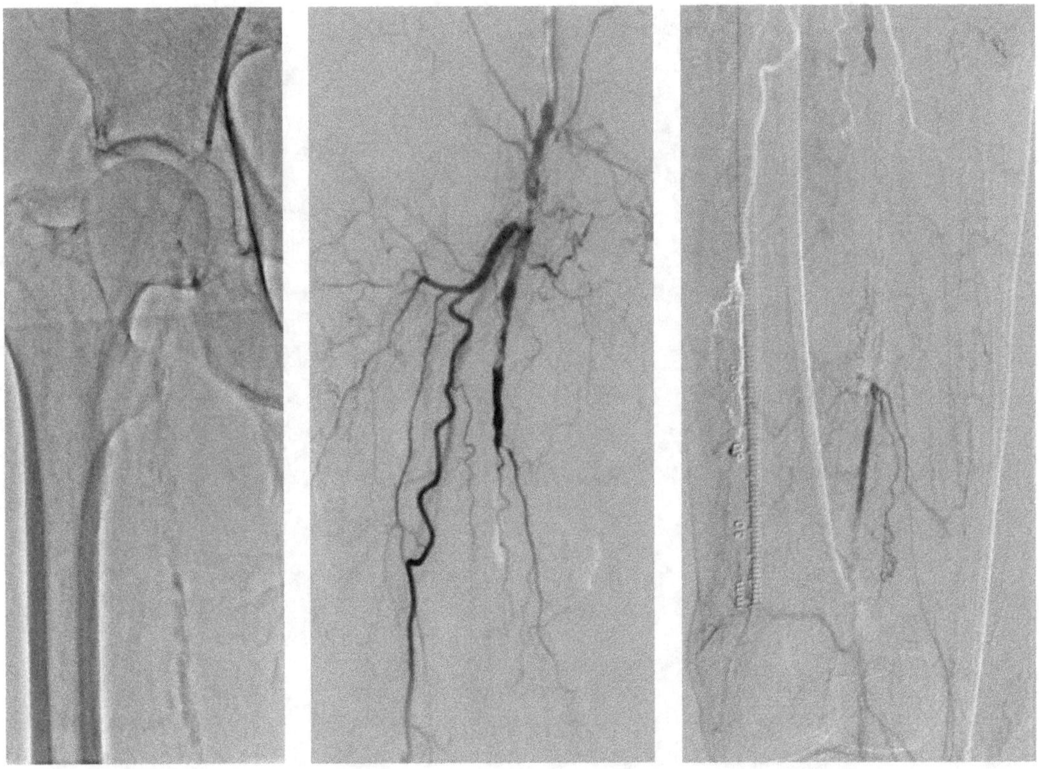

(a) (b) (c)

FIGURE 1: The first angiogram. (a) Digital angiography shows severe calcification of the right superficial femoral artery. (b) Digital subtraction angiography of the proximal part indicates the chronic total occlusion of the middle superficial femoral artery. (c) Digital subtraction angiography of the distal portion presents the puncturable distal superficial femoral artery.

2. Case Presentation

A 74-year-old male with hypertension, dyslipidemia, diabetes mellitus, coronary artery disease, and end-stage renal disease was transferred to our institution due to the bilateral intermittent claudication 6 months before admission. He had been given 75 mg of clopidogrel and 200 mg of cilostazol per day. His right ankle-brachial index was unmeasurable, and echography was suggestive of right SFA-CTO. Although this lesion was classified as class D based on the Transatlantic Inter-Society Consensus Document (TASC) [5], the patient refused surgical revascularization. Therefore, we chose endovascular therapy (EVT) and obtained a written informed consent from the patient. Since echography also indicated moderate stenosis of the bilateral iliac arteries, we initiated EVT in the right SFA-CTO using the contralateral approach. The first angiogram revealed the severely calcified SFA-CTO (Figure 1; Video Clip S1). The antegrade approach with the stiff CTO wire resulted in the subintimal wiring. Therefore, we used the bidirectional approach with direct distal-SFA puncture. Finally, the retrograde-antegrade rendezvous technique led to wire externalization (Figure 2; Video Clip S2). Regardless of the strong back-up force by wire externalization and child catheter support, no devices were able to pass the lesion by the antegrade and retrograde approaches and the thin balloon catheter was bent, Corsair microcatheter (ASAHI Intecc, Aichi, Japan) was fractured, Crosser system (C.R.Bard, NJ, USA) could not pass the lesion, and needle cracking technique [6] from outside and inside of the vessel could not modify the lesion fully. Despite using all these techniques, a minimal balloon could not pass the lesion (Figure 3). We consider abandonment and elective surgical conversion; however, bleeding from the retrograde puncture point and needle cracking techniques was uncontrollable. Therefore, we had to cross the lesion to perform balloon-assisted hemostasis.

Hence, we applied the ELA using the Turbo Elite 0.9 mm (Spectranetics, Co., USA). This device also could not pass the lesion; however, it modified the CTO entry-morphology (Figure 4(a)). After ELA ablation, the Caravel microcatheter (ASAHI Intecc) finally crossed the lesion using an antegrade approach with the BAlloon Deployment using FORcible Manner (BADFORM) technique [7] (Figure 4(b)), which enabled change of the wire from conventional the 0.014-inch wire to 0.009-inch RotaWire floppy (Boston Scientific) and RotaLink Plus 1.5mm burr ablation (Boston Scientific) (Figure 4(c)).

Thereafter, we dilated the entire SFA lesion with conventional balloons and simultaneously achieved hemostasis of the distal-SFA puncture point. A bare nitinol stent was deployed due to severe dissection of the partial SFA. The final angiography revealed acceptable result without delay in

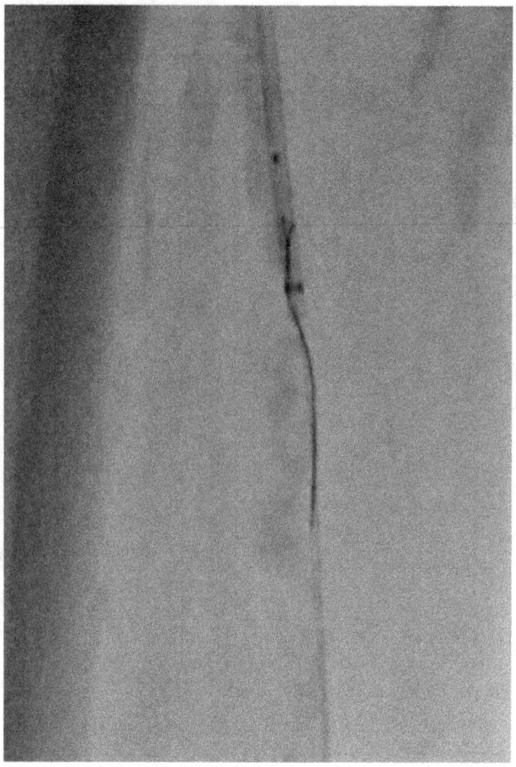

FIGURE 2: Rendezvous technique. The retrograde wire progresses into the antegrade child catheter.

blood-flow or bleeding complications (Figure 5; Video Clips S3 and S4).

Thereafter we treated the bilateral iliac arteries using the bare nitinol stents. The right ABI of the patient improved from being unmeasurable to 0.79, and his intermittent claudication disappeared. His ABI and symptom has remained satisfactory eight months after current EVT.

3. Discussion

The application of EVT is widespread with novel techniques and devices; however, severely calcified lesion is still a vulnerable point. To overcome this lesion, several atherectomy devices have been developed [8]. Most of these devices had relatively large diameters and posed problems with crossing the lesion. The combined strategy shown here could be superior in this point.

The application of ELA in EVT has been mainly limited to in-stent restenosis (ISR) lesions. The first prospective, multicenter study of 90 patients with ISR of nitinol stents in the femoropopliteal arteries treated by ELA and adjunctive percutaneous transluminal angioplasty (PTA) showed 97% procedural success, 7% residual stenosis, 2.2% 30-day major complication rate, and 64% 1-year freedom from target lesion revascularization [9]. A randomized control trial demonstrated the superiority of ELA with PTA versus PTA alone for treating femoropopliteal ISR in mid-term (6-month freedom from target lesion revascularization; 73.5% versus 51.8%, $p < 0.005$) [10]. With respect to imaging, intravascular ultrasound assessment indicated that ELA of peripheral artery lesions resulted in significant plaque debulking and increased lumen diameter with negligible degree of adventitial layer injury [11]. Angioscopy assessment also visualized the ELA effect of vaporization of thrombi in femoropopliteal in-stent lesions [12]. Thus, ELA was used as a debulking device. However, we herein used ELA as a modification or penetration device to cross the microcatheter to the distal CTO.

The application of high-speed RA in EVT section has been limited to a few case reports. Fukuda et al. reported a case of calcified SFA lesion after femoropopliteal bypass grafting treated by RA [13]. A guide wire and microcatheter crossed the lesion; however, a balloon catheter could not pass in their case. Hara et al. discussed the application of RA in heavily calcified CTO of the common iliac artery in a long-term hemodialysis patient. They had difficulties in passing the conventional microcatheter and used a Tornus microcatheter (ASAHI Intecc) instead [14]. The disadvantage of RA is the need for a dedicated 0.009-inch wire, which is cumbersome to control as a bare wire and requires microcatheter crossing.

Our case demonstrates a successful combination therapy of ELA and high-speed RA in severely calcified SFA-CTO. The modification of the CTO entry by ELA complemented the disadvantage of the need for the dedicated wire in RA and aided in crossing the microcatheter to the distal CTO. In fact, this combined strategy is known as the RASER (LASER and high-speed Rotational atherectomy) technique in coronary section [15, 16]. After the wire successfully crosses

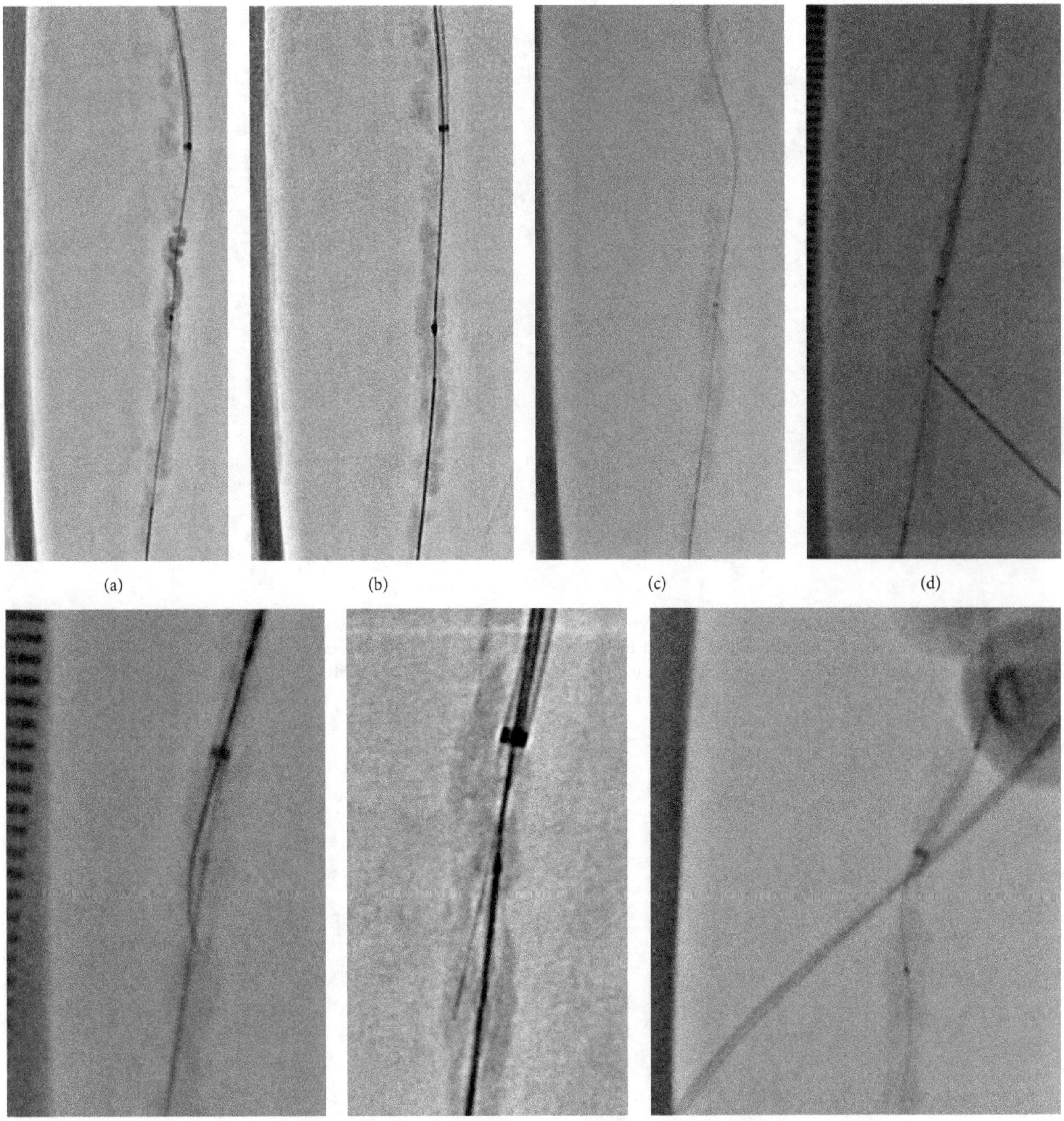

FIGURE 3: Devices that failed to cross the lesion. (a) The thin balloon is bent. (b) The Corsair PV microcatheter is fractured. (c) Crosser system cannot pass the lesion. (d) The needle cracking technique from outside of the vessel. (e) Needle cracking technique from inside of the vessel using the stiff wire. (f) Needle cracking technique from inside of the vessel using the tail of the wire. (g) The thin balloon cannot pass the lesion even after these devices and techniques.

the severely calcified lesion, a microcatheter often cannot pass the lesion. Subsequently, ELA ablates the only CTO entry. This modification enables the microcatheter to pass the lesion. RA can ablate the CTO body after retrieving a 0.014-inch conventional wire and crossing a 0.009-inch Rota-wire (Figure 6).

This is a treatment option for severely calcified lesions. To the best of our knowledge, the RASER technique in EVT section has not been reported in literature.

Although the above technique is technically feasible and beneficial, it should be considered as a last-resort technique in case of complications, like uncontrollable bleeding or

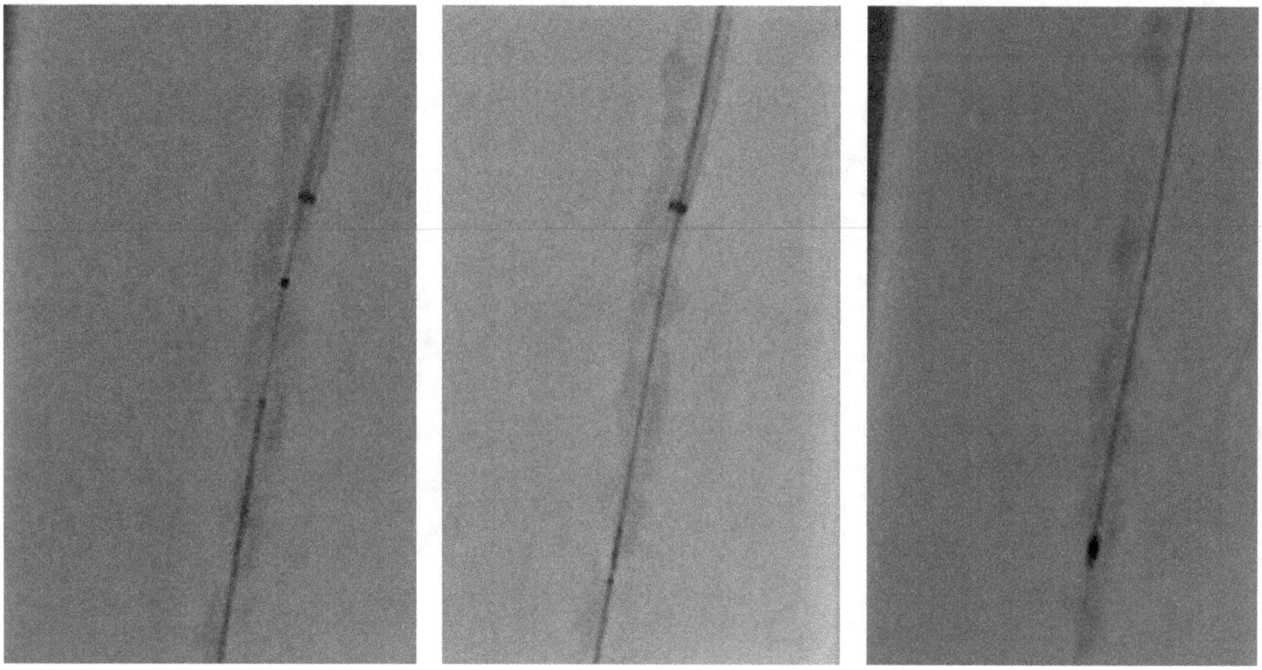

(a) (b) (c)

FIGURE 4: Combined strategy of the excimer laser atherectomy and high-speed rotational atherectomy. (a) The excimer laser catheter (Turbo Elite 0.9 mm) also cannot cross the lesion; however, it modifies the morphology of the chronic total occlusion lesion. (b) The Caravel microcatheter can pass the lesion. (c) Exchanging to the 0.009-inch Rota-wire from the conventional 0.014-inch wire, 1.5 mm burr ablation is performed.

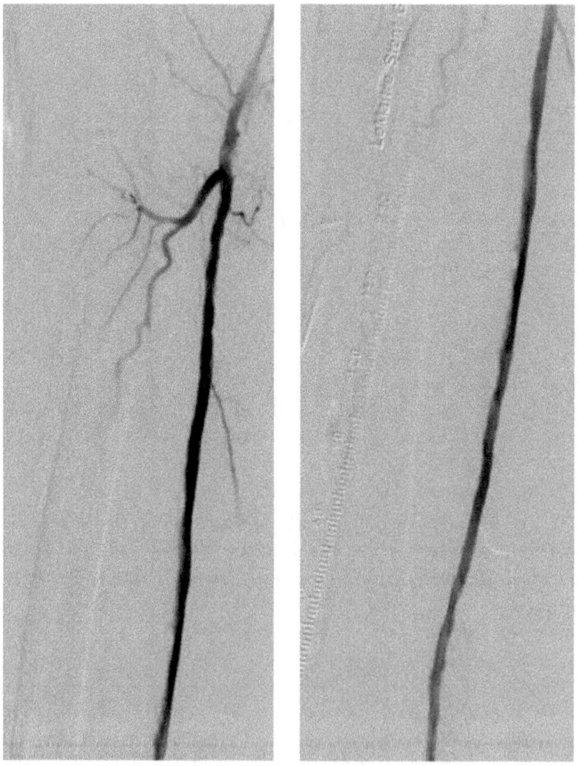

(a) (b)

FIGURE 5: The final angiogram. (a) Digital subtraction angiography of the proximal superficial femoral artery. (b) Digital subtraction angiography of the distal superficial femoral artery.

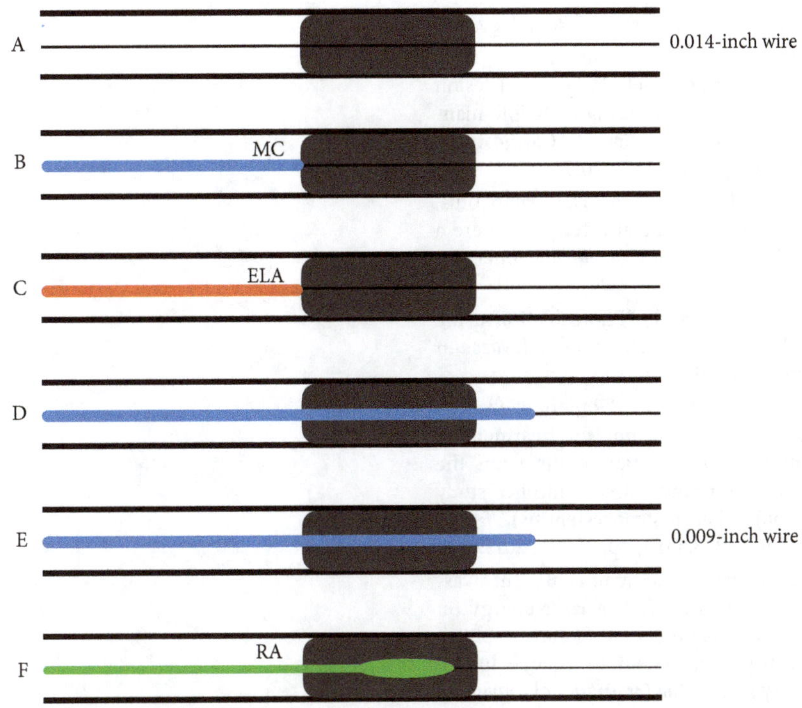

FIGURE 6: The schema of the "RASER" technique. A: conventional 0.014-inch wire crosses the severely calcified lesion. B: microcatheter often cannot pass the lesion. C: excimer laser catheter ablates and modifies the entry of the lesion. D: this modification enables a microcatheter to pass the lesion. E: exchanging to a 0.009-inch Rota-wire from a 0.014-inch conventional wire. F: high-speed rotational atherectomy is performed.

absolute contraindications of surgical revascularization, because both ELA and RA in EVT are considered off-label use in Japan.

4. Conclusion

Combined therapy with ELA and high-speed RA in EVT section is effective in CTO of the SFA and could be a useful option in managing severely calcified lesions.

Disclosure

This case was presented as an oral presentation in the Leipzig Interventional Course (LINC) National Meeting 2019. This research did not receive any specific grant from funding agencies in the public, commercial, or not-for-profit sectors.

Supplementary Materials

Video Clip S1: first angiogram. Digital angiography shows severe calcification of the right superficial femoral artery and the chronic total occlusion of the middle superficial femoral artery. Video Clip S2: rendezvous technique. The retrograde wire progresses into the antegrade child catheter. Video Clip S3: final angiogram of the proximal superficial femoral artery. Video Clip S4: final angiogram of the distal superficial femoral artery. *(Supplementary Materials)*

References

[1] P. A. Schneider, "Evolution and current use of technology for superficial femoral and popliteal artery interventions for claudication," *Journal of Vascular Surgery*, vol. 66, no. 3, pp. 916–923, 2017.

[2] M. R. Jaff, T. Nelson, N. Ferko, M. Martinson, L. H. Anderson, and S. Hollmann, "Endovascular interventions for femoropopliteal peripheral artery disease: a network meta-analysis of current technologies," *Journal of Vascular and Interventional Radiology*, vol. 28, no. 12, pp. 1617–1627, 2017.

[3] J. D. Garnic and A. S. Hurwitz, "Endovascular excimer laser atherectomy techniques to treat complex peripheral vascular disease: an orderly process," *Techniques in Vascular and Interventional Radiology*, vol. 8, no. 4, pp. 150–159, 2005.

[4] M. Abdel-Wahab, R. Baev, P. Dieker et al., "Long-term clinical outcome of rotational atherectomy followed by drug-eluting stent implantation in complex calcified coronary lesions," *Catheterization and Cardiovascular Interventions*, vol. 81, no. 2, pp. 285–291, 2013.

[5] J. B. Ricco, S. Parvin, M. Veller et al., "Statement from the european society of vascular inter-society consensus document (TASC) III and international standards for vascular care (ISVaC)," *European Journal of Vascular and Endovascular Surgery*, vol. 47, no. 2, p. 118, 2014.

[6] S. Ichihashi, T. Sato, S. Iwakoshi, H. Itoh, and K. Kichikawa, "Technique of percutaneous direct needle puncture of calcified plaque in the superficial femoral artery or tibial artery to facilitate balloon catheter passage and balloon dilation of calcified

lesions," *Journal of Vascular and Interventional Radiology*, vol. 25, no. 5, pp. 784–788, 2014.

[7] K. Nakabayashi, H. Ando, N. Kaneko et al., "A novel lesion crossing technique: balloon deployment using FORcible manner (BADFORM) technique," *Catheterization and Cardiovascular Interventions*, vol. 90, no. 7, pp. 1161–1165, 2017.

[8] K. Katsanos, S. Spiliopoulos, L. Reppas, and D. Karnabatidis, "Debulking atherectomy in the peripheral arteries: is there a role and what is the evidence?" *CardioVascular and Interventional Radiology*, vol. 40, no. 7, pp. 964–977, 2017.

[9] A. Schmidt, T. Zeller, H. Sievert et al., "Photoablation using the turbo-booster and PATENT study," *Journal of Endovascular Therapy*, vol. 21, no. 1, pp. 52–60, 2014.

[10] E. J. Dippel, P. Makam, R. Kovach et al., "Randomized controlled study of excimer laser atherectomy for treatment of femoropopliteal in-stent restenosis: initial results from the EXCITE ISR trial (EXCImer laser randomized controlled study for treatment of FemoropopliTEal in-stent restenosis)," *JACC: Cardiovascular Interventions*, vol. 8, no. 1, pp. 95–101, 2015.

[11] K. O. Kuku, H. M. Garcia-Garcia, E. Koifman et al., "Intravascular ultrasound assessment of the effect of laser energy on the arterial wall during the treatment of femoro-popliteal lesions: a CliRpath excimer laser system to enlarge lumen openings (CELLO) registry study," *The International Journal of Cardiovascular Imaging*, vol. 34, no. 3, pp. 345–352, 2018.

[12] A. Idemoto, N. Okamoto, A. Tanaka et al., "Impact of angioscopic evaluation for femoropopliteal in-stent restenosis before and after excimer laser atherectomy," *Vascular and Endovascular Surgery*, vol. 51, no. 5, pp. 335–337, 2017.

[13] K. Fukuda and Y. Yokoi, "Application of rotational atherectomy for a calcified superficial femoral artery lesion," *Cardiovascular Intervention and Therapeutics*, vol. 30, no. 4, pp. 351–355, 2015.

[14] M. Hara, M. Nishino, K. Matsuoka, and Y. Yamada, "Heavily calcified chronic total occlusion of common iliac artery successfully treated with Tornus microcatheter and rotational atherectomy," *Journal of Vascular Surgery*, vol. 48, no. 3, pp. 758–760, 2008.

[15] M. Egred, "RASER angioplasty," *Catheterization and Cardiovascular Interventions*, vol. 79, no. 6, pp. 1009–1012, 2012.

[16] D. B. McKenzie, S. Talwar, P. P. Jokhi, and P. D. O'Kane, "How should i treat severe coronary artery calcification when it is not possible to dilate a balloon or deliver a RotaWire™?" *EuroIntervention*, vol. 6, no. 6, pp. 779–783, 2011.

7

Endovenous Laser Ablation for Treatment of a Partially Thrombosed Proximal Great Saphenous Vein

Luca Spinedi,[1] Hans Stricker,[1] Daniel Staub,[2] and Heiko Uthoff[3]

[1] *Division of Angiology, Ospedale Regionale di Locarno, Locarno, Switzerland*
[2] *Division of Angiology, University Hospital Basel, University of Basel, Basel, Switzerland*
[3] *Gefässpraxis am See, Hirslanden Clinic St. Anna, Lucerne, Switzerland*

Correspondence should be addressed to Luca Spinedi; luca.spinedi@eoc.ch

Academic Editor: Konstantinos A. Filis

Introduction. Superficial vein thrombosis of the great saphenous vein near to the saphenofemoral junction is generally treated with anticoagulation or surgically. *Report.* We present the case of a 70-year-old man with varicosities and a partially thrombosed great saphenous vein near to the saphenofemoral junction, treated with endovenous laser ablation of the great saphenous vein. *Discussion.* The case illustrates an alternative treatment option for superficial vein thrombosis of the great saphenous vein, which permits avoiding a prolonged anticoagulation or surgical procedure.

1. Introduction

Different treatment modalities ranging from anticoagulation to surgery have been suggested and are performed to treat a superficial vein thrombosis (SVT) of the great saphenous vein (GSV) [1]. In this case report, we present a case of a thrombotic mass located in the GSV near to the saphenofemoral junction (SFJ), treated by endovenous laser ablation (EVLA).

2. Case Presentation

A 70-year-old man was evaluated for a long history of symptomatic varicose veins (pain and perimalleolar edema formation) on his left leg. Except for a dyslipidemia and arterial hypertension treated, respectively, with simvastatin and lisinopril, no other comorbidities were known. Personal and family history for prior venous thromboembolic events or neoplasia were negative. The physical examination revealed varicose veins in the area of the knee and lower leg mediodorsally, with perimalleolar edema on the left side. No varicose veins or local signs of inflammation were present in the groin. On the duplex ultrasound examination, an insufficient left GSV was disclosed, showing a long-lasting reflux (>2sec.) from the SFJ down to the ankle. The maximum diameter of the vein was 10mm in the thigh. Unexpectedly, a 10x10x8 mm isoechogenic mass with an hyperechogenic component could be detected in the region of the SFJ, in an eccentric dilated segment of the GSV adherent both to the terminal valve and to the vein wall. This mass was only partially obstructing the GSF (Figure 1). No color Doppler signals could be detected within the structure. The deep venous system of the left leg was patent and sufficient, without postthrombotic sequelae. Several characteristics, such as the location in a dilated segment of the vein, the echogenicity, and the absence of a Doppler signal within the mass, favored a diagnosis of focal thrombosis.

We started a thromboembolic prophylaxis with Rivaroxaban 10mg once daily. In addition, we discussed with the patient an accelerated EVLA of the GSV with the aim to treat the varicose veins, excluding at the same time the thrombotic mass. The outpatient-based intervention took place 7 days later. At that time, the thrombotic mass was still present and unchanged. A 1470nm wavelength radial fiber with a diameter of 600μm (ELVeS Biolitec Radial Laser) was inserted via a 21G introducer under echographic guidance from the mid third of the lower leg and pushed up to the SFJ. The thrombotic mass was passed under echographic guidance by maneuvering the tip laterally to the thrombotic

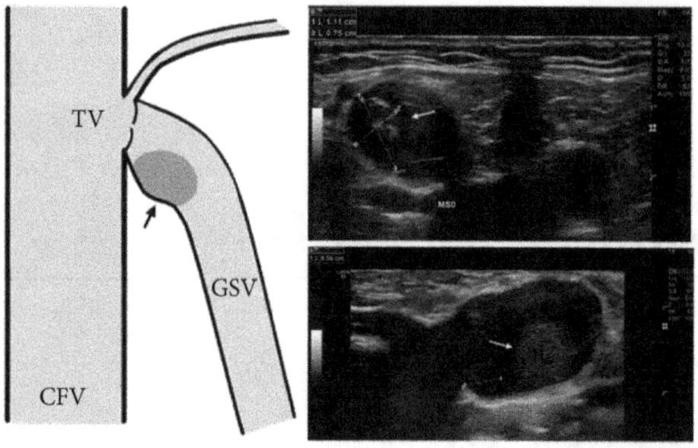

FIGURE 1: Partially obstructing, isoechogenic mass with hyperechogenic components (arrows) at the saphenofemoral junction in a medially situated eccentric dilatation of the great saphenous vein distally from the terminal valve.

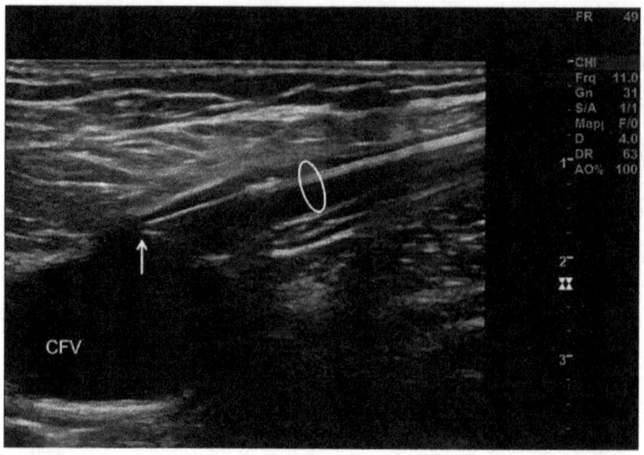

FIGURE 3: The tip of the laser fiber (arrow) is placed at the confluence between the great saphenous vein (white circle) and the common femoral vein (CFV).

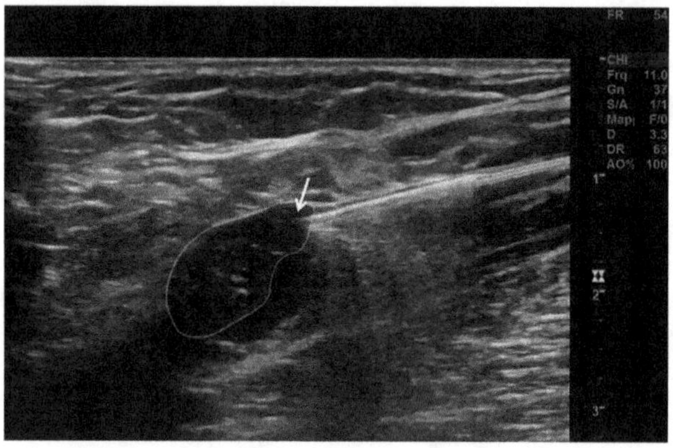

FIGURE 2: The tip of the laser fiber (white arrow) is stuck at the distal thrombotic mass (white-dashed line).

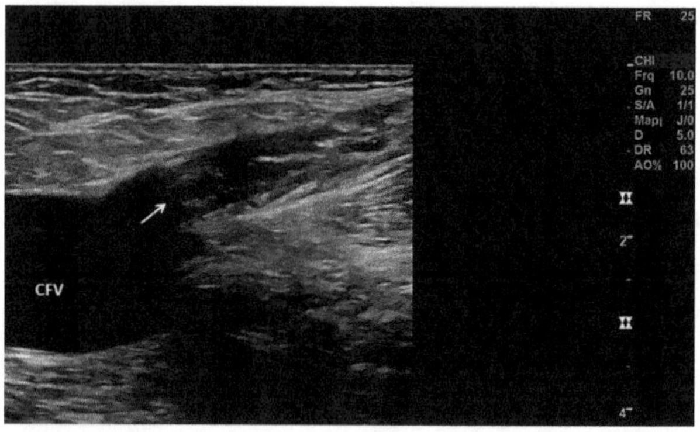

FIGURE 4: Result 13 days after endovenous laser ablation of the great saphenous vein (GSV) with exclusion of the thrombotic mass. The GSV (longitudinal view) is occluded up to the confluence (white arrow) between the great saphenous vein and the common femoral vein (CFV).

mass (Figure 2) without dislodging the thrombus (Figure 3) by gently steering the fiber, applying distal external manual pressure onto the laser fiber. The laser fiber was eventually placed at the confluence of the GSV with the common femoral vein without a safety distance in order to exclude the thrombotic mass. After tumescence anesthesia with diluted prilocaine and epinephrine, EVLA was performed (10W/100J proximally and 8W/80J distally, for a total energy of 6614 Joules and a treated length of 66cm). Subsequently, the tributaries were treated by miniphlebectomy. At the end of the procedure, an extrinsic compression with gauzes and elastic compression stocking (23-32 mmHg) were applied. Prophylactic anticoagulation with Rivaroxaban 10mg daily was continued for 5 days, according to our internal protocol after standard EVLA. Wound healing occurred without relevant complications, and the patient was asymptomatic during the follow-up.

Duplex ultrasound visits on day 1 and day 13, at 6 weeks, and one year after the intervention showed a permanent occlusion of the treated GSV up to the confluence without evidence of any thrombus propagation into the deep vein system (Figure 4). Particularly, no residual mass could be detected at the level of the SFJ.

3. Discussion

Deep venous thrombosis and pulmonary embolism (VTE) are potential complications that arise in 8% of patients affected by superficial venous thrombosis (SVT), particularly if the thrombus extends to the SFJ [2]. The treatment options of varicose vein thrombosis include compression therapy, pain control, anticoagulation, and surgical or endovascular interventions such as sclerotherapy, high ligation, vein stripping, phlebectomy, and thermal ablation [1]. The lack of consensus regarding the best care of this condition reflects the limited existing evidence as resumed in a 2013 published Cochrane review [3].

In our case, we used an accelerated EVLA to prevent VTE (obviating the need for a prolonged anticoagulation) and to treat the varicosities. Thermal ablation of the GSV in patients with SVT distally from the SFJ was already performed with success and described by Enzler [4], Bishara [5], and Gradma [6]. However, in our case, the thrombotic mass was located directly at the SFJ and could be excluded from the circulation by bypassing it with the laser fiber and treating the involved segment. Dislocation of the thrombus during placement of the laser fiber poses a potential risk. As the patient was generally healthy, the thrombotic mass was relatively small, and the patient had been anticoagulated during 7 days, the risk of a cardiopulmonal compromising lung embolism was deemed to be low. Furthermore, we expected an experienced operator, using a high-resolution ultrasound probe (6-15 MHZ), to be able to navigate the fiber tip past the wall adherent, nonocclusive thrombus quite safely.

Two potential alternative treatment options were discussed. First, a traditional surgical exploration and high ligation of the SFJ would have been possible. However, the risk of an embolization of the thrombotic mass by manual manipulation would still have been present. Therefore, also considering the less invasive nature of endothermal ablation as compared to surgery [7], we decided to use the endovenous approach. Alternatively, a prolonged (therapeutic) anticoagulation with an ultrasound follow up after 4-8 weeks to check for thrombus resolution, could have been chosen. However, as the treatment of the varicose veins would have been required later on anyway, the patient opted for the immediate exclusion of the GSV.

4. Conclusion

EVLA may be an alternative treatment option to anticoagulation or conventional surgery in the case of a partially thrombosed varicose GSV in the proximity of the SFJ, obviating the need for a prolonged therapeutic anticoagulation or a surgical procedure.

References

[1] A. Dua, J. A. Heller, B. Patel, and S. S. Desai, "Variability in the management of superficial venous thrombophlebitis across practitioners based in north america and the global community," *Thrombosis*, vol. 2014, Article ID 306018, 6 pages, 2014.

[2] H. Decousus, I. Quéré, E. Presles et al., "Superficial venous thrombosis and venous thromboembolism: a large, prospective epidemiologic study," *Annals of Internal Medicine*, vol. 152, no. 4, pp. 218–224, 2010.

[3] M. Di Nisio, I. M. Wichers, and S. Middeldorp, "Treatment for superficial thrombophlebitis of the leg," *Cochrane Database of Systematic Reviews*, vol. 4, Article ID CD004982, 2013.

[4] M. A. Enzler, D. Russell, and J. Schimmelpfennig, "Thermal ablation in the management of superficial thrombophlebitis," *European Journal of Vascular and Endovascular Surgery*, vol. 43, no. 6, pp. 726–728, 2012.

[5] R. A. Bishara, W. Taha, and A. I. Grace, "Endovenous great saphenous vein ablation for the treatment of superficial thrombophlebitis complicated by pulmonary embolism," *European Journal of Vascular and Endovascular Surgery*, vol. 47, no. 3, pp. 330-331, 2014.

[6] W. S. Gradman, "Endovenous saphenous vein ablation in patients with acute isolated superficial-vein thrombosis," *Phlebology*, vol. 30, no. 3, pp. 204–209, 2015.

[7] P. Gloviczki, A. J. Comerota, M. C. Dalsing et al., "The care of patients with varicose veins and associated chronic venous diseases: clinical practice guidelines of the society for vascular surgery and the american venous forum," *Journal of Vascular Surgery*, vol. 53, supplement 5, pp. 2S–48S, 2011.

8

A Case Study of Malrotated Kidneys with Asymmetric Multiple Renal Arteries, Variant Venous Drainage and Unilateral Ureteral Duplication

Martine Dunnwald and Marc A. Pizzimenti

Department of Anatomy and Cell Biology, Roy J. and Lucille A. Carver College of Medicine, University of Iowa, Iowa City, Iowa, USA

Correspondence should be addressed to Marc A. Pizzimenti; marc-pizzimenti@uiowa.edu

Academic Editor: Muzaffer Sindel

Variations in the arterial, venous, and ureteral patterning of the right (r) and left (l) kidneys are common; however, concomitant involvement with all three systems is rare. Specimens that demonstrate anatomic variation across multiple systems provide an opportunity to illustrate links between anatomic concepts, embryologic development, clinical practice, and education. During anatomic study of the abdominal cavity, a total of five major arteries (3l and 2r) emerged from the aortic and common iliac axes in a cadaveric donor. Through continued study, multiple contributing veins, of different caliber, coalesced into four major renal veins (2l and 2r) that returned blood from the kidneys to the inferior vena cava (IVC) at different locations. In addition, unilateral duplication of the kidney with concomitant ureters was evident on the right side. Both ureters continued inferiorly and independently entered the bladder, each with an observable orifice adjacent to the bladder trigone. Most evident in the specimen was the anteriorly directed hilum for both kidneys. Reported measures for each of the observed anatomic variations suggest that the current specimen has an estimated incidence of less than 0.3%. This comparatively rare specimen provides an example of important anatomic concepts that are relevant to educational and clinical practices.

1. Introduction

Although variations in the arterial, venous, and ureteral patterning of the kidneys are common, concomitant involvement of variant anatomy in all of these systems appears to be much rarer. Arterial variants that diverge from the generalized pattern of paired renal arteries emerging laterally from the aorta, inferior to the level of the superior mesenteric artery, have been observed in approximately 30% of individuals (e.g., [1, 2]). In the venous system, variations in the drainage pattern that diverge from the classically described paired vessels flowing into the inferior vena cava (IVC) have been well documented and can have an incidence rate similar to that of the arterial system (e.g., [3]). However, variation in the ureteral pattern is not as common as that found in the vascular system. Reports indicate that genetic factors contribute to ureteric variations [4, 5] which occur with an approximate incidence of 1% [6, 7].

The case study presented here demonstrates concomitant variation in the arterial, venous, and ureteric systems of the kidney. Collectively, this case provides examples of important anatomic considerations that relate the foundational anatomical science with educational practice. These include the generalized concept of anatomic variation, the process of renal morphogenesis with variant presentations, and considerations for clinical procedures with involved variant anatomy.

2. Case Report

During anatomic study of the abdominal cavity, additional renal branches from the aortic axis were revealed in a 97-year-old male Caucasian cadaveric donor. Continued dissection outlined notable anatomic variations in the arterial, venous, and ureteric patterns. No urologic or cardiovascular issues were reported by the donor or family at the time of enrolment in the Deeded Body Program. For this type of

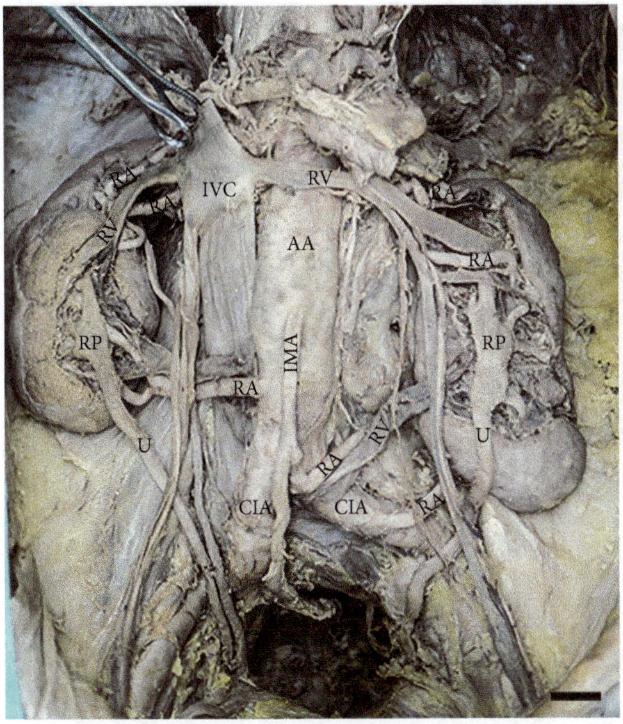

Figure 1: *Renal system in situ.* Macroscopic view of the renal system within the abdominal cavity of the donor. AA = abdominal aorta, CIA = common iliac artery, IMA = inferior mesenteric artery, IVC = inferior vena cava, RA = renal artery, RP = renal pelvis, RV = renal vein, U = ureter. Image scale bar = 2 cm.

study, Institutional Review Board approval is not required for research conducted with cadaveric specimens.

Both kidneys were retroperitoneal and similar in size with measurements of 12.3 cm (l) and 12.7 cm (r) in the craniocaudal direction. Despite the fact that the lengths were similar, there were marked differences in the relative positioning of the superior and inferior poles. The superior pole of the right kidney was situated more superiorly. The inferior pole of the left kidney was positioned near the superior border of the left common iliac artery. Although each kidney occupied an extended volume, neither kidney had a pelvic component. Hilar structures entered/exited the organs anteriorly, not with the typical medially projected hilum (Figure 1).

2.1. Arterial Pattern. A total of five major arteries (3l and 2r) emerged from the aortic and common iliac axes (Figures 2(a) and 2(b)). The superior left renal artery originated from the abdominal aorta and supplied the superior pole. This artery (5.2 mm diameter) branched into two vessels of similar caliber to supply the upper third of the organ. Supply to the left gonad originated from the more inferior of these two branches (Figures 2(b) and 3(b)). The middle left renal artery (6.1 mm diameter) originated from the iliac junction, just anterior to the median sacral artery (Figures 3(a) and 3(b)). The inferior left renal artery (5.4 mm diameter) originated from the common iliac artery, and coursed posteriorly to the kidney before entering the hilum anteriorly (from the lateral aspect of the organ), to supply the inferior pole (Figures 3(b), 3(c), and 3(d)). On the contralateral side, the vasculature to the right kidney consisted of only two renal arteries, both originating from the abdominal aorta. The superior renal artery (6.2 mm diameter) branched laterally from the aorta (at the same level as the left superior renal) and supplied the superior pole. As with the contralateral side, this artery also branched into two vessels of similar caliber, but supplied the superior half of the organ (Figures 4(a) and 4(b)). In contrast to the contralateral side, the right gonadal artery branched directly from the aorta at its generally observed position, just inferior to the (superior) renal artery. Arterial supply to the inferior pole (6.5 mm diameter) originated on the lateral aorta, at a level inferior to the inferior mesenteric artery, and branched into two arteries (Figures 4(b), 4(c), and 4(d)).

2.2. Venous Pattern. Multiple contributing veins, of different caliber, coalesced into four major renal veins (2l and 2r) that returned blood from the kidneys to the IVC (Figure 2(c)). The relative positioning of the superior renal veins followed the conventional pattern, entering the IVC through single vessels at a level just inferior to the superior mesenteric artery as it emerged from the aorta. On the right side, three major veins merged into a short segment (3 mm in length) to drain the superior 2/3 of the organ. The inferior 1/3 of the organ was drained through two primary contributors that merged into a single vein that ultimately drained into the IVC at the level of the previously described right inferior renal artery. A visible and substantive anastomotic connection was evident between the superior and inferior venous pathways (Figure 3(b)). On the left side, the superior renal vein received contributions from the suprarenal gland and the superior half of the kidney. Venous return from the left gonad ultimately merged into the most inferior branch of the three primary contributors to the superior renal vein (Figures 2(c) and 3(b)). The inferior renal vein drained directly into the anterior aspect of the IVC at the junction of the common iliac veins, posterior to the bifurcation of the aorta. The most inferior of the three primary contributors to the inferior renal vein emerged from the posterior lateral aspect of kidney and spanned the hilum to ultimately converge into the inferior renal vein. The middle contributor emerged from the parenchyma, but was unremarkable. As on the contralateral side, a visible and substantive venous anastomotic connection was evident between the superior and inferior aspects of the kidney (Figure 4(b)).

2.3. Ureteral Pattern. Unilateral duplication of the kidney with concomitant ureters was evident for the right side (Figure 2(d)). Aligned with the arterial pattern of this organ, the superior ureter demonstrated a discreet collecting system with well-formed minor and major calyces draining into a defined renal pelvis. The majority of the superior renal pelvis was positioned posterior to the vasculature (Figures 4(a) and 4(b)). At the inferior portion of the kidney, the hilum was more anteriorly directed with the calyces and renal pelvis more evident given their anterior position relative to the vasculature. Both ureters continued inferiorly and independently to enter the bladder (Figure 1). Histological

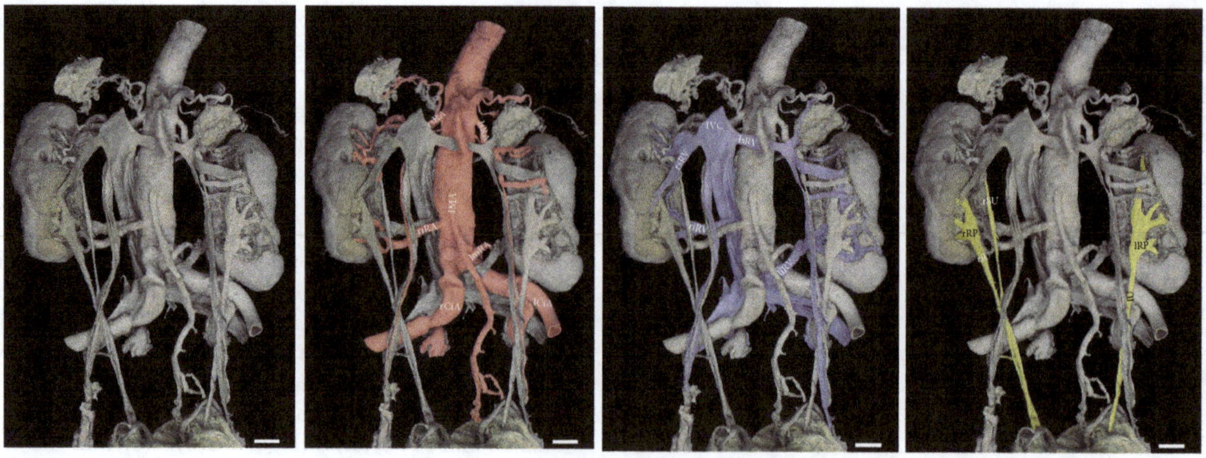

(a) (b) (c) (d)

Figure 2: *Ex situ renal system exhibits anatomical variations from normal pattern.* (a) Uncolorized renal system *ex situ.* (b) Arterial network pseudocolorized in red. rsRA = right superior renal artery, lsRA = left superior renal artery, IMA = inferior mesenteric artery, riRA = right inferior renal artery, lmRA = left middle renal artery, liRA = left inferior renal artery, rCiRA = right common iliac artery, lCiA = left common iliac artery. (c) Venous network pseudocolorized in blue. IVC = inferior vena cava, rsRV = right superior renal vein, lsRV = left superior renal vein, riRV = right inferior renal vein, liRV = left inferior renal vein. (d) Ureters pseudocolorized in yellow with rRP = right renal pelvis, lRP = left renal pelvis, rU = right ureters, lU= left ureter. Pseudocolorization created using Adobe Photoshop. Image scale bar = 2 cm.

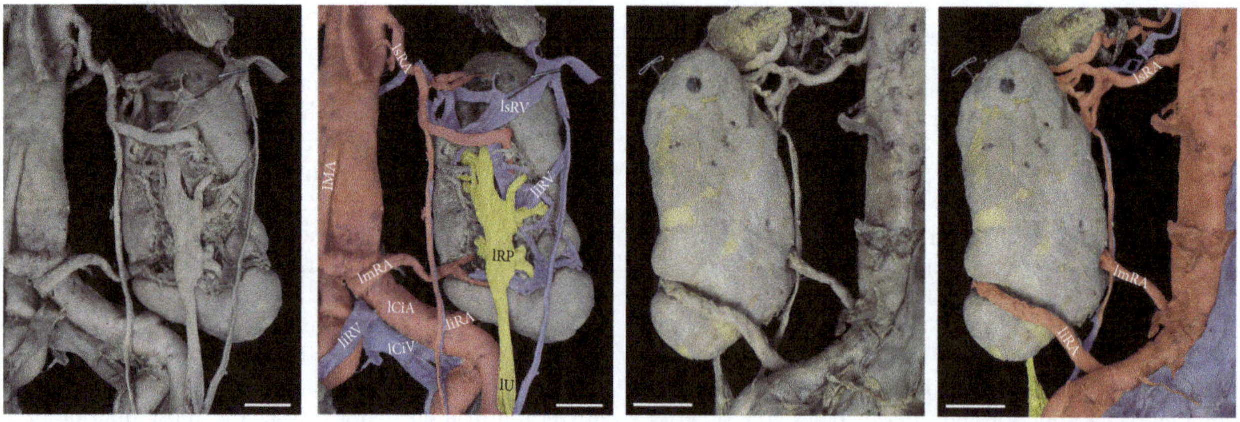

(a) (b) (c) (d)

Figure 3: *Ex situ left kidney exhibits anatomical variations.* Anterior (a, b) and posterior (c, d) views of the left kidney. Arterial, venous and ureteric systems (b, d) are pseudocolorized in red (arterial), blue (venous) and yellow (ureteric). Renal veins (lsRV, liRV) are reflected to better illustrate the arterial pattern. Image scale bar = 2 cm.

investigation of the ureterovesical junctions was not completed; however a distinct orifice near the bladder trigone was evident for each ureter. On the contralateral side, the single ureter emerged from a widened and anteriorly projected hilum (Figure 3(b)). Major calyces from the peripheral parenchyma were evident and these calyces contributed to an elongated renal pelvis. The remaining course of the left ureter was unremarkable.

3. Discussion

Rare case studies present opportunities to not only consider the observed morphological variations but also revisit underlying concepts in embryology and the associated educational implications. Variations in the arterial, venous, and ureteral patterning of the kidneys are common; however, involvement with all three systems is very rare. The current case demonstrates concomitant variation in the arterial, venous, and ureteral systems, which is conservatively estimated to have an incidence of less than 0.3%.

3.1. Anatomic Variation. Arterial variants have been observed in approximately 30% of individuals, although population specific incidences have been shown to vary considerably [1, 8]. Studies documenting the major renal branches, rather than the branching pattern into kidney parenchyma, suggest that arterial origins along the entire abdominal aortic axis are possible. Branches at or superior to the level of the superior mesenteric artery [9] and along the lumbar region [10–14] have been well documented. Arterial branching from

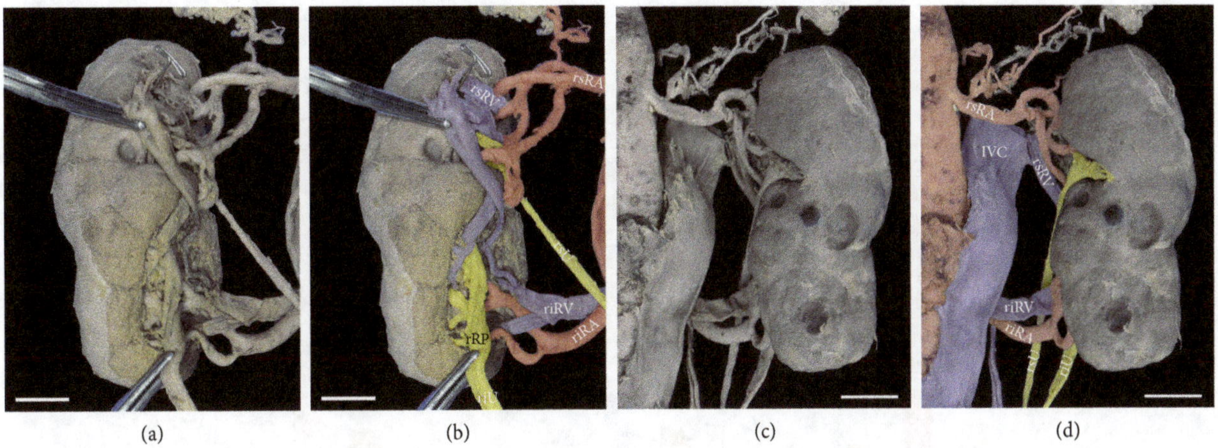

FIGURE 4: *Ex situ right kidney exhibits anatomical variations.* Anterior (a, b) and posterior (c, d) views of the right kidney. Arterial, venous, and ureteric systems (b, d) are pseudocolorized in red (arterial), blue (venous), and yellow (ureteric).

the iliac axis has also been documented, particularly in ectopic kidneys [15–17], however ectopic specimens without pelvic involvement have also demonstrated branches arising from the iliac region [14, 18]. Bilateral variation in the arterial patterning has been quantified with an incidence of approximately 10% [19] while unilateral arterial supply to the kidney arising from all of these regions has a suggested incidence of approximately 0.4% [20, 21].

Although early modern attempts to quantify patterning through direct patient (and/or cadaveric) observation (e.g., [22–24]) were compelling, more recent studies using imaging (e.g., [18, 19, 21]) have verified and improved our understanding of the incidence for these arterial patterns. They have been classified in Patterns (I-V) and Types (A-E) based on the number of vessels observed and the location from which the vessels arise, respectively. From these studies, the arterial distribution to the right kidney in the current specimen generally fits the description for Pattern II and Type D, where two arteries enter the kidney and the inferior renal segment is supplied directly from the aorta. This arterial pattern/type has an incidence rate of approximately 2%. The left kidney in the current specimen most closely demonstrates Pattern III, with 3-4 distinct arteries, but the Type descriptor falls outside of the general classification schema. Here, the current specimen is most similar to case studies presented through direct observation in cadaveric specimens [25] or visualized through CT-3D reconstruction [18]. Although Cases et al. did not include a reconstructed case in the analysis, the data set would suggest an hypothesized incidence for the current arterial pattern to be at minimum of 0.4%. However, a statistically sound meta-analysis that includes specific branching categories across studies has yet to be completed.

As with the arterial system, variation in renal vein patterning is not uncommon. Studies with large sample sizes (e.g., >100) suggest that variation in venous patterning has an incidence of 23.5-30%, as observed through computed tomography (CT) [3, 26–28]. This reported incidence has also been observed in 105 cases of horseshoe kidney [29]. Given the high incidence of renal vein variation, a recent study used CT to observe and classify these variations within a comparatively large sample size (1452 patients) [28]. In this classification system, the venous drainage of the right kidney in the current specimen could be described as Type 2A (0.3% incidence), with direct drainage into the IVC from two renal veins. The venous drainage of the left kidney could be described as Type IB (1.4% incidence), with drainage into the IVC and common iliac vein. What is unclear from these studies is if the incidence rates are applicable for bilateral variations.

Variation in ureteral patterning is not as common as that found in the vascular system, but reports indicate an approximate incidence of 1% [6, 7], with unilateral duplex kidney reported as high as 1.8% [30]. Incidence of ureteral duplication appears to have a familial pattern of inheritance [4, 5] that, for a duplex kidney, results from more than one ureteric bud outgrowth from the mesonephric duct during fetal development.

As outlined above, aspects of the variations described in the current case have been observed elsewhere. However, few of those cases have provided detailed descriptions and illustrations of concomitant involvement of each system. Collectively, this case appears to be rare given the low incidence rates for each (independent) system: arterial, 0.4%; venous, 0.3-1.4%; and ureteral, 1-1.8%. Based on this review of studies, and using the reported systems-related variation, the incidence rate for the current specimen is conservatively estimated at less than 0.3% of the population.

3.2. Educational and Embryological Considerations. Students who participate in dissection courses early in their training, or students rotating through their clinical training, learn the basic premise of anatomic variation—that organs/regions under study often do not appear, at least at first, as outlined in a referenced source. Distinguishing which variations have clinical significance requires both breadth and depth of training, particularly within each clinical specialty [31]. Although exposure to the concept of variation usually occurs early in training and primarily through dissection courses [31], many of the region/organ details are often revisited within clinical clerkships and during residency training [32].

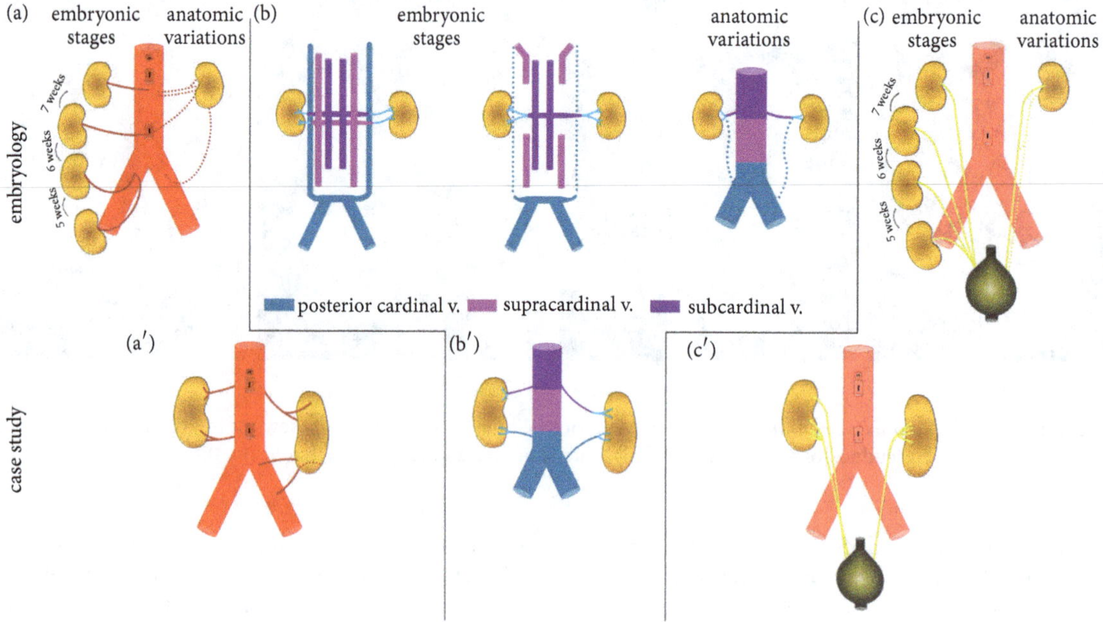

Figure 5: *Simplified schematic representation of renal development.* Around 5 weeks of fetal life, kidneys are formed from the metanephros. They are situated at the level of the pelvis and pelvic branches of the common iliac artery provide initial arterial blood supply. During the following 3 weeks, the kidneys ascend in the abdominal cavity (a) to their adult retroperitoneal location. As they move cranially and the metanephros coalesces, the lower arteries degenerate to, most often, leave a single renal artery as the main arterial supply. Occasionally, the temporary arteries (dotted lines (a)) do not degenerate leading to anatomical variations in the adult (a′). The cardinal systems contribute to the developing venous network of the kidney as it ascends (b). Persistence of some aspects of the developing venous network may lead to anatomical variations in the adult (dotted lines (b), (b′)). More than one ureteric bud may penetrate the metanephric mesoderm during ureteral development (c) that results in duplex kidney (left (c′)).

For example, variations in renal arterial patterning may have little clinical significance unless they are coupled with hypertension or require mapping for clinical procedures such as surgical resection (e.g., [33]), transplantation (e.g., [34]), or percutaneous access (e.g., [35]). Given the multisystem (i.e., arterial, venous, and ureteral) involvement, this case clearly demonstrates the anatomical aspect of this concept.

Collectively, the anatomic variations of the current case also reflect important concepts related to the morphological development of the kidney and its collecting system. During human development, three slightly overlapping renal systems are formed in a cranial to caudal fashion: pronephros, mesonephros and metanephros [36]. The pronephros is a temporary organ that regresses at the end of the fourth week of fetal life while the mesonephros contributes to Bowman's capsule and the Wolffian duct in adult kidneys. The metanephros appears in the fifth week of fetal life and will give rise to the adult kidney. The renal excretory units originate from the metanephric mesoderm and collecting ducts from the ureteric bud that penetrates the mesodermic tissue. While the primordial kidneys are initially located within the pelvis with their hila projected anteriorly to receive their arterial supply from a pelvic branch of the aorta, this orientation changes with development. Following growth and change in body length at the lumbar and sacral regions, the kidneys undergo a relative "ascent" in the abdomen as they shift to a more cranial position [37, 38]. This ascent is accompanied by a transitioning arterial supply originating from aortic branches at sequentially higher levels and medial rotation of the developing kidney, as schematically depicted in Figure 5(a). The lower vessels usually degenerate, but occasionally, some remain, leading to anatomical variations in the adult (Figures 2(b), 3(b), 3(c), 4(b), 4(d), and 5(a′)).

Unlike the arterial system, the venous system for the kidney arises from anastomotic connections between the developing cardinal veins [38]. Briefly, at 5-6 weeks of development the posterior and subcardinal veins exhibit anastomotic connections in a segment-like fashion that drain aspects of the early mesonephros. The subcardinal veins anastomose and coalesce in the midline, contributing to the prerenal portion of the IVC and what is generally considered the developed right renal vein. Supracardinal veins, like the other renal contributors, begin as bilaterally symmetric having segmental connections with the posterior cardinal veins. As development continues, the posterior cardinal veins degenerate, losing the segmental nature of the connections that were established earlier with the subcardinal and supracardinal network. Ultimately, the supracardinal system contributes to the postrenal segment of the IVC. This segment fuses with caudal posterior cardinal segment that, in turn, gives rise to the common iliac veins. Concomitantly, the supracardinal system on the left side loses connections with the developed left renal vein and the hemiazygos system. Even with this simplified overview of a very complex developmental process

(Figure 5(b)), the persistent connections between the venous cardinal networks (Figures 2(c), 3(b), 4(b), and 5(b′)) can be observed in the current specimen.

Development of the ureters arises from bud outgrowths of the mesonephric duct. For each kidney, the ureteric bud penetrates the metanephric mesoderm (metanephrogenic blastema) that forms a cap into which the renal pelvis, calyxes, and collecting tubules develop through branching morphogenesis [36]. The stalk of the ureteric bud elongates as the kidney undergoes its relative ascent resulting in the formed ureter by the ninth week of development (Figure 5(c)). The simultaneous morphogenesis of the vascular and ureteric structures influences the medial rotation of the hilum for each developing kidney. Details of the signaling pathways and the genes that regulate this entire process have been effectively summarized in the literature [39, 40] and are beyond the scope of this case study. These processes coupled with genetic factors may give rise to variations in the ureteric pattern (Figures 2(d), 4(b), 4(d), 5(c), and 5(c′)).

4. Conclusion

Anatomic variations in the systems of the developing kidney are common; however, concomitant involvement of the arterial, venous, and ureteric systems is rare. The current case study demonstrates a cadaveric specimen with anatomic variations having an estimated incidence of less than 0.3%. Collectively, this case illustrates examples of important anatomic concepts that are relevant for educational and clinical practice.

Authors' Contributions

Marc A. Pizzimenti contributed in project development, dissection, and manuscript writing. Martine Dunnwald contributed in dissection, illustrations, and manuscript writing.

Acknowledgments

The authors would like to thank the families of individuals who, through their most generous gift to the Deeded Body Program, allow us to continue studying the human body.

References

[1] E. Gulas, G. Wysiadecki, T. Cecot et al., "Accessory (multiple) renal arteries - Differences in frequency according to population, visualizing techniques and stage of morphological development," *Vascular*, vol. 24, no. 5, pp. 531–537, 2016.

[2] R. Bergman, S. Thompson, A. Afifi, and F. Saadeh, *Compendium of Human Anatomic Variation: Text, Atlas, and World Literature*, Urban & Scharzenberg, Inc., Baltimore, Munich, Germany, 1988.

[3] Z. Koc, S. Ulusan, L. Oguzkurt, and N. Tokmak, "Venous variants and anomalies on routine abdominal multi-detector row CT," *European Journal of Radiology*, vol. 61, no. 2, pp. 267–278, 2007.

[4] J. D. Atwell, P. L. Cook, C. J. Howell, I. Hyde, and B. C. Parker, "Familial incidence of bifid and double ureters," *Archives of Disease in Childhood*, vol. 49, no. 5, pp. 390–393, 1974.

[5] J. Whitaker and D. M. Danks, "A study of the inheritance of duplication of the kidneys and ureters.," *The Journal of Urology*, vol. 95, no. 2, pp. 176–178, 1966.

[6] V. Alberts, R. Minnee, K. van Donselaar-van der Pant et al., "Duplicated ureters and renal transplantation: a case-control study and review of the literature," *Transplantation Proceedings*, vol. 45, no. 9, pp. 3239–3244, 2013.

[7] R. Pollak, B. F. Prusak, and M. F. Mozes, "Anatomic abnormalities of cadaver kidneys procured for purposes of transplantation," *The American Surgeon*, vol. 52, no. 5, pp. 233–235, 1986.

[8] K. S. Satyapal, A. A. Haffejee, B. Singh, L. Ramsaroop, J. V. Robbs, and J. M. Kalideen, "Additional renal arteries: Incidence and morphometry," *Surgical and Radiologic Anatomy*, vol. 23, no. 1, pp. 33–38, 2001.

[9] C. Dalçik, T. Çolak, A. Özbek, and H. Dalçik, "Unusual origin of the right renal artery: a case report," *Surgical and Radiologic Anatomy*, vol. 22, no. 2, pp. 117-118, 2000.

[10] U. G. Rossi, M. Romano, and C. Ferro, "Seven renal arteries," *Clinical Anatomy*, vol. 19, no. 7, pp. 632-633, 2006.

[11] P. Mazengenya, "Multiple variations of the renal and testicular vessels: possible embryological basis and clinical importance," *Surgical and Radiologic Anatomy*, vol. 38, no. 6, pp. 729–733, 2016.

[12] K. Morishima, T. Miyaki, and H. Ito, "A rare case of a kidney with an (sic) widely opened hilus and supernumerary renal vessels," *Kaibogaku Zasshi. Journal of Anatomy*, vol. 71, no. 3, pp. 215–218, 1996.

[13] H. Narita, T. Tani, and Y. Tonosaki, "Associations between kidney position and surplus renal arteries in horseshoe kidney: Case report and analysis," *Okajimas Folia Anatomica Japonica*, vol. 89, no. 1, pp. 7–13, 2012.

[14] S. T. Patil, M. M. Meshram, and A. P. Kasote, "Bilateral malrotation and lobulation of kidney with altered hilar anatomy: a rare congenital variation," *Surgical and Radiologic Anatomy*, vol. 33, no. 10, pp. 941–944, 2011.

[15] S. Degani, Z. Leibovitz, I. Shapiro, and G. Ohel, "Variations of the origin of renal arteries in the fetus identified on power Doppler and 3D sonography," *Journal of Clinical Ultrasound*, vol. 38, no. 2, pp. 59–65, 2009.

[16] J. Singh, N. Singh, K. Kapoor, and M. Sharma, "Bilateral malrotation and a congenital pelvic kidney with varied vasculature and altered hilar anatomy," *Case Reports in Medicine*, vol. 2015, Article ID 848949, 3 pages, 2015.

[17] C. Krishnaveni and R. Kulkarni, "A right ectopic kidney with bilateral multiple anomalies of the renal vasculature – a case report," *Journal of Clinical and Diagnostic Research*, vol. 7, pp. 150–153, 2013.

[18] C. Cases, L. García-Zoghby, P. Manzorro et al., "Anatomical variations of the renal arteries: Cadaveric and radiologic study, review of the literature, and proposal of a new classification of clinical interest," *Annals of Anatomy - Anatomischer Anzeiger*, vol. 211, pp. 61–68, 2017.

[19] O. Kornafel, B. Baran, I. Pawlikowska, P. Laszczynski, M. Guzinski, and M. Sasiadek, "Analysis of anatomical variations of the main arteries branching from the abdominal aorta, with 64-detector computed tomography," *Polish Journal of Radiology*, vol. 75, pp. 38–45, 2010.

[20] F. J. B. Sampaio and M. A. R. F. Passos, "Renal arteries: anatomic study for surgical and radiological practice," *Surgical and Radiologic Anatomy*, vol. 14, no. 2, pp. 113–117, 1992.

[21] D. T. Tardo, C. Briggs, G. Ahern, A. Pitman, and S. Sinha, "Anatomical variations of the renal arterial vasculature: An Aus-

tralian perspective," *Journal of Medical Imaging and Radiation Oncology*, vol. 61, no. 5, pp. 643–649, 2017.

[22] J. R. Geyer and E. F. Poutasse, "Incidence of multiple renal arteries on aortography: report of a series of 400 patients, 381 of whom had arterial hypertension," *Journal of the American Medical Association*, vol. 182, no. 2, pp. 120–125, 1962.

[23] F. T. Graves, "The arterial anatomy of the congenitally abnormal kidney," *British Journal of Surgery*, vol. 56, no. 7, pp. 533–541, 1969.

[24] R. J. Merklin and N. A. Michels, "The variant renal and suprarenal blood supply with data on the inferior phrenic, ureteral and gonadal arteries: A statistical analysis based on 185 dissections and review of the literature," *Journal of the International College of Surgeons*, vol. 29, no. 1, pp. 41–76, 1958.

[25] A. H. Young and P. Thompson, "Abnormalities of the renal arteries, with remarks on their development and morphology," *Journal of Anatomy*, vol. 38, pp. 1–14, 1903.

[26] J.-P. Trigaux, S. Vandroogenbroek, J.-F. De Wispelaere, M. Lacrosse, and J. Jamart, "Congenital anomalies of the inferior vena cava and left renal vein: Evaluation with spiral ct," *Journal of Vascular and Interventional Radiology*, vol. 9, no. 2, pp. 339–345, 1998.

[27] S. Kawamoto, L. P. Lawler, and E. K. Fishman, "Evaluation of the renal venous system on late arterial and venous phase images with MDCT angiography in potential living laparoscopic renal donors," *American Journal of Roentgenology*, vol. 184, no. 2, pp. 539–545, 2005.

[28] J. Zhu, L. Zhang, Z. Yang, H. Zhou, and G. Tang, "Classification of the renal vein variations: a study with multidetector computed tomography," *Surgical and Radiologic Anatomy*, vol. 37, no. 6, pp. 667–675, 2015.

[29] T. Ichikawa, S. Kawada, J. Koizumi et al., "Major venous anomalies are frequently associated with horseshoe kidneys," *Circulation Journal*, vol. 75, no. 12, pp. 2872–2877, 2011.

[30] J. T. J. Privett, W. D. Jeans, and J. Roylance, "The incidence and importance of renal duplication," *Clinical Radiology*, vol. 27, no. 4, pp. 521–530, 1976.

[31] P. L. Willan and J. R. Humpherson, "Concepts of variation and normality in morphology: Important issues at risk of neglect in modern undergraduate medical courses," *Clinical Anatomy*, vol. 12, pp. 186–190, 1999.

[32] A. Raikos and J. D. Smith, "Anatomical variations: How do surgical and radiology training programs teach and assess them in their training curricula?" *Clinical Anatomy*, vol. 28, no. 6, pp. 717–724, 2015.

[33] N. Rani, S. Singh, P. Dhar, and R. Kumar, "Surgical importance of arterial segments of human kidneys: An angiography and corrosion cast study," *Journal of Clinical and Diagnostic Research*, vol. 8, pp. 1–3, 2014.

[34] S. Ersöz, A. Tüzüner, B. Erkek, S. Esen, and E. Anadol, "Double renal arteries in living-related kidney transplantation," *Transplantation Proceedings*, vol. 32, no. 3, p. 604, 2000.

[35] V. Ravery, O. Cussenot, F. Desgrandchamps et al., "Variations in arterial blood supply and the risk of hemorrhage during percutaneous treatment of lesions of the pelviureteral junction obstruction: report of a case of testicular artery arising from an inferior polar renal artery," *Surgical and Radiologic Anatomy*, vol. 15, no. 4, pp. 355–359, 1993.

[36] T. Sadler, "Urogenital system," in *Langman's medical embryology*, Lippinott Williams & Wilkins, Baltimore, MD, USA, 12th edition, 2012.

[37] K. L. Moore and T. V. N. Persaud, "The cardiovascular system," in *The Developing Human: Clinically Oriented Embryology*, pp. 330–335, Saunders, Philadelphia, Pa, USA, 7th edition, 2003.

[38] G. C. Schoenwolf, S. B. Bleyl, P. R. Brauer, and P. H. Francis-West, "Development of the vasculature," in *Larsen's human embryology*, pp. 385–432, Churchhill Livingstone, Philadelphia, Pa, USA, 4th edition, 2009.

[39] K. I. Glassberg, "Normal and abnormal development of the kidney: A clinician's interpretation of current knowledge," *The Journal of Urology*, vol. 167, no. 6, pp. 2339–2350, 2002, discussion 2350-2331.

[40] N. D. Rosenblum, "Developmental biology of the human kidney," *Seminars in Fetal and Neonatal Medicine*, vol. 13, no. 3, pp. 125–132, 2008.

9

Bilateral Hypothenar Hammer Syndrome Case Presentation and Literature Review

Andrés-Trasahedo Estíbaliz,[1] Labrador-Sánchez Eztizen,[1] Salazar-Asencio Osman-Alberto,[2] Flores-Robles Bryan-Josué,[1] Pinillos-Aransay Valvanera,[1] Laura Torrecilla Lerena,[1] and López-Martín Juan-Antonio[1]

[1]*Rheumatology Department, San Pedro Hospital, Logroño, La Rioja, Spain*
[2]*Neurosurgery Department, Son Espases University Hospital, Islas Baleares, Spain*

Correspondence should be addressed to Flores-Robles Bryan-Josué; aldolasa@hotmail.com

Academic Editor: Matthias Reinhard

Hypothenar hammer syndrome is a rare cause of vascular insufficiency. Generally, patients report a history of repetitive trauma to the hypothenar region of the hand. Symptoms often consist of cold intolerance, pain, paleness, and paresthesia due to digital ischemia. The severity of these symptoms will depend on the extent of ulnar artery occlusion and the presence or absence of collaterals between this artery's superficial and deep branches. It is a rare clinical entity, which on multiple occasions requires a surgical approach. We present a 63-year-old man with bilateral Raynaud's phenomenon secondary to hypothenar hammer syndrome successfully treated by vascular repair surgery. In patients with Raynaud's phenomenon, it is important to know that there are reversible causes such as hypothenar hammer syndrome.

1. Introduction

First described by Van Rosen in 1934, hypothenar hammer syndrome is an infrequent cause of Raynaud's phenomenon [1]. It usually occurs due to repeated microtraumas on the hypothenar eminence of the hand [2, 3]. The hook of the hamate strikes the superficial palmar branch of the ulnar artery in the Guyon space, leading to the development of (1) an aneurysmal dilation of the artery with subsequent distal embolization and (2) a local segmental occlusion of the ulnar artery [1]. Clinically, it is characterized by pain, intolerance to cold and cyanosis, paresthesias, digital ulcers, or palpable mass [1]. The gold standard for diagnosis is angiography since it provides information on the lesion's location, segment, and extent [1].

2. Case Presentation

A 63-year-old man, a medical doctor, and a cycling fan consulted for an episode of paleness and coldness affecting the fourth finger of the right hand, lasting three days. The patient reported that two months ago, he had presented the appearance of a tumor in the hypothenar region of the right hand. During the months of confinement due to the pandemic, he had been cycling as a sports activity. However, he did not report any symptoms suggestive of connective tissue disease.

His personal history included hypertension, dyslipidemia, and subarachnoid hemorrhage at age forty-five. He denied the use of tobacco, alcohol, or other toxic substances and was on regular treatment with aspirin, atorvastatin, ezetimibe, and telmisartan. Blood pressure was normal in both arms on physical examination, and cardiopulmonary auscultation did not show any relevant findings. Pulses in all four limbs were symmetrically palpable.

An analytical study including hemogram, biochemical profile, coagulation study, and autoimmune serology (ANA, ANCA, antiphospholipid antibodies) was performed, with normal values. In addition, an ultrasound study was performed in the vascular laboratory of the infrarenal aorta,

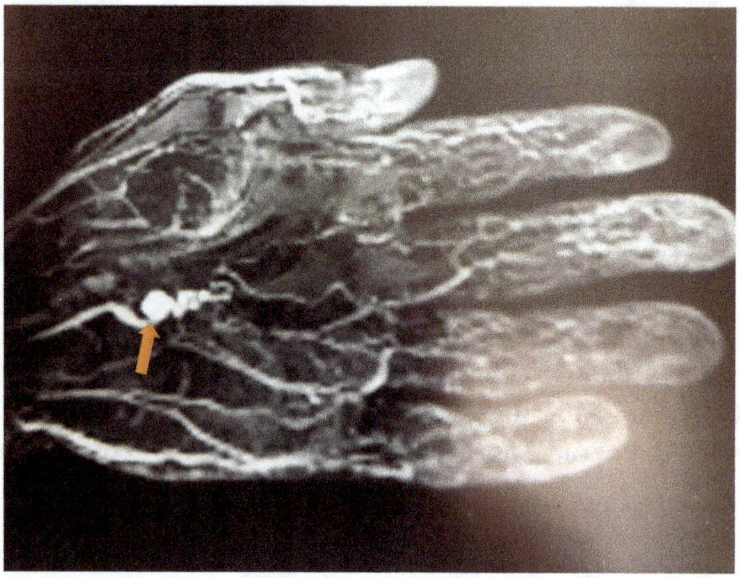

FIGURE 1: Angioresonance showing an aneurysm approximately 7 mm in diameter in the distal area of the ulnar artery, typical "corkscrew" image (red arrow).

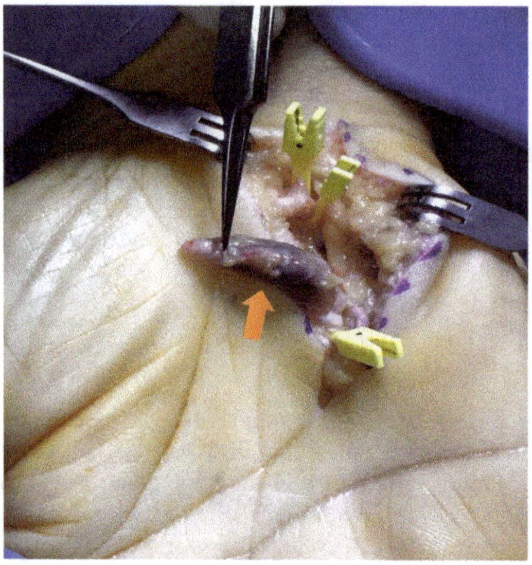

FIGURE 2: Vascular surgery repair with vein graft. The image shows the aneurysm of the ulnar artery (red arrow).

common iliac arteries, and popliteal arteries, which was also normal.

Magnetic resonance angiography was performed on both hands, showing an aneurysm in the distal area of the ulnar artery (approximately 7 mm in diameter in the left hand and an aneurysm of 4 mm in diameter in the right hand).

In both hands and distal to the aneurysm, a tortuous course of the ulnar artery referred to as a "corkscrew image" was observed, this being a typical finding of hypothenar hammer syndrome (Figure 1). The patient was referred to surgery and underwent vascular repair surgery with a vein graft in both hands (Figure 2). Four months after surgery, he is asymptomatic.

3. Discussion

Hypothenar hammer syndrome is one of the reversible causes of Raynaud's phenomenon [4, 5]. Its exact incidence is unknown and predominantly affects males [5]. It is common in people who use the volar surface of the hand as a hammer, although this history is not always documented [6]. It has also been linked to certain hobbies such as cycling, sport practiced by the patient. Repeated trauma to the hypothenar eminence of the hand leads to damage to the wall of the ulnar artery, with the consequent aneurysmal formation [2, 3]. Although it is usually unilateral, affecting the dominant hand, cases of bilateral involvement have also been described [2–18] (Table 1); in the case of the patient, the symptomatic hand was the right, although the left was asymptomatic, it presented the typical corkscrew lesion in the angiographic study. The presentation of symptoms is usually intermittent and persists for years. To date, its etiology is unknown, but it has been proposed that it is due to a preexisting abnormality in the ulnar artery, making it particularly sensitive to repetitive microtrauma damage [5].

The most commonly affected fingers are the third and fourth [7], like our case. Clinically, it is characterized by pain, intolerance to cold and cyanosis, paresthesias, digital ulcers, or palpable mass being less frequent (as in our case) [11]. The severity of symptoms depends on the extent of the occluded vascular segment and collateral circulation [8]. Regarding the diagnosis, the Allen maneuver is usually positive in most cases [7]. However, the gold standard for diagnosis is angiography since it provides information on the lesion's location, segment, and extent [1, 9]. Another technique that can be done is Doppler ultrasound that is used to assess blood flow and site of thrombus formation in the ulnar artery and the superficial palmar arch. This test is convenient but requires operator experience to carefully

Table 1: Literature review of bilateral Hypothenar hammer syndrome Cases [2–18].

Author (year)	Cases	Treatment
Williams et al. [4]	1	Vascular surgery
Wernick et al. [9]	1	Vascular surgery
Bhatla et al. [7]	1	Vascular surgery
Neill-Cage et al. [2]	1	Vascular surgery
Lambert et al. [3]	1	Vascular surgery
Ferris et al. [5]	12	Vascular surgery
Dethmers et al. [10]	2	Vascular surgery
Abudakka et al. [11]	1	Amputation
Facca et al. [12]	1	Vascular surgery
Temming et al. [13]	1	Vascular surgery
Larsen et al. [14]	6	Vascular surgery
Scharnbacher et al. [6]	5	No described
Sükrü et al. [8]	3	Vascular surgery
Niet et al. [15]	1	Vascular surgery
Endress et al. [16]	2	Vascular surgery
Kaji et al. [17]	5	Not described
Jin et al. [18]	1	Symptomatic
Flores-Robles et al. (2021)	1	Vascular surgery

map the arterial tree, and the patient must avoid movement during the entire examination. The benefit of Doppler mapping is that it does not induce vasospasm and may provide a demonstration of arterial hemodynamics [19].

The optimal treatment has not been determined to date since it is a rare disease, making challenging a comparison between different approaches [10–13]. Initially, conservative treatment is recommended, including calcium channel antagonists, beta-blockers, and botulinum toxin, among others [8]. The surgical approach is recommended if there are severe signs or symptoms [5]. Often decisions regarding surgical versus nonsurgical treatments are based on the acuteness of the symptoms and severity of the ischemia. Surgical options in this setting include the following: (1) arterial ligation (assuming an intact radial/palmar arch), (2) resection of thrombosed arterial segment or aneurysm with end-to-end anastomosis, and (3) resection and vascular reconstruction with vein or artery graft [5].

Surgery is not usually indicated for asymptomatic ulnar artery occlusion [5]. However, surgery is indicated in patients who present a "corkscrew" image on angiography with or without symptoms of digital ischemia to prevent the onset/recurrence of symptoms [5] like this case.

In conclusion, a patient with a bilateral hypothenar hammer syndrome is described as an uncommon cause of digital ischemia, thus demonstrating the importance of taking this clinical entity into account as a cause of reversible Raynaud's phenomenon.

References

[1] I. Marie, F. Hervé, E. Primard, N. Cailleux, and H. Levesque, "Long-term follow-up of hypothenar hammer syndrome: a series of 47 patients," *Medicine (Baltimore)*, vol. 86, no. 6, pp. 334–343, 2007.

[2] D. J. Neill-Cage, M. Rechnic, and R. M. Braun, "Bilateral thenar hammer syndrome as a result of cumulative trauma: a case report," *The Journal of Hand Surgery*, vol. 22, no. 6, pp. 1081–1083, 1997.

[3] M. Lambert, P. Y. Hatron, E. Hachulla, and B. Devulder, "Hypothenar hammer syndrome followed by systemic sclerosis," *The Journal of Rheumatology*, vol. 27, no. 10, pp. 2516-2517, 2000.

[4] W. V. Williams, A. Johnson, and D. Wilson, "Hypothenar hammer syndrome presenting as bilateral Raynaud's phenomenon," *Arthritis and Rheumatism*, vol. 30, no. 2, pp. 234-235, 1987.

[5] B. L. Ferris, L. M. Taylor Jr., K. Oyama et al., "Hypothenar hammer syndrome: proposed etiology," *Journal of Vascular Surgery*, vol. 31, no. 1, pp. 104–113, 2000.

[6] J. Scharnbacher, M. Claus, J. Reichert et al., "Hypothenar hammer syndrome: a multicenter case-control study," *American Journal of Industrial Medicine*, vol. 56, no. 11, pp. 1352–1358, 2013.

[7] A. Bhatla, I. S. Bulatao, and S. E. Walker, "Accelerated progressive systemic sclerosis in a patient with hypothenar hammer syndrome," *The Journal of Rheumatology*, vol. 23, no. 2, pp. 388–392, 1996.

[8] M. Ş. Şahin, T. Özyürekoğlu, and G. Çakmak, "Hypothenar hammer syndrome: a case series and literature review," *Eklem Hastalıkları ve Cerrahisi*, vol. 26, no. 1, pp. 11–15, 2015.

[9] R. Wernick and D. L. Smith, "Bilateral hypothenar hammer syndrome: an unusual and preventable cause of digital ischemia," *The American Journal of Emergency Medicine*, vol. 7, no. 3, pp. 302–306, 1989.

[10] R. S. Dethmers and P. Houpt, "Surgical management of hypothenar and thenar hammer syndromes: a retrospective study of 31 instances in 28 patients," *Journal of Hand Surgery*, vol. 30, no. 4, pp. 419–423, 2005.

[11] M. Abudakka, A. Pillai, and H. Al-Khaffaf, "Hypothenar hammer syndrome: rare or underdiagnosed?," *European Journal of Vascular and Endovascular Surgery*, vol. 32, no. 3, pp. 257–260, 2006.

[12] S. Facca and P. Liverneaux, "Robotic assisted microsurgery in hypothenar hammer syndrome: a case report," *Computer Aided Surgery*, vol. 15, no. 4-6, pp. 110–114, 2010.

[13] J. F. Temming, J. H. van Uchelen, and M. A. Tellier, "Hypothenar hammer syndrome: distal ulnar artery reconstruction with autologous descending branch of the lateral circumflex femoral artery," *Techniques in Hand & Upper Extremity Surgery*, vol. 15, no. 1, pp. 24–27, 2011.

[14] B. T. Larsen, W. D. Edwards, M. H. Jensen et al., "Surgical pathology of hypothenar hammer syndrome with new pathogenetic insights: a 25-year institutional experience with clinical and pathologic review of 67 cases," *The American Journal of Surgical Pathology*, vol. 37, no. 11, pp. 1700–1708, 2013.

[15] A. de Niet and J. H. Van Uchelen, "Hypothenar hammer syndrome: long-term follow-up after ulnar artery reconstruction with the lateral circumflex femoral artery," *Journal of Hand Surgery*, vol. 42, no. 5, pp. 507–510, 2017.

[16] R. D. Endress, C. H. Johnson, A. T. Bishop, and A. Y. Shin, "Hypothenar hammer syndrome: long-term results of vascular reconstruction," *Journal of Hand Surgery*, vol. 40, no. 4, pp. 660–665.e2, 2015.

[17] H. Kaji, H. Honma, M. Usui, Y. Yasuno, and K. Saito, "Hypothenar hammer syndrome in workers occupationally exposed to vibrating tools," *The Journal of Hand Surgery*, vol. 18, no. 6, pp. 761–766, 1993.

[18] K. Jin, Y. Matsuzaki, E. Akasaka et al., "Irreversible bilateral cyanosis of the hands caused by hypothenar hammer syndrome with systemic sclerosis," *European Journal of Dermatology*, vol. 28, no. 4, pp. 525-526, 2018.

[19] C. T. Ablett and L. A. Hackett, "Hypothenar hammer syndrome: case reports and brief review," *Clinical Medicine & Research*, vol. 6, no. 1, pp. 3–8, 2008.

10

Phlegmasia Cerulea Dolens in a Patient with Breast Cancer and Inferior Vena Cava Hypoplasia

A. Bianchi,[1] S. Pozza,[1] L. Giovannacci,[1] and Jos. C. van den Berg[2]

[1]*Department of Visceral and Vascular Surgery, Ospedale Regionale di Lugano-CH, Switzerland*
[2]*Department of Interventional Radiology, Ospedale Regionale di Lugano-CH, Switzerland*

Correspondence should be addressed to A. Bianchi; alessandro.bianchi13@gmail.com

Academic Editor: Tsung-I Peng

Background. No clear guidelines exist for the management of phlegmasia cerulea dolens. This case report shows how a hybrid approach might be successful. It also shows how rare pathologies can combine to create a life- and limb-threatening condition. *Case Presentation.* A 75-year-old man, known for nephrotic syndrome currently under investigation, presented to the emergency department with a 24-hour history of left leg swelling followed by intense pain. The left lower limb showed a phlegmasia cerulean dolens. Renal function, coagulation profile, and inflammatory parameters were normal; D-Dimers 5,6 mg/L. The CT scan showed juxtarenal thrombosis of the hypoplastic IVC, involving both renal veins, reaching the left iliac-femoral-popliteal axis, with collateralization to the pelvic and mesenteric veins, associated with bilateral segmental pulmonary embolisms. A suspected left breast nodule was also found. Intravenous heparin was immediately administered, and urgent hybrid procedure with surgical thrombectomy and venous angiography and thromboaspiration, liberating the iliolumbar collaterals, was performed. A lateral leg fasciotomy was mandatory due to the phlegmasia cerulea. Postoperative Doppler US showed a good venous compressibility of the left leg. Thrombophilia screening was negative. The breast nodule was biopsied showing an invasive ductal carcinoma. The patient was discharged with oral rivaroxaban and indication for left mastectomy and oncological therapy with aromatase inhibitors. *Conclusion.* This case highlights the dramatic consequence of different risk factors for venous thromboembolism as cancer and nephrotic syndrome in a patient with hypoplasia of the inferior cava vein. Venous thromboaspiration has been used in order to timely recanalize important collaterals. Phlegmasia cerulea dolens was resolved after the procedure and lateral calf fasciotomy. Further evidence is needed to clearly define the role of venous thromboaspiration in the treatment of complex proximal deep venous thrombosis of the lower extremity.

1. Case Presentation

We present the case of a 75-year-old healthy male patient, who arrived at our Emergency Department for excruciating pain and swelling of the left leg that, when measured, resulted 1,5 times bigger than the right one.

The pain started the day before and worsened during the day, as the diameter of the leg was also increasing. He did not report any previous trauma. The only relevant anamnestic data was a short flight 4 weeks before.

The patient's past medical history was characterized by type II diabetes, hypertension, COPD, and also a nephrotic syndrome, recently diagnosed and still under investigation. His cardiovascular risk factors were cigarette smoking and arterial hypertension.

At the clinical examination, the left leg presented typical signs of phlegmasia cerulea dolens (Figure 1): distal pulses were not palpable, and the calf was swollen, reddened, and painful, typical for a compartment syndrome.

An urgent angio-CT scan was performed and showed an extensive thrombosis of both renal veins, a hypoplasia of the inferior vena cava (Figure 2) extending from the renal veins to the diaphragm, and a complete thrombosis of the deep venous system of the left leg (Figure 3).

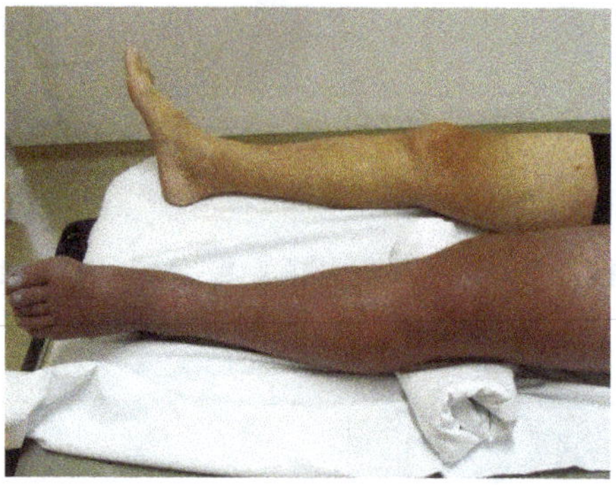

Figure 1: Picture showing the difference between the right normal leg and the left leg with a classic pattern of phlegmasia cerulea dolens.

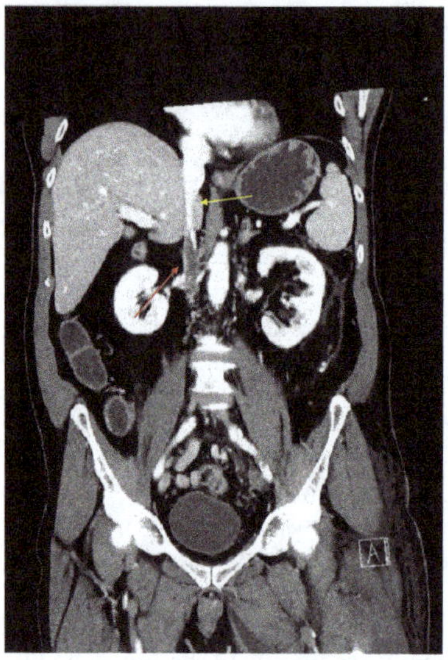

Figure 2: Angio-CT showing inferior vein cava thrombosis (red arrow) and inferior vein cava hypoplasia (yellow arrow).

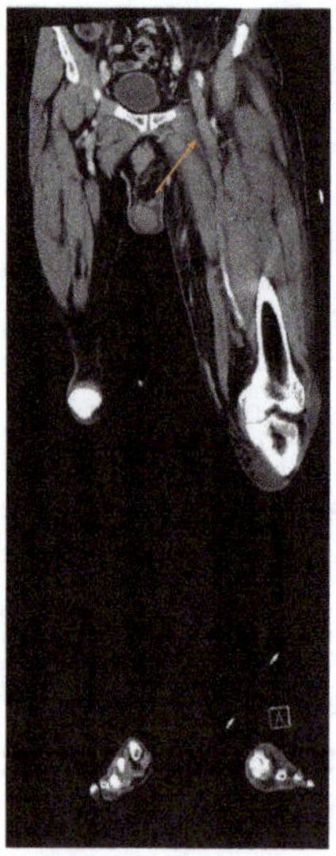

Figure 3: Angio-CT of the patient showing complete thrombosis of the left femoral vein (arrow).

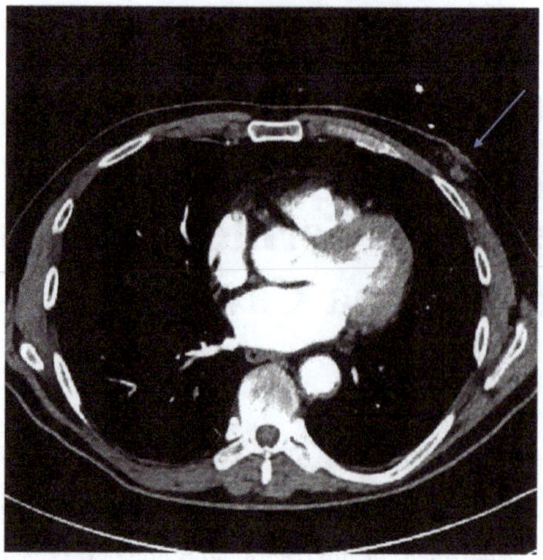

Figure 4: Angio-CT showing a left mammary mass (blue arrow).

The venous drainage was partially granted by collaterals, the major being a lumbar vein, which drained into the superior mesenteric vein.

The CT scan also showed a minimal bilateral basilar pulmonary embolism, a mass in the left mammary gland, and also an exceptionally big left inguinal hernia.

We decided to perform an iliofemoral venous thrombectomy associated with an intraoperative phlebography and venous PTA. The phlebography showed thrombotic material in the external iliac vein. The common iliac vein was occluded, determining a retrograde flux in the femoral vein. A thrombectomy with Fogarty catheter was performed, followed by a percutaneous angioplasty with the restoration of an anterograde flux. Due to the presence of good collateral circles, it was not necessary to liberate the renal veins. Because of the presence of a compartment syndrome, a fasciotomy of anterior and lateral compartments was also performed.

Postoperatively, the patient was transferred to the Intensive Care Unit and the clinical evolution was favorable.

At this point, the cause of this massive venous thrombosis had to be found, also considering the presence of a probable breast cancer (Figure 4).

The thrombophilia screening did not show any pathologic finding. The mammary lesion was on the inferior external quadrant of the left breast with retraction of the superimposed skin. After discussion with the OB/GYN specialist, a tru-cut biopsy was performed. The histopathological examination showed an invasive ductal carcinoma B.R.E. 2 with expression of estrogenic and progestin receptors at 90%, Ki-67 10%, C-erb-2 score 2+. Radical mastectomy was highly recommended, but the patient went back to his original country and we do not know if the operation was actually performed.

The hospital stay was regular, without any complication. A life-long oral anticoagulation with rivaroxaban 15 mg 1/day was started.

2. Discussion

This case gives us the chance to focus on three rare pathologies: phlegmasia cerulea dolens, inferior vena cava hypoplasia, and breast cancer in male patients.

Phlegmasia cerulean dolens is a rare condition, whose prevalence is unknown, and it represents the intermediate state between venous thrombosis and phlegmasia alba dolens. This condition was first described by Hildanus et al. in 1593 [1]. Etiopathogenesis was clarified in the first years of XX century by Crueveilhier [2] and Buerger [3]. The classical triad of symptoms, pain, swelling, and discoloration, was first described by Gregoire [4] in 1938. It is a severe condition which, even nowadays, is burdened by an amputation rate of 20-50% [5–7].

The literature about this condition is poor, and guidelines do not exist [8].

The prevalence is higher in men than in women, with a 1,5 : 1 ratio [9]. In 33% of cases [8], as in our case, a neoplastic disorder is found, which determines a paraneoplastic syndrome. In 50% of cases, a thrombophilic status, venous stasis, or oral contraceptives are found or used. In 16% of cases, the etiology is not found. Furthermore, for unknown reasons, the left leg is of interest in 45% of cases, while the right one only in 29%. Bilateral disease is found in 26%. One-third of the patients have a pulmonary embolism at admission.

Diagnosis is mainly clinical and the previously reported classic triad is preset. The radiological imaging of choice is a color Doppler ultrasound, eventually associated with angio-CT scan. Ultrasound is the exam of choice because it is widely available, not invasive, and without radiations. On the other hand, it is operator-related and is also difficult to find pelvic masses causing compression of venous axes.

Phlegmasia may be classified as not complicated, with incipient venous gangrene and with established venous gangrene. Morbidity and mortality increase as the clinical stage gets worse.

As already stated, no guidelines are available. As a consequence, the therapeutic choices are addressed to thrombus reduction and limb salvage. Two other main goals are the prevention of thrombus propagation and the maintenance of the venous axis patency.

Initial treatment is based on general support treatment and heparin infusion [9] in therapeutic range, which means that the aPTT has to be two times higher than normal reference values. Platelet count is mandatory to surveil heparin-induced thrombocytopenia (HIT syndrome).

If no clinical improvement occurs within few hours, normally 12 [9], a more aggressive treatment is needed. In this kind of pathology, as in the rest of the vascular surgery, there is a clear augmentation of endovascular procedures, both lysis or stenting, to the detriment of open venous thrombectomy. Open approach has the advantage to be a fast resolution of venous hypertension and also reduces thrombus propagation. However, this is a major invasive procedure, which needs general anesthesia and it is at high risk of rethrombosis. Endovascular approach, both lysis or mechanical thrombectomy, is less invasive and may grant a major permeability of micro circulation. The major disadvantage is the risk of pulmonary embolism due to clot fragmentation.

Vena cava anomalies have an incidence of 0,05-8,7% [10] in Caucasian population, sometimes associated with other vascular anomalies. Agenesis or hypoplasia of the inferior vena cava has a prevalence of 0,0005%. This condition is a risk factor for deep venous thrombosis: in fact, deep venous thrombosis in patient younger than 30 is 5%, largely superior to 0,5% of the health population of the same age. This difference is attributable to rheological phenomena, as stated by Virchow's triad.

Breast cancer in men has an incidence of 0,5-1% in Caucasian population [11], different from some areas of Central Africa where it shows an incidence up to 6% [11].

Hormonal imbalance between estrogens and androgens may play a major role in this rare condition. Hormonal alterations may be caused by a genetic condition, as in Klinefelter syndrome, or by acquired conditions, as in hepatic diseases, thyroid dysfunction, and obesity. A relationship exists between testicular pathology and mammary neoplasia: the most accredited hypothesis in literature is that diseases such as orchitis, retained testicles, and testicular lesions cause a reduction in androgen production and a consequent increase of estrogen production.

Breast cancer is associated with 9-14% increase of thrombophilia due to an increase in endogenous carbon monoxide production, known to enhance plasmatic coagulation both in vivo and in vitro, determining a higher risk for thrombosis in affected patients [12].

The severe condition presented by the patient is due to the combination of two strong risk factors for venous thrombosis, such as hypoplastic vena cava and breast cancer, that determined a rare clinical presentation.

3. Conclusion

To summarize, the treatment of phlegmasia cerulea dolens is still not codified by precise protocols. A recent review points out some milestones:

(1) Early anticoagulation

(2) Unclogging, if possible, the major venous axes

(3) Active research of thrombophilia causes, especially neoplasia, and treatment

In the reported case, our treatment was coherent with those principles, aimed at avoiding limb amputation, which is still the major complication of phlegmasia, with an estimate rate of 20%.

In the future, especially if we analyze actual trend in vascular surgery, we shall see a major use of endovascular procedures, thanks to new drugs and new devices, at the expense of the traditional open techniques. Nowadays, clear evidences in the literature are yet to be found.

Authors' Contributions

The author and the coauthor performed the same kind of work.

References

[1] H. Haimovici, "Gangrene of the extremities of venous origin," *Circulation*, vol. 1, no. 2, pp. 225–240, 1950.

[2] J. Crueveilhier, *Traite de pathologie generale*, vol. 228, Tome IV Paris, 1862.

[3] L. Buerger, *The Circulation Disturbances of the Exteremity*, WB Saunders, Philadelphia, 1924.

[4] R. Gregoire, *La phlebite bleue (phlegmasia cerulea dolens)*, vol. 46, no. 71, 1938Press Med., 1938.

[5] J. M. T. Perkins, T. R. Magee, and R. B. Galland, "Phlegmasia caerulea dolens and venous gangrene," *The British Journal of Surgery*, vol. 83, no. 1, pp. 19–23, 1996.

[6] J. M. Stallworth, G. B. Bradham, R. R. Kletke, and R. G. Price, "Phlegmasia cerulea dolens: a 10-year review," *Annals of Surgery*, vol. 161, no. 5, pp. 802–811, 1965.

[7] S. Bhatt, C. Wehbe, and V. S. Dogra, "Phlegmasia cerulea dolens," *Journal of Clinical Ultrasound*, vol. 35, no. 7, pp. 401–404, 2007.

[8] K. Chinsakchai, K. ten Duis, F. L. Moll, and G. J. de Borst, "Trends in management of phlegmasia cerulea dolens," *Vascular and Endovascular Surgery*, vol. 45, no. 1, pp. 5–14, 2011.

[9] F. A. Weaver, P. W. Meacham, R. B. Adkins, and R. H. Dean, "Phlegmasia cerulea dolens: therapeutic considerations," *Southern Medical Journal*, vol. 81, no. 3, pp. 306–312, 1988.

[10] L. Man, N. Hendricks, and H. Maitland, "IVC agenesis: a rare cause of deep vein thrombosis," *Journal of Thrombosis and Thrombolysis*, vol. 41, no. 3, pp. 541–543, 2016.

[11] R. L. Siegel and K. D. Miller, "Cancer statistics, 2017," *CA: a Cancer Journal for Clinicians*, vol. 67, no. 1, pp. 7–30, 2017.

[12] V. G. Nielsen, M. L. Ley, A. L. Waer, P. W. Alger, R. W. Matika, and E. B. Steinbrenner, "Plasmatic hypercoagulation in patients with breast cancer: role of heme oxygenase-1," *Blood Coagulation & Fibrinolysis*, vol. 24, no. 8, pp. 809–813, 2013.

11

Use of Edoxaban for the Treatment of Heparin-Induced Thrombocytopenia

Ryo Kanamoto, Shinichi Hiromatsu, Tomoyuki Anegawa, Kanako Sakurai, Shohei Yoshida, Yusuke Shintani, Hiroyuki Otsuka, Satoru Tobinaga, and Hiroyuki Tanaka

Department of Surgery, Kurume University School of Medicine, Fukuoka, Japan

Correspondence should be addressed to Ryo Kanamoto; kanamoto_ryou@med.kurume-u.ac.jp

Academic Editor: Matthias Reinhard

Heparin-induced thrombocytopenia (HIT) is a life-threatening adverse drug reaction of heparin therapy, which increases a patient's risk of developing venous and/or arterial thromboembolism. HIT should be treated through discontinuation of heparin and administration of nonheparin anticoagulants such as argatroban. For long-term anticoagulation, parenteral nonheparin anticoagulants are generally converted to oral treatment with a vitamin K antagonist such as warfarin. Although administration of warfarin is recommended to overlap with a nonheparin anticoagulant for a minimum of 5 days, overlapping with argatroban and warfarin presents high risks of bleeding. We describe a case of HIT treated with edoxaban. A 78-year-old man underwent surgery for esophageal cancer and was administered heparin perioperatively. After surgery, he was diagnosed with HIT and venous thromboembolism. We immediately stopped heparin and initiated parenteral argatroban. The patient was subsequently started on edoxaban without any overlap between the two drugs. The treatment was successful. The treatment of edoxaban following argatroban for HIT could reduce bleeding complications and shorten the length of hospital stay. To the best of our knowledge, this is the first report of the use of edoxaban for HIT treatment.

1. Introduction

Heparin-induced thrombocytopenia (HIT) is a life-threatening and limb-threatening adverse drug reaction that can lead to venous thromboembolism (VTE), which includes pulmonary embolism (PE) and deep vein thrombosis (DVT). HIT may also lead to arterial thromboembolism, which includes limb ischemia, acute myocardial infarction, and stroke. HIT results from the antibodies against complexes of platelet factor 4 (PF4) and heparin following exposure to unfractionated or low-molecular-weight heparin.

In HIT patients, heparin should be discontinued immediately and replaced with nonheparin anticoagulants such as argatroban, danaparoid, bivalirudin, or fondaparinux. Parenteral anticoagulation treatment is generally converted to oral treatment with a vitamin K antagonist (VKA), such as warfarin, for long-term anticoagulation [1, 2]. Recently, several studies have reported the use of direct oral anticoagulants (DOACs), such as the direct factor Xa inhibitors, rivaroxaban, apixaban, and edoxaban, or the direct thrombin inhibitor, dabigatran, instead of warfarin, as a new treatment option for HIT patients. However, to date, HIT treatment using edoxaban has not been reported [2]. Here, we report the case of an HIT patient with VTE who was successfully treated with edoxaban. To the best of our knowledge, this is the first report that describes the use of edoxaban for HIT treatment.

2. Case Report

A 78-year-old man was admitted to our hospital for the surgical treatment of esophageal cancer. He had been administered oral clopidogrel for a previous cerebral infarction. His medical history did not show previous venous thromboembolic events. Oral clopidogrel treatment was switched to continuous intravenous unfractionated heparin (UFH) administration (10000 IU once daily) during the preoperative period. Four days after the surgical treatment of esophageal cancer, the administration of UFH was resumed. The patient's platelet count was $197 \times 10^3/\mu L$ prior to surgery and $158 \times 10^3/\mu L$ immediately after surgery. However, his platelet count decreased to approximately $35 \times 10^3/\mu L$ on postoperative day seven. We suspected HIT and immediately stopped treatment with UFH and initiated treatment with intravenous argatroban. Argatroban was initially administered at an infusion rate of 0.35 μg/kg/min because of the risk of bleeding after major surgery. The infusion rate of argatroban was increased to 0.7 μg/kg/min upon monitoring activated partial thromboplastin time (aPTT) (target aPTT is 1.5–2.0× the patient's baseline value; the reagent we used in this case is Coagpia APTT-N, SEKISUI MEDICAL CO., LTD., Tokyo, Japan). Four days after UFH withdrawal, the patient complained of right leg swelling. Contrast computed tomography (CT) revealed bilateral PE and proximal DVT in the right leg (Figure 1). His plasma D-dimer value was 20.3 μg/mL. He underwent placement of a retrievable inferior vena cava (IVC) filter (Günther Tulip Vena Cava Filter, Cook Medical, Bloomington, USA) because of the occurrence of a new PE event during anticoagulant therapy. The 4T's score was 6, and levels of anti-PF4/heparin antibodies were >5.0 U/mL according to the results of the HemosIL® HIT-$Ab_{(PF4\text{-}H)}$ latex immunoturbidimetric assay (Instrumentation Laboratory, Bedford, MA). Eleven days after UFH withdrawal and initiation of argatroban treatment, the platelet count gradually increased to $268 \times 10^3/\mu L$ and the D-dimer value decreased to 11.4 μg/mL. Because the IVC filter did not capture the thrombus, we removed it 1 week after its placement. Twenty-one days after UFH withdrawal, the platelet count was $268 \times 10^3/\mu L$ and the D-dimer value was 8.1 μg/mL. We then stopped the treatment with argatroban and gave the patient edoxaban (30 mg once a day) without any overlap in treatment with the two drugs. As the patient experienced no bleeding complications after 5 days of edoxaban (30 mg) administration, we increased the dose of edoxaban to 60 mg/day. Although the patient suffered from bleeding of the colon diverticulum 38 days after the initial treatment with edoxaban, we performed endoscopic hemostasis and the patient recovered. Later, he did not experience further bleeding complications during edoxaban treatment. We continued his anticoagulant therapy for 6 months to treat cancer-associated thrombosis. Six months after UFH withdrawal, we discontinued treatment with edoxaban because the D-dimer value normalized, PE and DVT disappeared according to the follow-up contrast CT, and there was no evidence of cancer recurrence in any follow-up examinations (Figure 2). At a follow-up appointment 3 years after stopping edoxaban treatment, the patient had experienced neither recurrent thromboembolism nor other complications.

3. Discussion

For the treatment of HIT, heparin treatment should immediately be changed to parenteral treatment with a nonheparin anticoagulant. Argatroban is the only parenteral nonheparin anticoagulant that has been approved for the treatment of HIT in Japan. The 9th guideline of the American College of Chest Physicians (ACCP) recommends that argatroban be administered initially at an infusion rate of 2 μg/kg/min for patients with normal organ function and at 0.5–1.2 μg/kg/min for those with heart failure, liver dysfunction, and severe anasarca or patients recovering from cardiac surgery [2]. Conversely, Miyata et al. recommend that the initial infusion rate of argatroban should be reduced to 0.7 μg/kg/min for Japanese patients with normal organ function and to 0.2 μg/kg/min for those with liver dysfunction or having a high risk of bleeding. This has been recommended because Japanese patients treated with a dose the same as that recommended by the ACCP often experience serious bleeding accompanied by a rapid increase of aPTT [3]. When long-term anticoagulative treatment for treating HIT-associated thromboembolism is necessary, parenteral nonheparin anticoagulant treatment is usually converted to treatment with a VKA (e.g., warfarin) after platelet recovery [1, 2]. Because it takes a median of 50–85 days until HIT-related antibodies in the serum to decrease to negative levels [4], it is recommended that HIT patients without thromboembolism receive alternative anticoagulants until platelet recovery. This treatment recommendation is similar to that of HIT patients with thromboembolism. Additionally, the risk of HIT-related thrombosis is high until 2–4 weeks after the beginning of treatment; therefore, the administration of alternative anticoagulants or warfarin should be continued for at least 4 weeks [5]. Because HIT is considered to be a transient risk factor for developing VTE, at least 3 months of anticoagulant therapy is recommended in HIT patients with thrombosis. This treatment recommendation is similar to that of VTE associated with transient provoking risk factors [1, 4, 5]. Therefore, HIT patients with thrombosis require a switch to oral anticoagulants from parenteral nonheparin anticoagulants. However, an early transition to oral VKA treatment or treatment with VKA alone should be avoided because of the risk of thrombotic complications. These complications include venous limb gangrene and warfarin-induced skin necrosis, which is caused by a faster reduction of protein C than that of vitamin K-dependent clotting factors including II, VII, IX, and X [1, 6]. The 9th ACCP guideline recommends that the administration of VKA be overlapped with nonheparin anticoagulant treatment for at least 5 days [1]. However, overlapping treatment with argatroban and warfarin often causes increase in the international normalized ratio and increases the risk of major bleeding [7]. We believe that two major issues associated with HIT treatment in Japan include the possibility of prolonged hospital stay and bleeding complications due to overlapping treatment with argatroban/warfarin.

Several studies have proposed the use of DOACs as new treatment options for HIT. HIT treatment with DOACs offers the following advantages: (1) DOACs have no potentially deleterious immunological interactions with HIT antibodies [8]; (2) DOACs do not reduce the levels of protein C activity, meaning that there is a lower risk of developing venous limb gangrene compared with conventional VKA therapy; and (3) DOACs have a more rapid onset compared with warfarin and could be useful for shortening hospitalization and lowering costs [2]. Warkentin et al. reported their experience with DOACs for HIT treatment in addition to a literature review. The progression or recurrence of thrombosis occurred in 2.2% (1 of 46), 0% (0 of 12), and 9.1% (1 of 11)

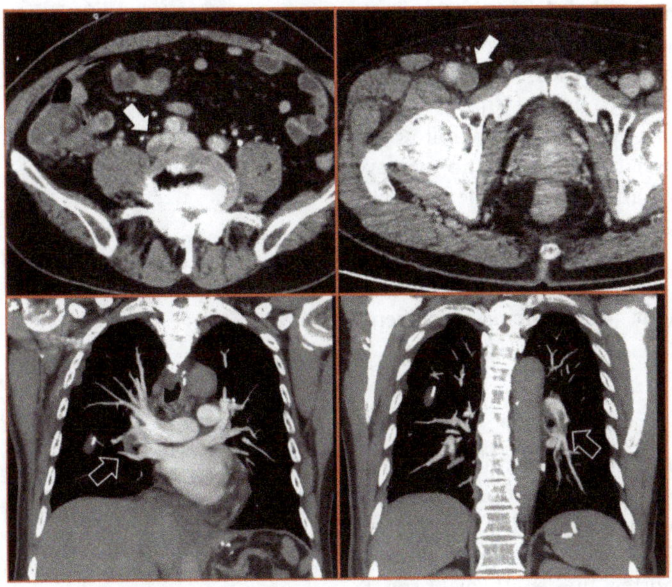

FIGURE 1: Contrast computed tomography imaging. White arrows indicate the region from the right iliac to the common femoral vein that was occluded by deep vein thrombosis, whereas black arrows indicate the bilateral pulmonary artery thromboembolism.

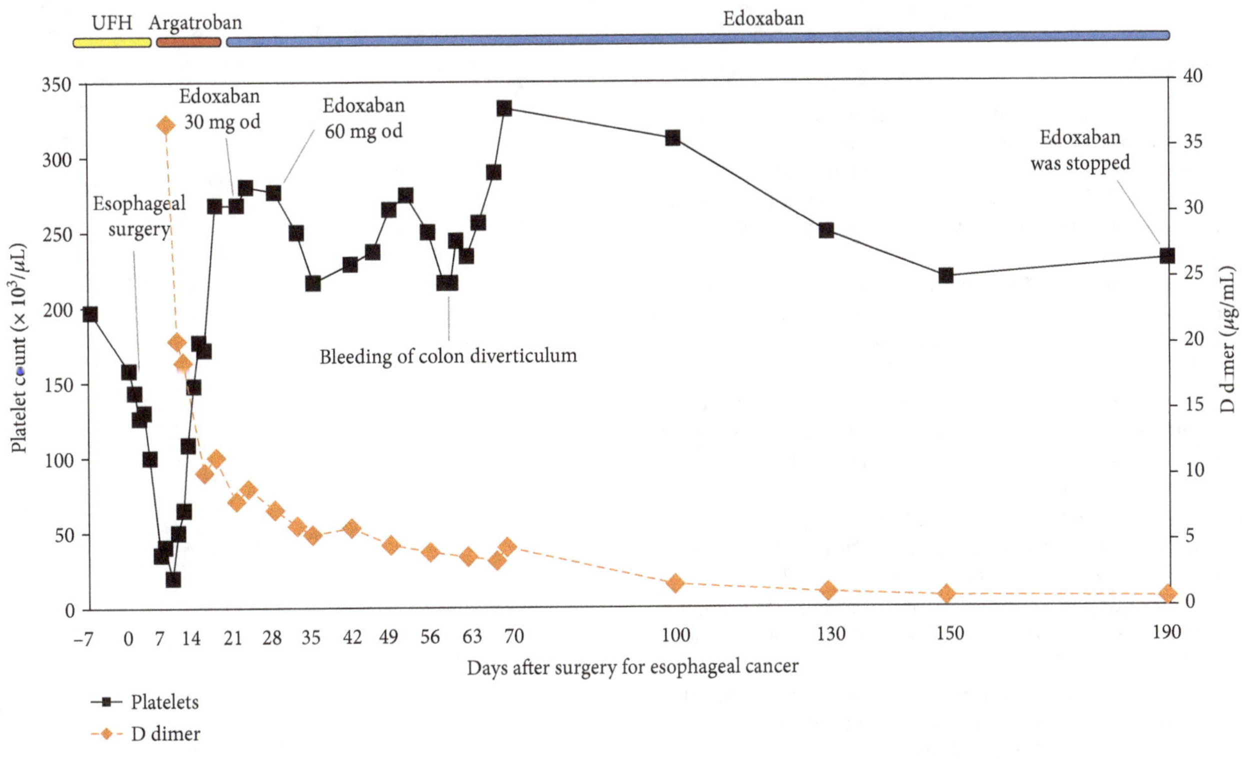

FIGURE 2: Platelet count and D-dimer value during the administration of anticoagulants in a patient with heparin-induced thrombocytopenia after surgery for esophageal cancer. UFH: unfractionated heparin.

of HIT patients treated with rivaroxaban, apixaban, and dabigatran, respectively. No major bleeding occurred in any of the patients treated with these DOACs. In these results, although efficacy and safety of rivaroxaban, apixaban, and dabigatran for HIT treatment were suggested, the data regarding the use of edoxaban for HIT treatment were not included [2].

In the Hokusai-VTE study (a randomized, double-blind clinical trial for the treatment of VTE with edoxaban), the efficacy and safety of the use of edoxaban for treating VTE were indicated, which were similar to those of other DOACs [9]. Therefore, favorable outcomes regarding the use of edoxaban to treat HIT are also expected. It is recommended that edoxaban be administered at a dose of 60 mg or 30 mg (for patients with a creatinine clearance rate of 15–50 mL/min or bodyweight below 60 kg) once per day following initial therapy with parenteral anticoagulants for at least 5 days without overlapping the treatments of the two drugs [10].

The advantages of edoxaban administration following parenteral argatroban are a lower bleeding risk, no overlap between a parenteral and an oral anticoagulant, the possibility of switching to oral anticoagulation therapy earlier, and no anticoagulant monitoring. Our patient encountered diverticulum bleeding but was treated endoscopically and had been doing well without experiencing recurrent thrombosis.

4. Conclusion

We successfully and safely treated a patient with HIT in the present study. To the best of our knowledge, this is the first report on the use of edoxaban for HIT treatment. The administration of edoxaban following argatroban could reduce bleeding complications and shorten the length of hospital stay. However, appropriately designed clinical studies are required to assess the effectiveness and safety of DOACs for HIT treatment.

References

[1] L. A. Linkins, A. L. Dans, L. K. Moores et al., "Treatment and prevention of heparin-induced thrombocytopenia. Antithrombotic therapy and prevention of thrombosis, 9th ed: American College of Chest Physicians evidence-based clinical practice guidelines," *Chest*, vol. 141, no. 2, pp. e495S–e530S, 2012.

[2] T. E. Warkentin, M. Pai, and L. A. Linkins, "Direct oral anticoagulants for treatment of HIT: update of Hamilton experience and literature review," *Blood*, vol. 130, no. 9, pp. 1104–1113, 2017.

[3] S. Miyata, H. Yamamoto, M. Kamei et al., "Heparin-induced thrombocytopenia clinical studies and the efficacy of argatroban in Japan," *Seminars in Thrombosis and Hemostasis*, vol. 34, no. S1, pp. 37–47, 2008.

[4] T. E. Warkentin and J. G. Kelton, "Temporal aspects of heparin-induced thrombocytopenia," *The New England Journal of Medicine*, vol. 344, no. 17, pp. 1286–1292, 2001.

[5] G. M. Arepally and T. L. Ortel, "Heparin-induced thrombocytopenia," *New England Journal of Medicine*, vol. 355, no. 8, pp. 809–817, 2006.

[6] J. R. Bartholomew, "Transition to an oral anticoagulant in patients with heparin-induced thrombocytopenia," *Chest*, vol. 127, no. 2, pp. 27S–34S, 2005.

[7] J. R. Bartholomew and M. J. Hursting, "Transitioning from argatroban to warfarin in heparin-induced thrombocytopenia: an analysis of outcomes in patients with elevated international normalized ratio (INR)," *Journal of Thrombosis and Thrombolysis*, vol. 19, no. 3, pp. 183–188, 2005.

[8] K. Krauel, C. Hackbarth, B. Fürll, and A. Greinacher, "Heparin-induced thrombocytopenia: in vitro studies on the interaction of dabigatran, rivaroxaban, and low-sulfated heparin, with platelet factor 4 and anti-PF4/heparin antibodies," *Blood*, vol. 119, no. 5, pp. 1248–1255, 2012.

[9] The Hokusai-VTE Investigators, "Edoxaban Versus Warfarin for the Treatment of Symptomatic Venous Thromboembolism," *New England Journal of Medicine*, vol. 369, no. 15, pp. 1406–1415, 2013.

[10] LIXIANA, *Summary of product characteristics*, Daiichi Sankyo Europe GmbH, 2020.

12

Bilateral Popliteal Artery Entrapment Syndrome: An Approach to Diagnosis and Salvage

Aman Berry Williams

The Townsville Hospital and Health Service, Australia

Correspondence should be addressed to Aman Berry Williams; amanbw@gmail.com

Academic Editor: Nilda Espinola-Zavaleta

Popliteal artery entrapment syndrome (PAES) is a rare cause of limb-threatening vascular disease. Usually, it arises from aberrant embryological development or acquired dysfunctionality of the popliteal artery and its surrounding musculotendinous structures in the popliteal fossa. Here, we present a case report of a young woman with relatively sudden-onset short-distance claudication and paraesthesia affecting her right leg primarily. She had no recent traumatic history and no atherosclerotic risk factors and was otherwise previously very active. She had a feeble right popliteal artery pulse and no foot pulses. Nerve conduction studies demonstrated no electrophysiological abnormalities. Following computed tomography angiography and magnetic resonance imaging, it was determined she had type 2 PAES. Subsequently, the patient underwent surgical division of a lateralised head of her medial gastrocnemius, resection of her fibrosed popliteal artery, and repair with a reversed long saphenous vein interposition graft. Following surgery, her symptoms resolved, and she remains on aspirin and ultrasound surveillance.

1. Full Case Report

A 28-year-old woman was referred by her local general practitioner to the vascular surgical department with intermittent claudication, predominantly affecting her right leg. The claudication had gradually worsened over a 9-month period, now limiting her to a walking distance of 30 metres—relieved by 10-15 minutes of rest. Though denying rest pain, she also described some numbness and pins and needles in her right foot and occasionally had similar sensations in her left. Ultimately, her symptoms were impacting her ability to work, where as a teacher, she found it difficult to walk between classrooms. She denied any previous lower limb trauma, though previously regularly exercised by running. She had no relevant personal or family past medical history, with no significant risk factors for atherosclerotic disease given she was a nonsmoker, nondiabetic, and without hypertension or hypercholesterolemia.

On physical examination, she appeared generally well. A pulse examination demonstrated that she had a feebly palpable right popliteal artery pulse (in comparison to her left) and no palpable pedal pulses. Despite this, she had a normal capillary return, with no lower limb ulceration.

Initially, the patient was referred for Doppler ultrasound, which demonstrated a normal right popliteal vein; however, it did demonstrate a short popliteal artery occlusion with notable large collateral vessels. For completion, blood tests were collected including a vasculitic screen and a thrombophilia screen, both of which were negative. Nerve conduction studies were also then performed, which demonstrated no electrophysiological abnormalities.

To quantify her disease further, computed tomography angiography (CTA) was conducted confirming in-fact bilateral short-segment popliteal artery disease, with a total occlusion on the right, a high-grade stenosis on the left, and three vessel run-offs bilaterally (Figure 1). Magnetic resonance (MR) angiography was then performed, demonstrating an abnormal medial deviation of bilateral popliteal arteries secondary to an unusually lateral insertion of the medial heads of the gastrocnemius at the superior aspect of the intercondylar notches (Figure 2). Radiographically, this demonstrated a type 2 PAES using the Whelan and Love classification [1].

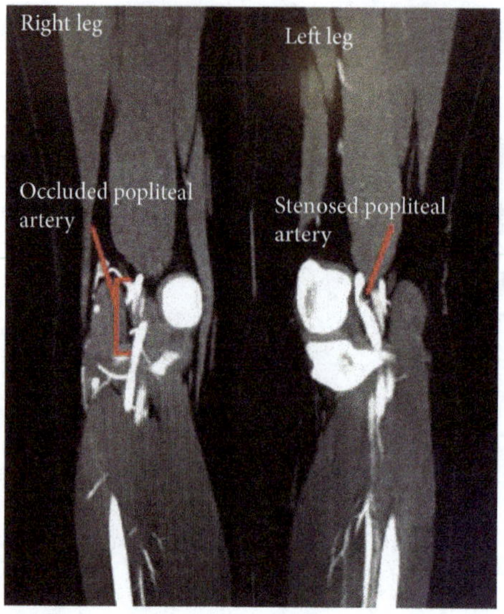

FIGURE 1: Computed tomography angiography demonstrating a coronal view of the behind knee popliteal arteries, with labelled total occlusion of the right popliteal artery and tight stenosis of the left popliteal artery.

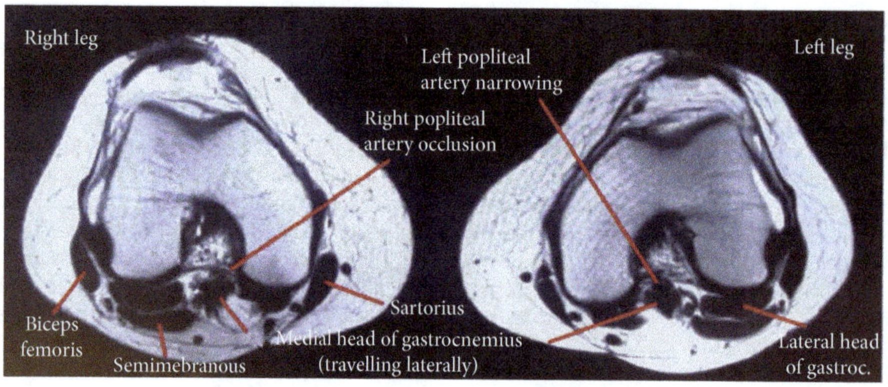

FIGURE 2: Magnetic resonance imaging demonstrating an axial view of bilateral knees. Note the lateral travel of the medial head of gastrocnemius, resulting in a right popliteal artery occlusion and left popliteal artery high-grade stenosis.

There was no evidence of popliteal vein entrapment, and the popliteus muscles appeared normal.

Following an anaesthetic evaluation, the patient was taken to theatre. Under general anaesthetic, a left leg long saphenous vein harvest was performed, followed by repositioning the patient prone. A lazy-S incision was made over the right popliteal fossa, with appreciation and preservation of the tibial nerve and popliteal vein. The popliteal artery was dissected free, noting a tough muscular band of the medial head of the gastrocnemius travelling laterally over the popliteal artery causing extrinsic compression (Figure 3). This band was divided, and the now released but occluded and fibrosed segment of the popliteal artery was resected. Vessel repair concluded with end-to-end anastomosis of a reversed long saphenous vein interposition graft. Postsurgery, the patient recovered well and after a period of rehabilitation was discharged on aspirin alone. Clinical and ultrasound surveillance monitoring took place at 6 weeks and 3 and 6 months postdischarge, and she now remains on annual graft surveillance. Fortunately, her minor left leg symptoms have completely resolved following participation in a self-motivated claudication walking program.

2. Discussion

Popliteal artery entrapment syndrome (PAES) is a rare cause of potentially limb-threatening vascular disease. Typically, it arises from aberrant embryological development or acquired traumatic dysfunctionality of the popliteal artery secondary to surrounding musculotendinous structures in the popliteal fossa [2]. Usually affecting physically active and younger patients (under age 30), common symptoms on presentation include intermittent claudication, paraesthesia, and cold or discoloured peripheries—characteristically relieved by rest [3]. Though usually devoid of other cardiovascular risk factors, as a result of repetitive injury, these patients are prone to further complications such as popliteal artery stenosis, thrombosis, aneurysmal change, and distal lower limb thromboembolic shower—ultimately with potential for acute limb ischaemia [4].

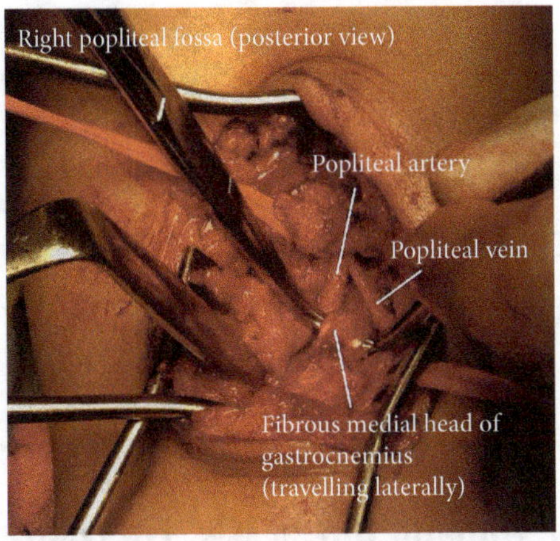

FIGURE 3: Intraoperative posterior approach of the right popliteal fossa, demonstrating the culprit fibrous muscular band of the medial head of the gastrocnemius.

Whether acquired or embryological in nature, given that PAES is generally complex in its development, the potential anatomical variations have been described in a multitude of classification systems—the Whelan and Love system (see [2]), as mentioned earlier, being the most popular. Imaging utility varies greatly with modality. Ultrasound and CTA provide gross arterial perfusion and flow distributions, whereas MR has proved particularly useful in defining extrinsic extra-arterial disease and guiding surgical approach [5]. Furthermore, CTA and MR are particularly pertinent in screening and identifying bilateral disease, where up to 60% of patients with symptomatic PAES will have demonstrable contralateral disease [3].

A high suspicion for PAES should be held when assessing young patients presenting with intermittent claudication, particularly in the absence of other atherosclerotic risk factors. In conjunction with a thorough history and examination, a targeted imaging assessment should be conducted to assist in narrowing the differential diagnosis, as well as prompt for early operative salvage from potential limb-threatening complications.

References

[1] T. J. Whelan and J. Love, "Popliteal artery entrapment syndrome," in *Vascular Surgery, Principles and Techniques*, H. Haimovici, Ed., pp. 557–567, McGraw-Hill, New York, NY, 2nd edition, 1986.

[2] H. Henry, L. Szolomayer, B. Sumpio, and K. Sutton, "Popliteal artery entrapment syndrome: bilateral lower extremity involvement," *Orthopedics*, vol. 41, no. 2, pp. e295–e298, 2018.

[3] S. Sinha, J. Houghton, P. J. Holt, M. M. Thompson, I. M. Loftus, and R. J. Hinchliffe, "Popliteal entrapment syndrome," *Journal of Vascular Surgery*, vol. 55, no. 1, pp. 252–262.e30, 2012.

[4] F. C. F. Carneiro Júnior, E. N. A. Carrijo, S. T. Araújo, L. C. U. Nakano, J. E. de Amorim, and D. G. Cacione, "Popliteal artery entrapment syndrome: a case report and review of the literature," *American Journal of Case Reports*, vol. 19, pp. 29–34, 2018.

[5] H. K. Kim, M. J. Shin, S. M. Kim, S. H. Lee, and H. J. Hong, "Popliteal artery entrapment syndrome: morphological classification utilizing MR imaging," *Skeletal Radiology*, vol. 35, no. 9, pp. 648–658, 2006.

13

Iatrogenic Fistula in Hemodialysis Patients: An Alternative Approach to Thrombectomy of Arteriovenous Graft (AVG) Thrombosis

Ramanath Dukkipati,[1,2,3] Alexandre M. Benjo,[4] Antonio Jimenez,[5] Ivo Lukitsch,[6] Gift C. Echefu,[7] and Damodar R. Kumbala[8]

[1]Harbor-UCLA Medical Center, Torrance, California, USA
[2]Lundquist Research Institute, Torrance, California, USA
[3]UCLA School of Medicine, Westwood, California, USA
[4]Lake Side Heart and Vascular Center, Lake Havasu, Arizona, USA
[5]Puerto Rico Vascular Center, Puerto Rico, USA
[6]Division of Nephrology, Ochsner Medical Center, New Orleans, Louisiana, USA
[7]Baton Rouge General Medical Center, Internal Medicine Program, Baton Rouge, Louisiana, USA
[8]Renal Associates of Baton Rouge, Baton Rouge, Louisiana, USA

Correspondence should be addressed to Gift C. Echefu; gift.echefu@brgeneral.org

Academic Editor: Hiroyuki Nakajima

Arterial venous (AV) fistula is the first choice of vascular access to perform hemodialysis in the vast majority of suitable patients followed by arteriovenous grafts (AVG). An iatrogenic fistula can occur when a second vein adjacent to the graft is punctured and the needle traverses the vein. In normal circumstances, this has no clinical repercussions and does not need correction, and in prior reports, it has helped to maintain the patency of partially occluded grafts but rarely can lead to thrombosis of the graft due to reduced flow and pressure in the graft lumen. We report here what we believe is a unique approach to perform thrombectomy of an occluded graft in a 71-year-old patient on hemodialysis to avoid placement of tunneled hemodialysis catheters and complications associated with catheters. When the outflow of basilic vein in this patient was thrombosed and could not be traversed, we successfully used an iatrogenic fistula as main outflow vein for the graft and created an alternative vein for drainage thus avoiding placement of a tunneled catheter for hemodialysis.

1. Introduction

The basilic vein is the larger vein in diameter compared to the cephalic vein. It is a commonly used vein for creation of arteriovenous fistula (AVF) in the upper extremity [1]. Basilic vein is also used as the outflow vein for arteriovenous grafts (AVG). Cephalic arch stenosis and thrombosis are a complication seen in patients with brachial artery-cephalic vein fistulas [2]. Thrombosis of these two upper extremity fistulas requires urgent endovascular intervention to salvage them to avoid the associated complications associated with tunneled hemodialysis catheters in the event thrombectomy of the fistula is unsuccessful. According to the 2019 KDOQI guidelines, the selection of a specific hemodialysis access is an individualized shared decision-making process aimed at providing the right access for the right patient, with a focus on vessel preservation, access creation, contingency, and succession plans [3]. Arteriovenous fistula is considered the first line choice for permanent vascular access in hemodialysis (HD) patients while AV graft is a second line option [4]. Innovative approaches for salvage of thrombosed AVF's to extend their life span are urgently needed. We present an innovative endovascular approach to salvage a thrombosed basilic vein fistula that extended the use of this fistula to receive HD for our patient. Salvage of thrombosed AVF or AVG avoids complications related to tunneled dialysis catheters.

2. Case Presentation

We present a 71-year-old male with ESRD on hemodialysis for 6 months who was deemed not suitable for creation of a fistula due to his suboptimal vein size and therefore had surgical creation of right brachial-basilica AV graft. Eight months after placement of the AVG, he presented with complete loss of thrill over the AVG. A few weeks prior to that adequacy of hemodialysis access was declining during the InterAccess flow monitoring which was below 500 ml/min. Patient was referred for a fistulogram but was unable to follow up prior to thrombosis of access. An ultrasound duplex scan demonstrated thrombosis in the AVG and therefore patient was referred to us for declotting.

We cannulated the graft in antegrade direction. Angiogram showed that the basilic vein was thrombosed (Figure 1). We could not cross the basilic vein occlusion in both antegrade and retrograde direction with soft and stiff 0.18 and 0.35 mm wires, and, therefore, we opted to attempt thrombectomy of the cephalic vein and outflow. Initially, we passed a 0.35 mm soft and angled hydrophilic (Terumo) wire in to the outflow performing rheolytic aspiration followed by balloon maceration of the remaining thrombus burden. We also noted a completely thrombosed basilic vein (Figure 1) during the first injection of radiocontrast and a partially clotted cephalic vein which was draining from the graft that drained the graft flow (Figure 2). Angioplasty of the cephalic arch stenosis was performed (Figures 3 and 4). A severe outflow lesion with subclavian vein stenosis was also observed. Additionally, we performed balloon angioplasty of the subclavian vein stenosis which was followed by declotting the arterial limb with a 5.5 French size Fogarty catheter. We were able to establish optimal flow with excellent back flow, normal thrill, and absence of pulsations. To ensure patency of this iatrogenic fistula, we placed a covered stent 7 mm × 5 cm stent (Viabahn) at the site where the graft drains into the cephalic vein, and angiogram showed good flow from the graft into the cephalic vein (Figure 5). Postoperatively, he underwent successful hemodialysis through access. We electively brought the patient two months later for readdressing the basilic vein thrombosis as the clot burden was much larger than the clot seen in the cephalic vein (Figure 6). Once the outflow was established for the graft through the cephalic vein with creation of the iatrogenic fistula, we observed spontaneous resolution of the basilic vein thrombosis and we did angioplasty of the basilic vein (Figures 7 and 8). Angiogram after the angioplasty of the basilic vein showed excellent flow in the basilic vein all the way into the central veins (Figure 8). The patient had successful cannulation of the graftula (one needle in the graft and the other in the vein) for hemodialysis on the next day using the graft segment for arterial needle placement and the stent area for venous needle placement. He has received hemodialysis without any problems with optimal blood flow or cannulation problems for several months following our intervention.

3. Discussion

An iatrogenic fistula is a conduit created between the arteriovenous graft and nearby vein(s), described as a consequence of repetitive traumatic cannulation of the AV graft, which leads to establishment of an alternative pathway of venous outflow of the graft. The repeated cannulations can lead to a hematoma in the surrounding tissue. This results in creation of a fistula with near native veins and can remain asymptomatic and nonfunctioning. Thrombosis of the graft leads to increased intragraft pressure in the venous arm of the AV graft which leads to increased blood flow through the iatrogenic fistula [5, 6]. The iatrogenic fistula could lead to AV graft dysfunction and decreased blood flow through the graft and may lead to thrombosis of the venous arm of the graft [6]. Most cases of iatrogenic fistulas do not require an intervention but with appropriate management at the correct time they resolve on their own. In this unique case, we were unsuccessful in establishing the patency of the basilic vein (the main outflow of the AV graft in this patient) due to severe stenosis and large clot burden, and, therefore, we used iatrogenic fistula as an alternative outflow vein. A stent was placed where the graft is draining to the cephalic vein to maintain patency as vein-graft interface segment stenosis is the leading cause of graft thrombosis. This resolution of outflow obstruction made it possible for this patient to continue his dialysis without the need for placement of a tunneled dialysis catheter. This prevented our patient from the complications associated with placement of vascular catheters for hemodialysis. This intervention allowed adequate time to lapse for spontaneous resolution of the basilic vein thrombosis.

Common complications of fistulas and grafts in hemodialysis patients include thrombosis, infection, steal syndrome, pseudoaneurysms with risk of bleeding, venous hypertension, seromas, and heart failure. Thrombosis and infection occur more frequently with grafts than with fistulas but the patency advantage of fistulas over grafts is not found in people who are 65 years and older [7–9]. Thrombosis of AV grafts in HD patients is most often due to stenosis at the anastomosis of the graft to vein and is one of the most common cause of vascular access malfunction, typically in the range of 0.6 to 1.2 per patient-year [10–12]. The goal of chronic vascular access is to offer repetitive access to blood circulation with minimal complications. Difficulties in vascular access generate significant problems to the healthcare providers, the healthcare system, and especially the patients with end-stage renal disease where a failing access is the leading cause of hospitalizations for patients on HD. An autogenous AV fistula using the patient's native tissues is still the preferred form of permanent vascular access, but when creation of a fistula is not possible, a graft should be considered [13]. Greater than 80 percent of thrombosed grafts have a stenotic lesion and often the site of lesion is in the anastomosis segment of the outflow vein to the graft. Risk factors for graft thrombosis are presence of stenotic lesion, infection, pseudoaneurysm, hypotension, hypovolemia, excessive compression, hypercoagulable state, and trauma [14]. Potential complications during percutaneous

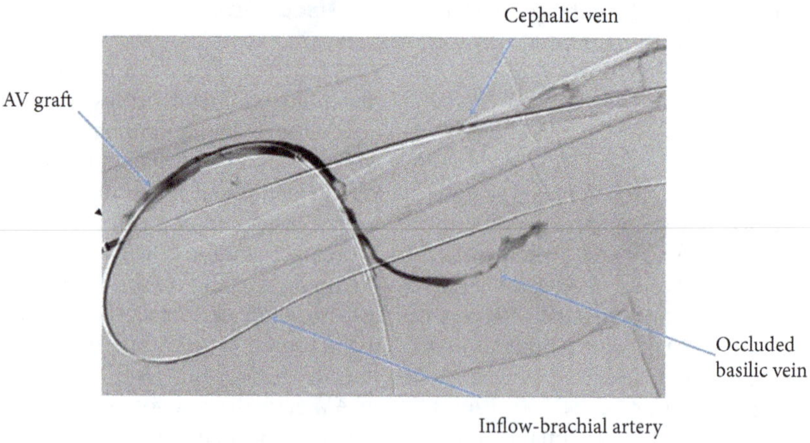

Figure 1: Thrombosed basilic vein.

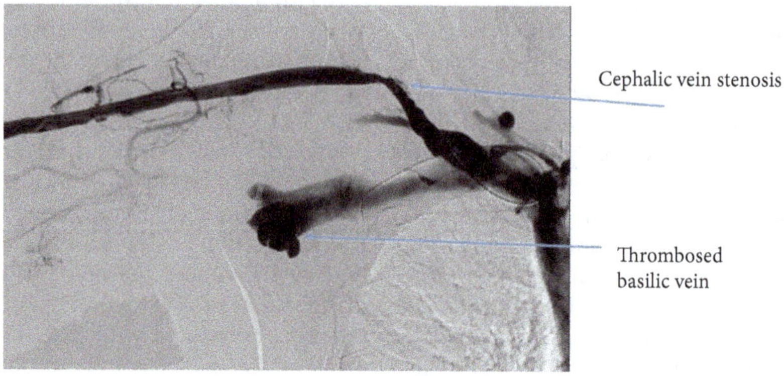

Figure 2: Outflow obstruction—cephalic vein stenosis and basilic vein thrombosis.

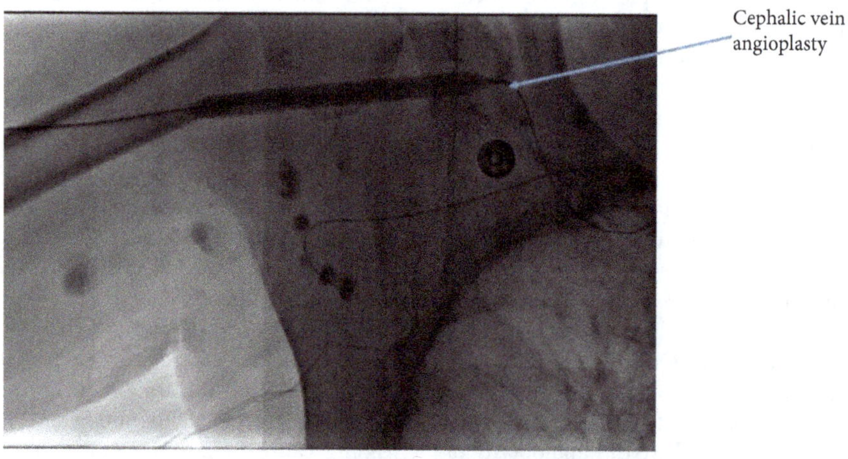

Figure 3: Outflow angioplasty.

thrombectomy include pulmonary emboli, distal arterial embolization, and rupture of the AV access.

In our case, the cause of thrombosis we suspect could be that the graft-to-vein fistula reducing intraluminal pressure in the graft played a key role in causing graft thrombosis [15]. We suspect that the fistula formed after repeated inadvertent concomitant cannulations of the vascular graft and the adjacent cephalic vein during hemodialysis. In the presence of other risk factors, the graft-to-vein fistula can predispose to graft thrombosis by steal phenomenon. Consistent with the scenario, especially in the presence of venous stenosis at the anastomosis site, significant amount

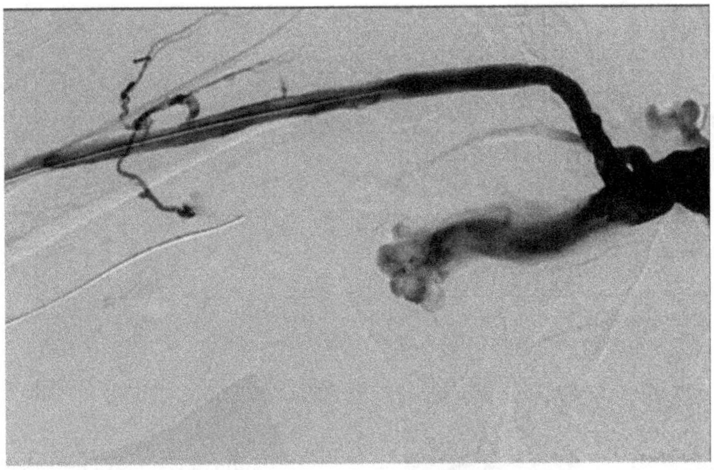

Figure 4: Outflow final result.

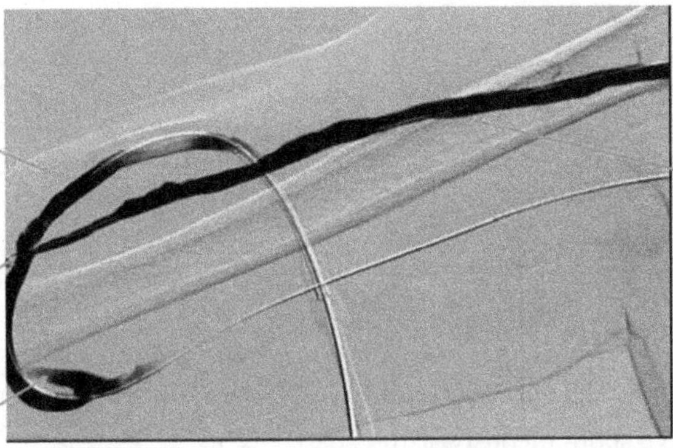

Figure 5: Post cephalic vein thrombectomy/percutaneous angioplasty.

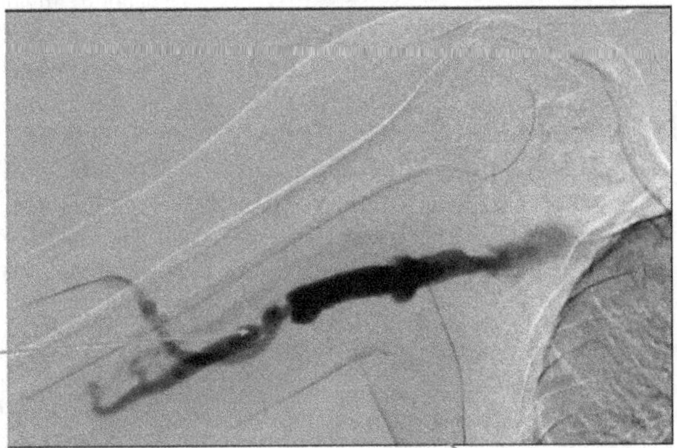

Figure 6: Relook after 2 months—self recanalization of basilic vein with significant stenosis.

of blood steal through the iatrogenic fistula can decrease blood flow in the venous limb of graft and may leaded to thrombosis.

The iatrogenic fistula formation between AV graft and an adjacent vein is a rare but a reported cause of graft thrombosis. The prevalence of this complication is not well established, but the major contributing factor is repeated inadvertent concomitant cannulation of AV graft and adjacent vein in the presence of venous outflow stenosis. Careful selection of cannulation site and proper cannulation technique is extremely important to prevent this rare complication. Early detection and resolution of venous outflow stenosis are of high importance in preventing and treating this complication. These iatrogenic fistulas only manifest during periods of elevated graft pressure. Once the graft pressure is normalized, these fistulas have minimal

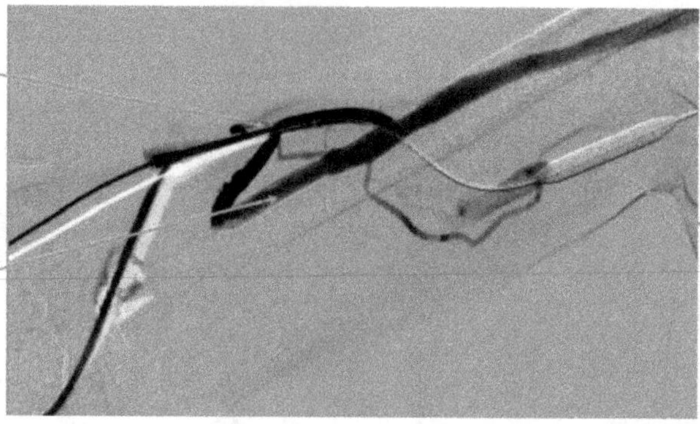

FIGURE 7: Patent graft to cephalic vein stent and basilic vein angioplasty.

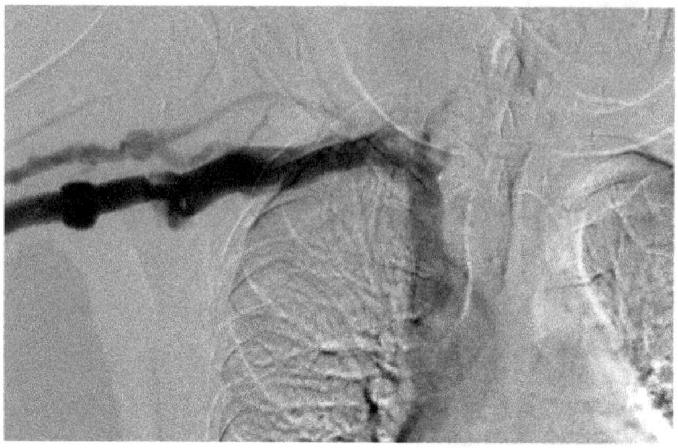

FIGURE 8: Basilic vein postangioplasty.

hemodynamic effect, and some resolve spontaneously without the need of any specific treatment [16].

In conclusion, although a traumatic graft-to-vein fistula is not a common hemodialysis access complication to occur, it can lead to graft thrombosis. Careful cannulation technique is important to prevent the development of iatrogenic fistulas. Endovascular techniques can be utilized to salvage this type of thrombotic traumatic AV fistulas using different outflow vein than the original vein the graft was anastomosed to.

References

[1] R. Dukkipati, C. de Virgilio, T. Reynolds, and R. Dhamija, "Outcomes of brachial artery–basilic vein fistula," *Seminars in Dialysis*, vol. 24, no. 2, pp. 220–230, 2011.

[2] R. Dukkipati, L. Lee, N. Atray, R. Kajani, G. Nassar, and K. Kalantar-Zadeh, "Outcomes of cephalic arch stenosis with and without stent placement after percutaneous balloon angioplasty in hemodialysis patients," *Seminars in Dialysis*, vol. 28, no. 1, pp. E7–E10, 2015.

[3] C. E. Lok, T. S. Huber, T. Lee et al., "KDOQI clinical practice guideline for vascular access: 2019 update," *American Journal of Kidney Diseases*, vol. 75, no. 4, Supplement 2, pp. S1–S164, 2020.

[4] R. Dukkipati, M. Peck, R. Dhamija et al., "Biological grafts for hemodialysis access: historical lessons, state-of-the- art and future directions," *Seminars in Dialysis*, vol. 26, no. 2, pp. 233–239, 2013.

[5] R. Y. Kanterman, T. M. Vesely, T. K. Pilgram, B. W. Guy, D. W. Windus, and D. Picus, "Dialysis access grafts: anatomic location of venous stenosis and results of angioplasty," *Radiology*, vol. 195, no. 1, pp. 135–139, 1995.

[6] B. A. Standage, E. S. Schuman, S. F. Quinn, J. W. Ragsdale, and R. C. Sheley, "Single limb patency of polytetrafluoroethylene dialysis loop grafts maintained by traumatic fistulization," *Annals of Vascular Surgery*, vol. 12, no. 4, pp. 364-369, 1998.

[7] R. K. Dhingra, E. W. Young, T. E. Hulbert-Shearon, S. F. Leavey, and F. K. Port, "Type of vascular access and mortality in U.S. hemodialysis patients," *Kidney International*, vol. 60, no. 4, pp. 1443-1451, 2001.

[8] M. R. Chan, R. J. Sanchez, H. N. Young, and A. S. Yevzlin, "Vascular access outcomes in the elderly hemodialysis population: a USRDS study," *Seminars in Dialysis*, vol. 20, no. 6, pp. 606-610, 2007.

[9] L. Coentrão, W. Van Biesen, I. Nistor et al., "Preferred haemodialysis vascular access for diabetic chronic kidney disease patients: a systematic literature review," *The Journal of Vascular Access*, vol. 16, no. 4, pp. 259–264, 2015.

[10] Z. J. Haskal, S. Trerotola, B. Dolmatch et al., "Stent graft versus balloon angioplasty for failing dialysis-access grafts," *New England Journal of Medicine*, vol. 362, no. 6, pp. 494–503, 2010.

[11] M. F. Fillinger, E. R. Reinitz, R. A. Schwartz et al., "Graft geometry and venous intimal-medial hyperplasia in arteriovenous loop grafts," *Journal of Vascular Surgery*, vol. 11, no. 4, pp. 556–566, 1990.

[12] B. S. Rifkin, U. C. Brewster, J. E. Aruny, and M. A. Perazella, "Percutaneous balloon cryoplasty: a new therapy for rapidly recurrent anastomotic venous stenoses of hemodialysis grafts?," *American Journal of Kidney Diseases*, vol. 45, no. 2, pp. e27–e32, 2005.

[13] R. K. Kerlan Jr. and J. M. LaBerge, "Fistula first, stent graft second," *New England Journal of Medicine*, vol. 362, no. 6, pp. 550–552, 2010.

[14] J. C. Harms, S. Rangarajan, C. J. Young, J. Barker-Finkel, and M. Allon, "Outcomes of arteriovenous fistulas and grafts with or without intervention before successful use," *Journal of Vascular Surgery*, vol. 64, no. 1, pp. 155–162, 2016.

[15] S. K. Min, Y. H. Park, H. H. Lee et al., "Iatrogenic fistula between prosthetic haemodialysis access graft and autogenous vein: unusual cause of graft thrombosis," *Nephrology, Dialysis, Transplantation*, vol. 19, no. 10, pp. 2647–2649, 2004.

[16] L. M. Moist, D. N. Churchill, A. A. House et al., "Regular monitoring of access flow compared with monitoring of venous pressure fails to improve graft survival," *Journal of the American Society of Nephrology*, vol. 14, no. 10, pp. 2645–2653, 2003.

14

Thrombosed Aneurysm of Superficial Epigastric Vein Simulating Inguinal Hernia: Report of Two Cases

Eleni Skandalou,[1] Panagiotis Papadopoulos,[2] Marianthi Kavelidou,[2] Stavros Kalfadis,[3] Theodoros Tzigkalidis,[4] and Ioannis Skandalos[2]

[1]*Internal Medicine Department, General Hospital "G. Papanikolaou", Thessaloniki, Greece*
[2]*Surgical Department, General Hospital "Agios Pavlos", Thessaloniki, Greece*
[3]*B΄Surgical Department General Hospital "G. Papanikolaou", Thessaloniki, Greece*
[4]*Pathology Department, General Hospital "Agios Pavlos", Thessaloniki, Greece*

Correspondence should be addressed to Eleni Skandalou; skandaloueleni@gmail.com

Academic Editor: Ayman El-Menyar

Aim. Presentation of two cases of superficial epigastric vein aneurysm simulating inguinal hernia. To our knowledge, only one other case is reported in the literature. *Case presentation.* The first case was a 34-year-old female with left inguinal pain and swelling which was clinically diagnosed as inguinal hernia. The second case was a 28-year-old female with inguinal pain and swelling, depicted with triplex ultrasonography and computed tomography, and was suspected to have inguinal hernia or enlarged inguinal lymph node. During the surgical exploration, both patients were found to have thrombosed aneurysm of the superficial epigastric vein. During the surgical exploration, both patients were found to have thrombosed aneurysm of the superficial epigastric vein. The superficial epigastric vein was ligated, and the venous aneurysms ($6 \times 4 \times 3$ and $2 \times 3 \times 2.5\,cm$, respectively) were excised. Histological examination of the thrombosed aneurysm showed complete replacement of the vascular wall by fibrous tissue, thrombosis, and an inflammatory reaction. There were no postoperative complications, and both patients were discharged on the second postoperative day. The 3-month and 1-year follow-up examination, respectively, was uneventful. *Conclusion.* Although venous aneurysms in the inguinal area are rare, they should be included in the differential diagnosis of a groin swelling.

1. Introduction

Venous aneurysms are usually uncommon. Venous aneurysms were first identified in autopsy studies by Osler in 1915 (1). Venous aneurysms can be caused by trauma, inflammation, connective tissue abnormalities, and degenerative changes (2). Superficial venous aneurysms in the inguinal region may be misdiagnosed soft tissue masses or inguinal or femoral hernias (3, 4). Herein, we describe two cases of a thrombosed aneurysm of the superficial epigastric vein simulating an inguinal hernia. To our knowledge, only one other case of inferior epigastric vein aneurysm is reported in the literature, and it is not clear if this is an aneurysm of the superficial or the deep inferior epigastric vein (5).

2. Case Presentation

First case: a 34-year-old female patient was admitted for an extensive painful swelling along her left inguinal area during the past 6 months. She was a nonsmoker, there was no trauma, use of oral contraceptive pills, infection, inflammatory disease, and recent travel in her medical history while review of systems was unremarkable. The patient had a medical history of left saphenectomy 8 years ago. Physical examination revealed a nonpulsating, immobile, and painful swelling along her left groin. The results of electrocardiography, routine biochemistry, and blood analysis were normal. The patient was clinically diagnosed with a left inguinal hernia, while an ultrasonic scan, unfortunately, had not been previously performed.

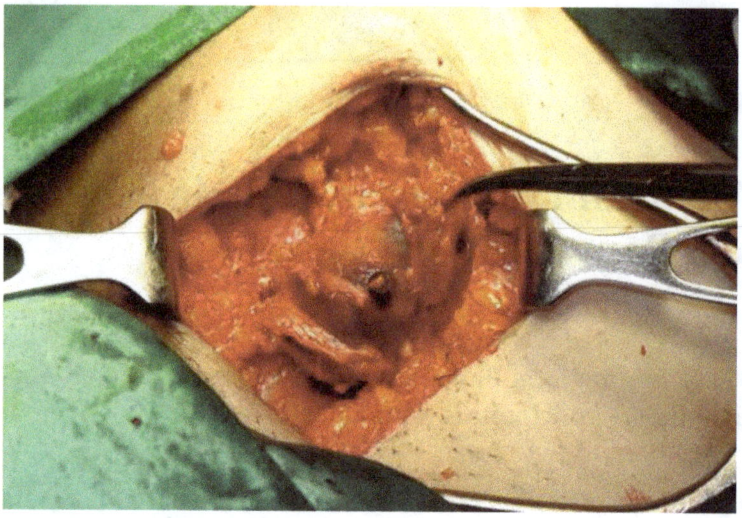

FIGURE 1: Surgical field: thrombosed aneurysm of the left superficial epigastric vein.

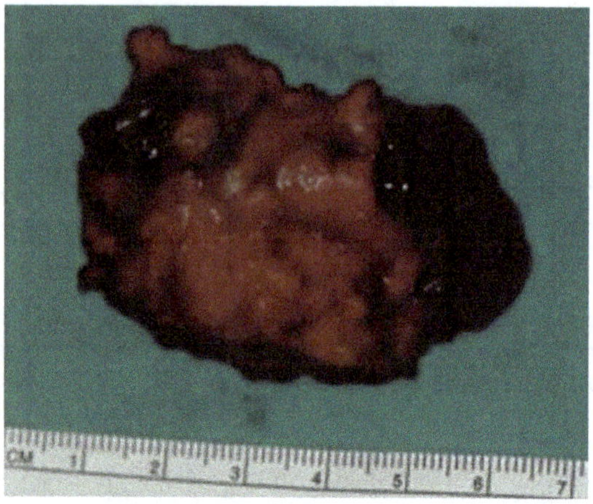

FIGURE 2: Surgical specimen: resected thrombosed superficial epigastric venous aneurysm (6 × 4 × 3 cm).

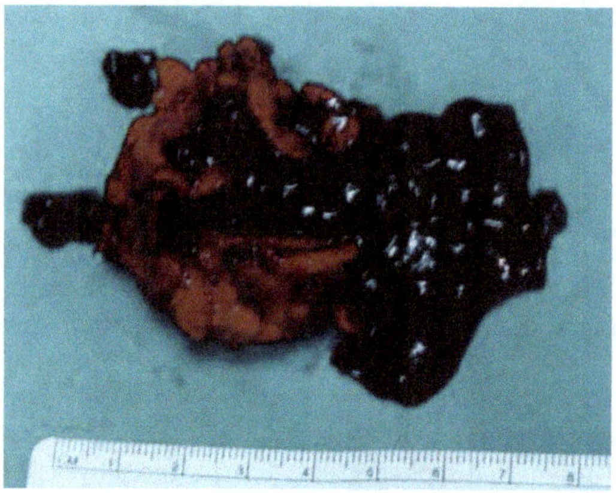

FIGURE 3: Surgical specimen: esected thrombosed superficial epigastric venous aneurysm (6 × 4 × 3 cm).

The patient was operated under spinal anesthesia, and a left oblique inguinal incision was performed. A large blue mass, due to a thrombosed fusiform aneurysm of the superficial epigastric vein, was found (Figure 1). The superficial epigastric vein was ligated flat to saphenous stump, and the venous aneurysm ($6 \times 4 \times 3\,cm$) was excised (Figures 2 and 3).

The second case: a 28-year-old female patient was admitted for mild painful swelling along the left inguinal area over the past 2 months. There were no remarkable findings in the patient's history of the predisposing factors, and the review of the systems was unremarkable. Physical examination revealed an inconsolable, immobile, and painful swelling along the left groin. The imaging examination with triplex ultrasonography (left inguinal hernia) (Figure 4) and computed tomography (inguinal lymph node enlargement) (Figure 5) was not diagnostic. The results of electrocardiography, biochemistry routine, and blood analysis were normal.

The differential diagnosis preoperatively was left inguinal hernia and inguinal lymph node enlargement. The patient was operated under spinal anesthesia, and a left oblique inguinal incision was performed. A large blue mass, due to a thrombosed saccular aneurysm of the superficial epigastric vein, was found (Figure 6). The superficial epigastric vein was ligated flat to saphenous stump, and the venous aneurysm ($2 \times 3 \times 2.5\,cm$) was excised (Figure 7).

3. Results

Histological examination of the thrombosed aneurysm showed complete replacement of the vascular wall by fibrous tissue, thrombosis, and an inflammatory reaction (Figure 8). There were nopostoperative complications, and both patients were discharged on the second postoperative day. The 3-month and 1-year follow-up examination, respectively, was uneventful.

4. Discussion

Venous aneurysms are rare vascular malformations that occur throughout the body and vessels at various sites can be affected as in the internal jugular vein, superior vena cava,

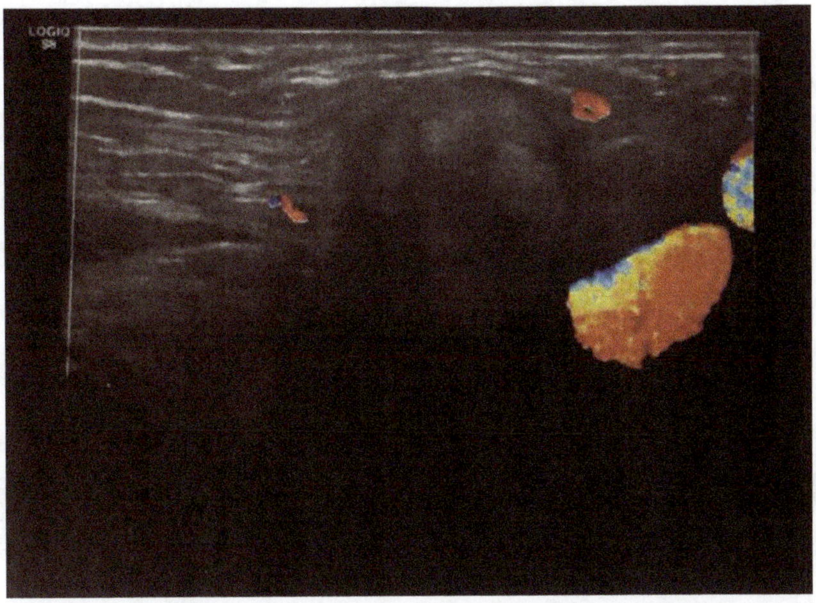

FIGURE 4: Tripplex ultrasonography: ultrasound findings suggesting left inguinal hernia (arrow).

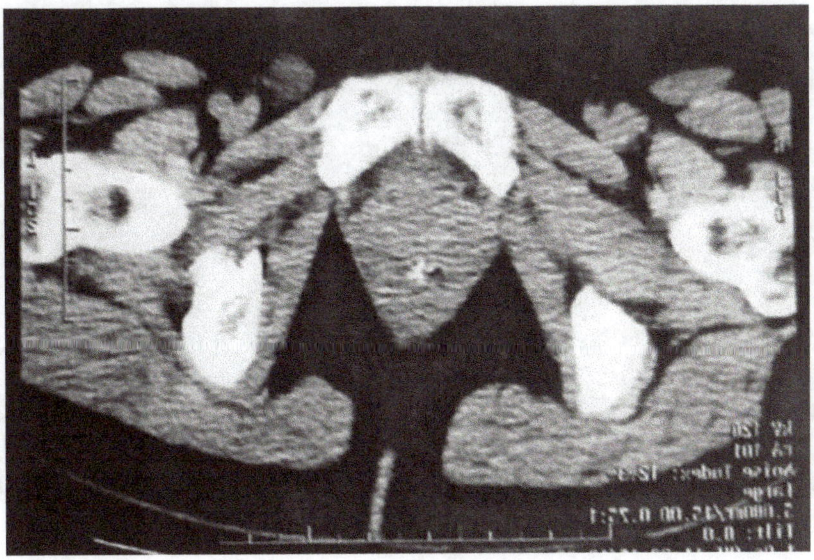

FIGURE 5: Computed tomography: in the inguinal region, a clearly demarcated formation diameter of 2 cm, with solid and cystic elements, is showed (swollen lymph node?) (arrow).

inferior vena cava, superior mesenteric vein, and also veins of the extremities (6, 7). Primary venous aneurysms are morphologically divided into two subgroups, saccular and fusiform (8). In literature, there are cases of venous aneurysms in all ages with equal distribution between both sexes (9). Primary venous aneurysms are usually congenital or develop from defective venous wall tissue (10). Secondary or acquired venous aneurysms are usually found in adults and are associated with trauma, inflammation, stretch injury, or altered venous hemodynamics. The previously reported case of superficial epigastric vein thrombosed aneurysm (5) and our two cases occurred in women of young age.

Histologically, there is replacement of three normal vascular wall layers by fibrous tissue with thrombosis and inflammatory infiltration (11). In both of our cases, the histological findings, due to aneurysm thrombosis, were complete replacement of the vascular wall by fibrous tissue, thrombosis, and an inflammatory reaction.

The causing symptoms are due to disfigurement, rupture, fistulation, or compression. Deep venous aneurysms present with pain or pulmonary embolism, while superficial venous aneurysms are usually asymptomatic; so, venous aneurysms located in the inguinal region,could be misdiagnosed as soft tissue lesions (6, 12) or as inguinal hernias (3, 4). Patients often complain of pain and a gradually

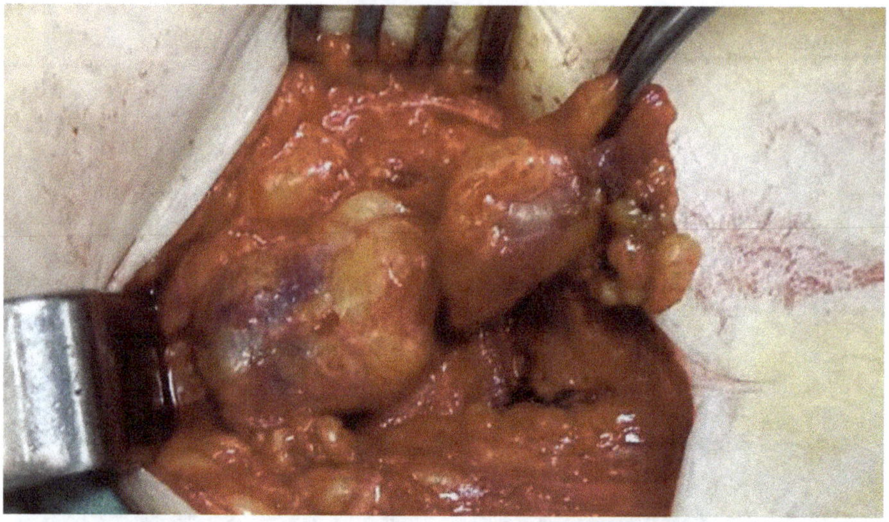

FIGURE 6: Surgical field: thrombosed superficial epigastric venous aneurysm (white arrow) and lymph node (black arrow).

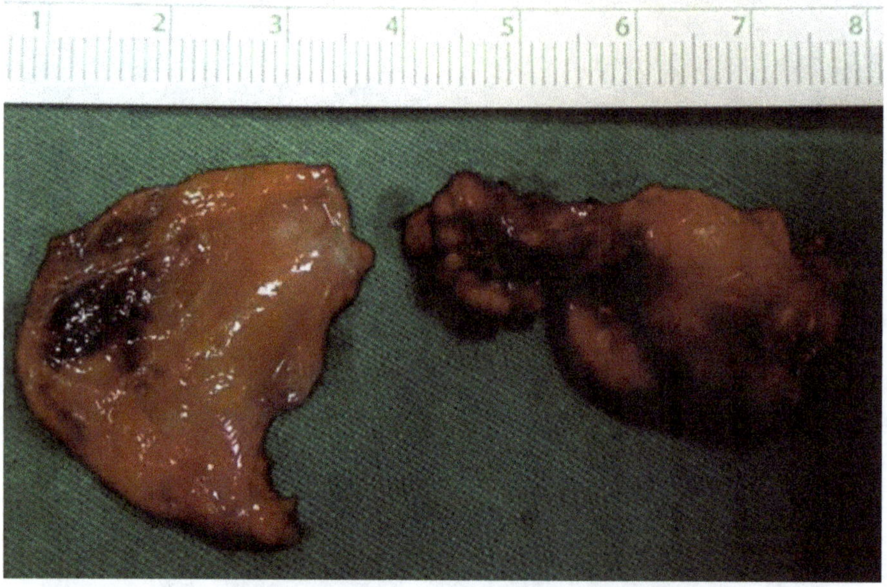

FIGURE 7: Surgical specimen: thrombosed superficial epigastric venous aneurysm ($2 \times 3 \times 2.5$ cm) (white arrow) and lymph node (black arrow).

increasing swelling (12). Because of the confusing symptoms and the unknown clinical entity, our patients were clinically misdiagnosed as having an inguinal hernia instead of the correct diagnosis.

Venous aneurysms can generally be diagnosed mainly by color Doppler imaging (12), as well as by computed tomography (CT) or magnetic resonance imaging (MRI). Our second patient was misdiagnosed by imaging examination with triplex ultrasonography (left inguinal hernia) and computed tomography (inguinal lymph node enlargement), due to the rarity and not considering of the diagnosis of superficial epigastric vein aneurysm.

The anatomic position of the venous aneurysm defines the best surgical approach. The indication for surgical treatment of superficial, neck, and face venous aneurysms is usually cosmetic. Asymptomatic nonenlarging venous aneurysms can be safely followed up, due to their high surgical morbidity and mortality. Abdominal venous aneurysms are at high risk of becoming painful or bleeding, and thus surgery should be considered for low risk patients (7, 13). As deep venous aneurysms of the extremities are at high risk of thromboembolic complications despite anticoagulant therapy, surgery may be the optimal management in terms of tangential aneurysmectomy and lateral venorrhaphy (9). Endovascular techniques continue to lack a defined role in their management (6). A superficial epigastric venous aneurysm is a rare entity. It should be suspected in cases of an inguinal mass, and it can be safely resected, because it is a superficial vein.

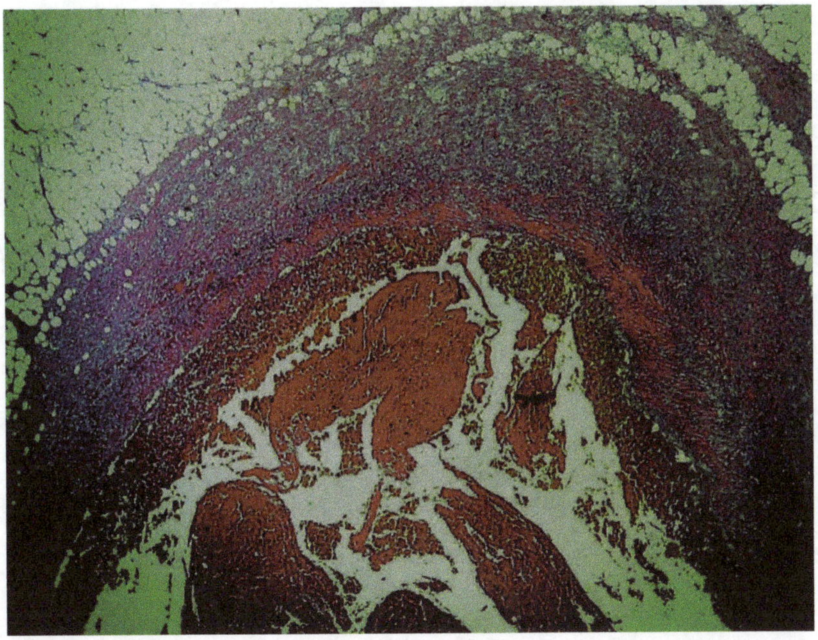

Figure 8: Complete replacement of three normal wall layers by fibrous tissue (white arrow), with thrombosis (blue arrow) and inflammatory reaction (black arrow) (H&E ×20).

5. Conclusion

We report two rare cases of a thrombosed venous aneurysm of the superficial epigastric vein, simulating an inguinal hernia. Although venous aneurysms in this region are rare, they should be included in the differential diagnosis of a groin swelling.

Consent

Written informed consent was obtained from the patients for publication of their personal data.

References

[1] J. M. Castle and E. J. Arous, "Femoral vein aneurysm: a case report and review of the literature," *Cardiovascular Surgery*, vol. 3, no. 3, pp. 317–319, 1995.

[2] M. D. Sarap and W. E. Wheeler, "Venous aneurysms," *Journal of Vascular Surgery*, vol. 8, no. 2, pp. 182-183, 1988.

[3] J. S. de Miranda, S. H. Damous, M. P. Júnior et al., "Great saphenous vein aneurysm: a differential diagnosis of femoral hernia and review," *International Journal of Surgery Case Reports*, vol. 8, pp. 154–157, 2015.

[4] C. Tschuor, D. Dindo, P. A. Clavien, and D. Hahnloser, "A challenging hernia: primary venous aneurysm of the proximal saphenous vein," *Hernia*, vol. 17, no. 1, pp. 111–113, 2013.

[5] N. Bhasin, M. J. Weston, and D. J. A. Scott, "Inferior epigastric vein aneurysm: an unusual cause of groin pain," *EJVES Extra*, vol. 6, no. 1, pp. 22-23, 2003.

[6] K. A. Teter, T. M. Maldonado, and M. A. Adelman, "A systematic review of venous aneurysms by anatomic location," *Journal of Vascular Surgery. Venous and Lymphatic Disorders*, vol. 6, no. 3, pp. 408–413, 2018.

[7] M. Uematsu, M. Okada, and M. Uematsu, "Primary venous Aneurysms," *Angiology*, vol. 50, no. 3, pp. 239–244, 1999.

[8] P. Nana, C. Korais, A. Mpouronikou, V. Lachanas, K. Spanos, and G. Kouvelos, "Management of an external jugular vein aneurysm in a young patient," *Journal of Vascular Surgery. Venous and Lymphatic Disorders*, vol. 8, no. 5, pp. 861–863, 2020.

[9] J. Majeski, "Surgical repair of primary saphenous vein aneurysm of the proximal leg after initial presentation as an inguinal hernia," *The American Surgeon*, vol. 68, pp. 999–1002, 2002.

[10] M. Yasumoto, H. Shibuya, Y. Goto, T. Saitoh, K. Nakajima, and S. Suzuki, "Primary saphenous venous aneurysms presenting in a child," *Clinical Nuclear Medicine*, vol. 12, pp. 29-30, 1987.

[11] S. H. Seo, M. B. Kim, K. S. Kwon, C. W. Kim, and C. K. Oh, "Primary venous aneurysms of the superficial venous system," *Angiology*, vol. 59, no. 5, pp. 593–598, 2008.

[12] H. Y. Lee, S. H. Cho, T. Y. Ko et al., "Saccular aneurysm of the external jugular vein: A Case report," *The Korean Journal of Thoracic and Cardiovascular Surgery*, vol. 47, no. 2, pp. 171–173, 2014.

[13] A. Siani, I. Flaishman, A. Schioppa, A. Zaccaria, and E. Baldassarre, "Jugular venous phlebectasia: uncommon in children, anecdotical in adults," *American Journal of Surgery*, vol. 195, no. 3, pp. 419-420, 2008.

15

A Spontaneous Isolated Superior Mesenteric Artery Dissection Associated with Cocaine Abuse: A Pathomechanistic Association

Rayan S. El-Zein,[1] **Jeffrey Sobecki**,[1] **Roy Greenberg**,[1] **Michael Keleher**,[2] **and Robert A. Palma**[1]

[1]*Department of Internal Medicine, OhioHealth Doctors Hospital, 5100 W Broad St, Columbus, OH 43228, USA*
[2]*Department of Interventional Radiology, OhioHealth Doctors Hospital, 5100 W Broad St, Columbus, OH 43228, USA*

Correspondence should be addressed to Rayan S. El-Zein; rayan.el-zein@ohiohealth.com

Academic Editor: Antonio Silvestro

Spontaneous isolated superior mesenteric artery dissection (SISMAD) is a rare potentially fatal disease. We present a case of cocaine-related SISMAD in a patient with abdominal pain. A 38-year-old African American male with hypertension and alcohol, cocaine, and tobacco abuse presented with abdominal pain and recent cocaine use. A CT angiogram revealed SISMAD; he was treated with conservative management. Cocaine and SISMAD share similar pathophysiologic mechanisms pertaining to vascular smooth muscle cell apoptosis and increased shear stress at fixed vascular positions. Our report emphasizes the need to consider cocaine abuse in SISMAD pathophysiology, risk stratification, and treatment algorithms in future studies.

1. Introduction

Initially reported by Bauersfeld in 1947, spontaneous isolated superior mesenteric artery dissection (SISMAD) is a rare but potentially fatal arterial disease with an incidence of 0.06% from a cohort of 6666 autopsies [1]. Prior to 2001, only 46 cases were reported; since 2016, more than 622 cases have been reported [2] reflecting the advancement of imaging rather than prevalence. Multiple risk factors have been suggested such as arteriopathy (connective tissue diseases, cystic medial necrosis, etc.), tobacco use, atherosclerosis, alcohol abuse, obesity, heavy weight lifting, and pregnancy [3]. While cocaine use has been associated with other mesenteric pathology (ischemia, perforation), cocaine-related SISMAD remains a rare finding.

2. Case Report

A 38-year-old African American male with a history of hypertension and alcohol, cocaine, and tobacco use presented with recurrent abdominal pain. Three days prior, he was admitted with abdominal pain and hypertensive urgency. Cocaine and cannabinoids were found in his urine. A computed tomography (CT) scan of the abdomen with IV contrast demonstrated atherosclerosis of the aortoiliac system. With conservative management, the patient was diagnosed with cocaine-induced vasospasm and was discharged after two days.

The following day, he returned with recurrence of his abdominal pain and reported continued cocaine use. He described his symptoms as crampy in nature localizing to the upper right and left quadrants. He denied any associated nausea, vomiting, diarrhea, melena, or hematochezia. On arrival, his blood pressure was 190/120 mmHg. His abdomen was soft and flat with diffuse abdominal tenderness to soft and deep palpation with no guarding, organomegaly, rebound tenderness, or peritoneal signs.

Results of laboratory tests revealed a serum lactic acid of 2.7 mmol/L. A CT angiogram (CTA) of the abdomen and pelvis revealed a SISMAD within the proximal-to-mid SMA

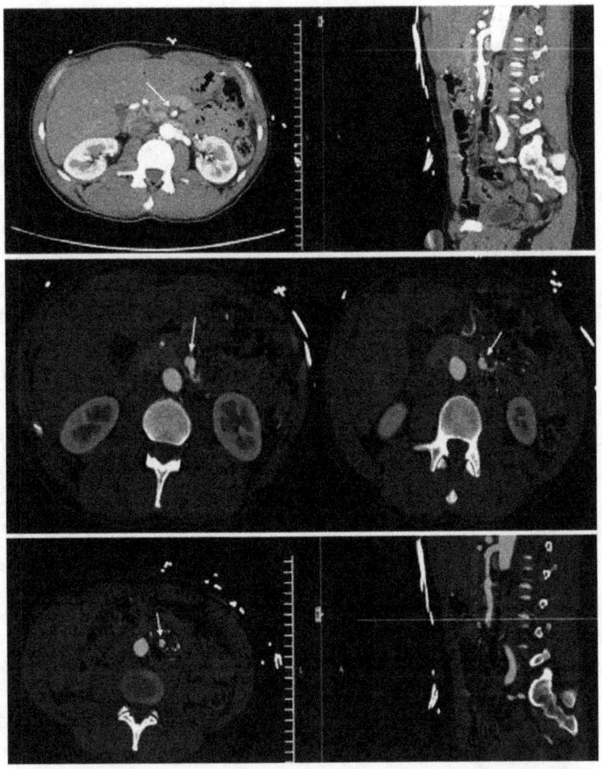

FIGURE 1: SISMAD within the proximal-to-mid SMA with a 3 cm segment along the proximal SMA with thrombosis of the false lumen extending craniocaudally; 70% stenosis of the proximal SMA; an intimal flap was seen intermittently below this level extending to the major bifurcations of the middle colic artery.

with a 3 cm thrombosis of the proximal false lumen and distal false lumen patency; 70% stenosis of the proximal SMA was noted secondary to this process (Figure 1). There was no evidence of abdominal ischemia. He was admitted to a medical/surgical floor with telemetry and was treated with conservative management. In addition to pain control and bowel rest, his home amlodipine 5 mg daily and hydrochlorothiazide 12.5 mg daily were restarted with the addition of as-needed hydralazine for a strict systolic blood pressure target of <140. In conjunction with the vascular surgery team, he was started on antiplatelet monotherapy with aspirin 325 mg daily. Two days after presentation, a repeat CT angiogram showed stabilization of the SMA dissection and the patient was safely discharged. The patient did not have any further abdominal imaging after discharge.

3. Discussion

SISMAD is rare with <1000 reported cases [2, 3]. Clinical presentations can range from an asymptomatic incidental finding to severe abdominal pain from bowel ischemia or fatal aneurysmal rupture. The severity of the pain has been shown to correlate with the length of dissection [4]. CTA is considered the gold standard [5].

Five classifications have been proposed by Sakamoto et al., Yun et al., Zerbib et al., Luan et al., and Li et al. [6]. Yun's classification based on dissection entry and reentry points, length, patency, and degree of luminal stenosis has become the most commonly used due to its simplicity [4]. The SISMAD in our case is classified as a combination of type 2a and type 2b. The proximal false lumen is thrombosed; however, there is a visible false lumen distal to thrombosis without an obvious reentry site. Previously, Park et al. published a series in which they found that Yun type 2 (2a or 2b) dissections were more likely to undergo complete remodeling [7].

Although the precise pathogenesis of SISMAD remains uncharacterized, it is suggested to be related to arterial wall dysfunction involving atherosclerosis, vasculitis, cystic medial necrosis, segmental arteriolar mediolysis, fibromuscular dysplasia, and connective tissue diseases [3, 8, 9]. Histopathological and hemodynamic components have also been established which point towards a relationship with cocaine. Cocaine is associated with several arterial dissections: coronary [10], aortic [11], carotid [12], and renal artery dissections [13]. The sympathomimetic action of cocaine leads to significantly increased shear stress resulting in intimal tear, especially in fixed vascular positions (e.g., ligamentum arteriosum) as seen in aortic dissections [11]. Approximately 1-3 cm from the SMA ostium, the SMA transitions from a fixed retropancreatic segment to an unfixed mesenteric segment where most SISMADs originate. Flow dynamic studies revealed greater shear stress at this point along the anterior convex portion of the SMA [14, 15]. In a study by Bigi et al. [16], chronic cocaine use (average 10 years) was associated with impairment of elastic properties of the aorta; another study on cultured rat aortic vascular smooth muscle cells (VSMCs) demonstrated that aortic VSMCs undergo rapid apoptosis in response to cocaine [17]. Concurrently in SISMAD, elastic fiber fragmentation and loss of smooth muscle cells are seen histologically thus reflecting increased wall weakness and decreased distensibility [3].

In our case, we postulated that our patient's chronic cocaine abuse along with other risk factors (atherosclerosis, tobacco, and alcohol) has likely resulted in gradual SMA wall dysfunction forming a nidus for subsequent dissection. His recent acute cocaine use may have produced a significant shear stress elevation leading to dissection. Therefore, with the aforementioned mechanisms, our patient's cocaine use played a significant role in his disease development.

No prospectively randomized clinical trial has been published regarding treatment guidelines of SISMAD. Treatment options range from conservative management with or without antithrombotic therapy (anticoagulation or antiplatelet), endovascular SMA stenting, or open surgery. In a recent meta-analysis of 25 selected studies, conservative medical treatment was successful in 397 of 447 of cases, irrespective of anticoagulation or antiplatelet therapy, and 50 underwent conversion to endovascular therapy or open surgery [18]. Park et al. showed that 41% treated conservatively had improvement on surveillance CTA and 15% of patients had complete remodeling [7]. There has been no difference in outcomes with the use of anticoagulants or antiplatelet agents, as anticoagulation may prevent false lumen thrombosis and promote dissection propagation [4]. Persistent abdominal pain or significant stenosis (>80%) indicates endovascular stenting whereas hemorrhage or bowel ischemia necessitates open surgery [3]. It is reasonable to apply current recommendations for patients with SISMAD unrelated to cocaine to patients with cocaine-related SISMAD. This report emphasizes the need to consider cocaine in SISMAD risk stratification, pathophysiology, and treatment algorithms in future studies.

References

[1] A. G. Foord and R. D. Lewis, "Primary dissecting aneurysms of peripheral and pulmonary arteries: dissecting hemorrhage of media," *Archives of Pathology*, vol. 68, pp. 553–577, 1959.

[2] J. Y. Luan, X. Guan, X. Li et al., "Isolated superior mesenteric artery dissection in China," *Journal of Vascular Surgery*, vol. 63, no. 2, pp. 530–536, 2016.

[3] M. J. Dougherty and D. A. Troutman, "Mesenteric arterial dissection," in *Rutherford's Vascular Surgery and Endovascular Therapy. 2*, pp. 1771–1779, Elsevier, Philadelphia, 9th edition, 2019.

[4] W. S. Yun, Y. W. Kim, K. B. Park et al., "Clinical and angiographic follow-up of spontaneous isolated superior mesenteric artery dissection," *European Journal of Vascular and Endovascular Surgery*, vol. 37, no. 5, pp. 572–577, 2009.

[5] G. Subhas, A. Gupta, M. Nawalany, and W. F. Oppat, "Spontaneous isolated superior mesenteric artery dissection: a case report and literature review with management algorithm," *Annals of Vascular Surgery*, vol. 23, no. 6, pp. 788–798, 2009.

[6] Z. Jia, J. Tu, and G. Jiang, "The classification and management strategy of spontaneous isolated superior mesenteric artery dissection," *Korean Circulation Journal*, vol. 47, no. 4, pp. 425–431, 2017.

[7] Y. J. Park, K. B. Park, D. I. Kim, Y. S. Do, D. K. Kim, and Y. W. Kim, "Natural history of spontaneous isolated superior mesenteric artery dissection derived from follow-up after conservative treatment," *Journal of Vascular Surgery*, vol. 54, no. 6, pp. 1727–1733, 2011.

[8] M. N. Tameo, M. J. Dougherty, and K. D. Calligaro, "Spontaneous dissection with rupture of the superior mesenteric artery from segmental arterial mediolysis," *Journal of Vascular Surgery*, vol. 53, no. 4, pp. 1107–1112, 2011.

[9] H. E. Garrett Jr., "Options for treatment of spontaneous mesenteric artery dissection," *Journal of Vascular Surgery*, vol. 59, no. 5, pp. 1433–1439.e2, 2014.

[10] I. Merinopoulos, D. Bloore, and P. Read, "A 'sniff' away from death: a case of cocaine-induced coronary artery dissection," *Oxford Medical Case Reports*, vol. 2017, no. 10, article omx058, 2017.

[11] A. Singh, A. Khaja, and M. A. Alpert, "Cocaine and aortic dissection," *Vascular Medicine*, vol. 15, no. 2, pp. 127–133, 2010.

[12] B. D. Jaffe, T. M. Broderick, and C. V. Leier, "Cocaine-induced coronary-artery dissection," *The New England Journal of Medicine*, vol. 330, no. 7, pp. 510-511, 1994.

[13] D. A. Edmondson, J. B. Towne, D. W. Foley, M. Abu-Hajir, and M. S. Kochar, "Cocaine-induced renal artery dissection and thrombosis leading to renal infarction," *WMJ*, vol. 103, no. 7, pp. 66–69, 2004.

[14] Y. J. Park, C. W. Park, K. B. Park, Y. N. Roh, D. I. Kim, and Y. W. Kim, "Inference from clinical and fluid dynamic studies about underlying cause of spontaneous isolated superior mesenteric artery dissection," *Journal of Vascular Surgery*, vol. 53, no. 1, pp. 80–86, 2011.

[15] Z. Wu, J. Yi, H. Xu et al., "The significance of the angle between superior mesenteric artery and aorta in spontaneous isolated superior mesenteric artery dissection," *Annals of Vascular Surgery*, vol. 45, pp. 117–126, 2017.

[16] M. A. B. Bigi, A. Aslani, and M. Mehrpour, "Effect of chronic cocaine abuse on the elastic properties of aorta," *Echocardiography*, vol. 25, no. 3, pp. 308–311, 2008.

[17] J. Su, J. Li, W. Li, B. T. Altura, and B. M. Altura, "Cocaine induces apoptosis in primary cultured rat aortic vascular smooth muscle cells: possible relationship to aortic dissection, atherosclerosis, and hypertension," *International Journal of Toxicology*, vol. 23, no. 4, pp. 233–237, 2004.

[18] Y. Zhu, Y. Peng, M. Xu et al., "Treatment strategies and outcomes of symptomatic spontaneous isolated superior mesenteric artery dissection: a systematic review and meta-analysis," *Journal of Endovascular Therapy*, vol. 25, no. 5, pp. 640–648, 2018.

16

A Tumultuous Course of Exogenous Testosterone by a Bodybuilder Causing a Catastrophic Hypercoagulable State in the Surgical Intensive Care Unit

Kevin Lee,[1] **Sophia Toraby**,[2] **Robert Cotterman**,[2,3] **Babatunde Oriowo**,[2,4] **and John Fish**[2,4]

[1]*Department of Anesthesiology, The University of Toledo Medical Center, Toledo, OH, USA*
[2]*Department of Surgery, The University of Toledo Medical Center, Toledo, OH, USA*
[3]*Department of Critical Care and Trauma Surgery, ProMedica Toledo Hospital, Toledo, OH, USA*
[4]*Department of Vascular Surgery, ProMedica Toledo Hospital, Toledo, OH, USA*

Correspondence should be addressed to Kevin Lee; kevin.lee2@utoledo.edu

Academic Editor: Muzaffer Sindel

Present literature demonstrates an equivocal relationship between testosterone and thrombogenicity. Herein, we describe a case in which a patient used an unspecified amount and duration of exogenous testosterone injections, subsequently developing thrombotic events in his: right radial artery, right iliac artery, superficial femoral artery, splenic artery and a bilateral lower lobe pulmonary embolism. As a result, clinicians should consider exogenous testosterone use as a potential risk factor when the etiology of a patient's thrombotic events are not clear. We also completed a literature review of the molecular mechanisms in which testosterone can increase the clot burden through an increases human platelet thromboxane A2 receptor density and an increase in erythropoiesis.

1. Introduction

The use of performance enhancing drugs (PEDs), particularly the use of androgens, is a way for some bodybuilders and non-athletes to increase muscle mass, improve performance, and enhance physical attractiveness. In fact, the use of androgenic steroids has become a global epidemic in which the overall global lifetime prevalence in men is 6.4 percent and in women is 1.6 percent [1]. The use of exogenous androgens does not come without consequences as acne, gynecomastia, liver toxicity, cardiac dysfunction, and psychiatric symptoms are known side effects which have been well documented in the literature [2]. While the association between testosterone use and venous thromboembolism in men remains dubious, we present a case in which a 32-year-old Caucasian male developed multiple venous and arterial thromboembolisms likely secondary to his exogenous testosterone use. Though there is no clear relationship between testosterone use and hypercoagulability as per a recent Systematic Review and Meta-Analysis in 2018 by Mayo Clinic, several molecular mechanisms have been proposed to explain such [3]. The first being that testosterone increases human platelet thromboxane A2 receptor density and aggregation response which could increase the thrombogenicity [4]. Secondly, testosterone stimulates erythropoiesis, which increases hemoglobin and hematocrit in a dose-dependent manner ultimately increasing the propensity of a thrombotic event [5]. As the prevalence of androgenic steroids continues to rise, further investigation for establishing testosterone as a risk factor for thrombogenicity is warranted.

2. Case History/Examination

A 32-year-old, Caucasian, morbidly-obese (BMI of 42.96 kg/m^2), male with a past medical history of hypertension, obstructive sleep apnea was transferred from an outside facility with complaints of worsening cyanosis, paresthesias, numbness, and weakness in his right upper extremity. The patient's only home medication was 10 mg of Lisinopril daily for which his blood pressure was controlled. It should also be noted that the patient had no documented history of hyperlipidemia as a lipid profile was drawn four months prior which showed a total cholesterol level of 157 mg/dl (100–199 mg/dl), triglyceride level of 76 mg/

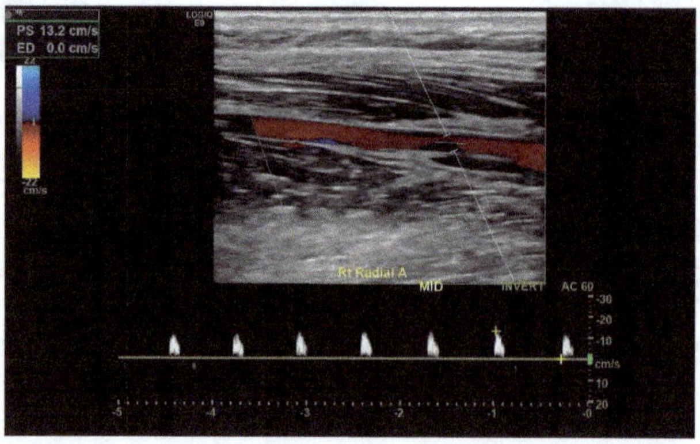

FIGURE 1: Vascular arterial duplex of the right mid radial artery with pre-occlusive "thump" waveforms. Spectral waveforms with normal triphasic diastolic flow were noted in the subclavian, axillary, brachial and ulnar artery without significant color flow disturbance.

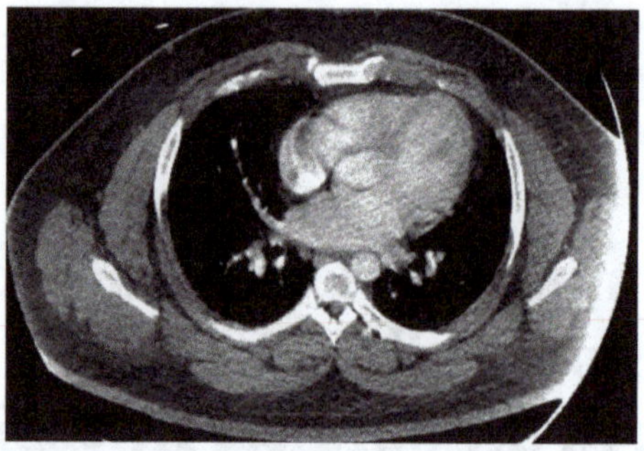

FIGURE 2: CT angiogram chest with intravenous contrast shows small to moderate left lower lobe pulmonary emboli. A 2 cm pleural-based right lower lobe nodular density can also be seen. It should be noted that evaluation of the pulmonary arteries is suboptimal secondary to patient body habitus and under opacification of the pulmonary vessels.

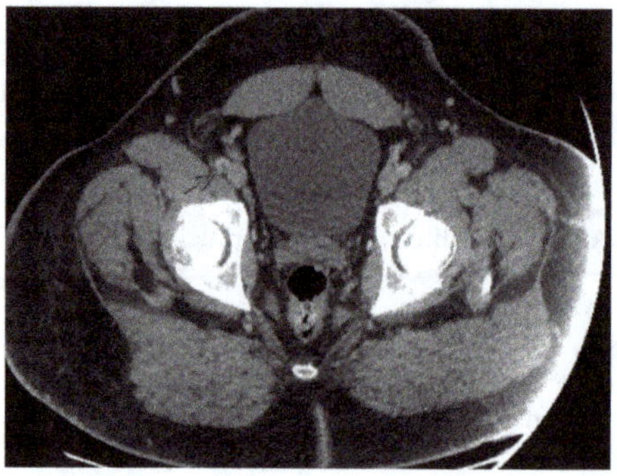

FIGURE 3: CT angiogram abdominal aorta with right lower extremity runoff shows a nonoccuslive longitudinal filling defect in the distal right external iliac artery and tibioperoneal trunk suggestive of a thrombus. There, however, are Patent common femoral artery, profunda, and SFA. Left lower extremity runoff showed a patent common femoral artery, profunda, popliteal artery and SFA. The abdominal aorta is widely patent and measures 2.3 cm the celiac, 2 cm at the SMA, and 1.7 cm below the renal arteries.

dl (100–199 mg/dl), HDL level of 39 mg/dl (<40 mg/dl) and LDL level of 103 (<100 mg/dl). Prior to the patient's initial presentation, he had been experiencing this symptomatology three weeks prior which was managed conservatively with pain medication and steroids by his primary care physician. The patient was also fully mobilize and active placing him at minimal risk of venous stasis. At the outside facility, the patient had a CT angiogram of his right upper extremity which showed a thrombotic occlusion of the right radial artery just proximal to the wrist and a right upper extremity. Right upper extremity arterial Doppler ultrasound showed monophasic flow and was flat-line at the index finger and thumb with a preocclusive waveform in the mid radial artery and subsequent distal radial artery occlusion, as seen in Figure 1.

The patient denied any personal or family history of thrombosis. Upon review of his social history, the patient did admit to using exogenous testosterone in the past. The exact dose and duration of his testosterone use was not fully clarified with the patient directly. He also admitted to being a former smoker with an undocumented duration prior to experiencing any symptoms in his right upper extremity.

Upon presentation, the patient was started on a continuous heparin infusion and was admitted to the vascular surgery service for acute limb ischemia. The following day, the patient had a right radial artery catheterization via cut-down technique, thrombectomy of the radial artery, intra-arterial tPA into the distal radial artery and he was continued on a heparin infusion. The patient also had an echocardiogram which was negative for a cardioembolic event and the patient had no known history of cardiac arrhythmia or disease which was also not present on cardiac monitoring.

However, the next two days, the patient had developed increased swelling and pain in his right upper extremity. The orthopedic surgery team was consulted for evaluation and management for concerns of compartment syndrome and had subsequent right hand thenar and hypothenar fasciotomies. The patient also had IR angiography performed that day which showed occlusion of the mid and distal right radial artery to the level of the arch with occlusions of the interdigital arteries involving the thumb and the index finger. He was continued on a heparin infusion and started on an epoprostenol infusion. TEE was unremarkable and CBC and renal and hepatic function remained normal.

Prior to the patient being transferred to the medical-surgical floor, SICU nursing staff expressed that they could not identify a pulse in the right dorsalis pedis pulse and the extremity was cold to palpation. CTA of the chest and CTA of the abdomen were ordered and showed small to moderate, bilateral lower lobe, pulmonary emboli and a thrombus in the right external iliac artery as seen in Figures 2 and 3.

Of particular clinical significance, the CTA of the chest also showed a 2 cm pleural-based right lung nodular density. He was placed on tPA for catheter directed thrombolysis for four days in conjunction with heparin and epoprostenol. Heparin was also switched to bilvarudin due to subtherapeutic Heparin-Xa levels. The patient was not thrombocytopenic or profoundly anemic and both heparin inducted thrombocytopenia and disseminated intravascular coagulation were both ruled out.

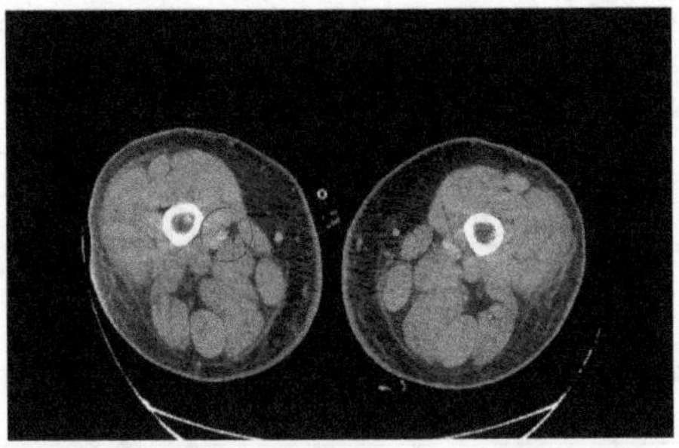

FIGURE 4: CT angiogram abdominal aorta with right lower extremity runoff shows a globular filling defect at the mid and distal segment of the right SFA most consistent with an arterial embolus. The right profunda artery is grossly unremarkable. There is grossly adequate 3 vessel runoff. Left superficial femoral artery is grossly patent as well as popliteal artery with 3 vessels runoff. Both external iliac arteries are grossly patent. Both common femoral arteries are grossly patent.

Repeated CTA of the abdomen with runoff showed a splenic infarct, and a filling defect at the mid and distal right superficial femoral artery, as seen in Figure 4, both consistent with underlying emboli.

The patient had a full hypercoagulable workup which was unremarkable and included: a hemolysis workup, homocysteine level, Heparin PF4, antiphospholipid antibodies, monoclonal protein, paroxysmal nocturnal hemoglobinuria, JAK2 mutation, Factor V Leiden mutation, and Prothrombin mutation as seen in Table 1. Initial testosterone and luteinizing hormone levels were not drawn on presentation or during admission as this was a diagnosis of exclusion, at the time, because of the lack of clear relationship between testosterone use and hypercoagulability in previous studies. The decision was made to not order Protein C, Protein S, Antithrombin 3, and lupus anticoagulant studies, per the oncology team, because the patient was already on anticoagulation and the values would be confounding.

During the patient's hospital course, the patient also developed septic shock secondary to *A. baumannii* complex, aspiration pneumonia, and C diff colitis. He went into Acute Respiratory Distress Syndrome as a manifestation of his septic shock and eventually required tracheostomy and percutaneous endoscopic gastrostomy due to severe decompensated respiratory status.

Upon improvement of the patient's clinical status, he was transitioned to a long-term acute care facility. He was discharged on warfarin with INR goal of 2.5–3.5, ticagrelor and baby aspirin and he was instructed to follow up with vascular medicine as an outpatient. Despite, no clear etiology for the patient's hypercoagulable state, it is suspected that the patient's exogenous testosterone use prompted his profound hypercoagulable state among other risk factors. It should be noted that the patient did initially present with a hematocrit of 51.6%. As an outpatient, the patient continued to be evaluated by vascular medicine for thrombophilia, which was negative for standard genetic and acquired conditions. Presently, the patient symptomatically has some mild residual weakness in his right upper and lower extremities.

TABLE 1: Initial hematologic studies which indicate an unremarkable coagulopathic evaluation.

Initial hematologic labs	Reference range and units	Result
Hemoglobin	13.1–17.3 g/dl	15.0
Hematocrit	39–49%	44.4
Platelets	150–450 × 10^9/L	330
Heparin anti-xa unfractioned	0.30–0.70 IU/mL	0.36
Protime	9.5–12.6 sec	12.3
Inr	0.9–1.2	1.1
Anticardiolipin IgA	0–19.9 APL	0.5
Anticardiolipin IgM Ab	0–19.9 MPL	0.5
Anticardiolipin IgG	0–19.9 GPL	<1.6
Beta-2 gp1 IgA	0–19.9 u/mL	<0.6
Beta-2 gp1 IgM	0–19.9 u/mL	0.5
Beta-2 gp1 IgG	0–19.9 u/mL	<1.4
Homocysteine	5.90–16.00 mcmol/L	14.64
Collagen/ epinipherine	0–179 sec	112
Collagen/adp	0–114 sec	91
Heparin pf4 antibody (hit)	<0.4 OD	0.168
JAK2 exon 12 mutation detection	—	Negative. No pathogenic genetic alterations were detected in JAK2, exons 12–15.
Pnh by flow cytometry	—	No evidence of paroxysmal nocturnal hemoglobinuria detected by flow cytometry.
Factor V leiden R506Q gene mutation		Negative. The patient does not have the Factor V leiden mutation.
Prothrombin G20210A gene mutation		Negative. The patient does not have the prothrombin G20210A mutation.

3. Discussion

While there have been previous documented case reports that have highlighted an association between exogenous testosterone use and pulmonary embolus, we present a unique case in which our patient developed diffuse multi vessel arterial and venous thrombotic events [6]. During our patient's 43 day hospital course, we treated the patient for thrombotic events in his right radial artery, right iliac artery, superficial femoral artery, splenic artery, and a bilateral lower lobe pulmonary emboli. The patient did have several risk factors to develop a thrombotic event including obesity and a smoking history, however, the acuity and recurrence of thrombotic events in a short timeframe make these risk factors an unlikely sole contributor. The patient did have a 2 cm pleural-based right lung nodular density seen on imaging. Given the presence of multi organ failure during this patient's hospital admission, it was recommended by our hematology/oncology team that this be evaluated further as an outpatient. Given the negative hypercoagulable workup, we felt that the patient's clot burden was most likely associated with his recent exogenous testosterone use as he did not present with any other plausible risk factors.

Multiple studies have not established a clear relationship between thrombogenicity and exogenous testosterone use [7]. Thromboxane A_2 (TXA_2), a major arachidonic acid metabolite of platelets, acts through membrane surface receptors to aggregate platelets and constrict vascular smooth muscle. A study done by Ajayi, et al. demonstrated that testosterone increases platelet TXA_2 receptor density and aggregation responses in both in vitro and in vivo studies. Specifically, they found that testosterone treatment significantly increased the human platelet TXA_2 receptor density with a peak effect at 4 weeks and a return to baseline at 8 weeks [4]. Further, results show that the increase in platelet TXA_2 receptor density was significantly ($P < 0.001$) greater in the testosterone-treated group than in the placebo group or its own baseline. Given the timeframe that Ajayi, et al. [4] established between testosterone and peak effect of TXA_2 receptor, it would be reasonable to suspect that our patient's testosterone use for five weeks prior would have placed him at a greater propensity toward clot formation.

Testosterone has also been well documented in the literature to stimulate erythropoiesis. A study done by Bachman, et al. demonstrates that increases in hemoglobin and hematocrit are due to testosterone stimulating erythropoietin (EPO) and reducing ferritin and hepcidin concentrations. As a result, this recalibrates the set point of EPO in relation to hemoglobin and by increasing iron utilization for erythropoiesis [5]. The authors found that the testosterone plays two pivotal roles in increasing red cell mass. First, the testosterone inhibits BMP-Smad signaling in hepatocytes leading to suppression of hepcidin transcription [5]. Secondly, the testosterone stimulates renal secretion of EPO, stimulating erythropoiesis which could then further suppress hepcidin. This causes a cascade which subsequently upregulates the expression of GATA-1- and GATA-dependent genes, which could also increase EPO sensitivity and stimulate stress erythroposis [5]. Testosterone is then converted to estradiol and can regulate hepcidin transcription. In our patient, his serum ferritin level (12–300 ng/mL) was elevated to 668 ng/mL and his erythropoietin level (2.6–18.5 mIU/mL) was 104.4 mIU/mL which was drawn approximately two weeks later. A potential explanation for an elevated ferritin level seen in our patient as opposed to a decreased ferritin level as Bachman, et al. describes in their cascade is that the ferritin level was drawn early in the patient's hospital course. Therefore, the dualistic stimulation of the patient's platelets through the TXA_2 pathway and increased erythropoiesis likely explains this patient's arterial thrombi.

TABLE 2: Correlation between INR levels and Factor X and Factor II levels as a manifestation of an undescribed effect from exogenous testosterone use.

	Reference range and units	3/15/19	4/18/19
Protime	9.5–12.6 sec	18.9	37.4
Inr	0.9–1.2	1.6	3.2
Factor X activity	70–150% act	93	11
Factor II activity	79–131% act	63	29

In regards to the underlying mechanism for the patient's venous thromboembolism, it can certainly be explained by a provoked event related to the patient's ICU stay and sepsis. However, more interestingly, we propose that the patient's exogenous testosterone use may have had an undescribed effect on the activation of clotting factors. The patient was discharged on warfarin with an INR goal of 2.5–3.5, ticagrelor and baby aspirin but required an INR as high as 4.32 in order to achieve Factor II and Factor X suppression. Table 2 is a correlation between the INR levels and Factor II and Factor X levels. The decision to manage the patient initially with an INR of 2.5–3.5 was made because the patient's factor inhibition on warfarin within the INR range of 2.0–3.0 was not adequate in the less than 30% range, despite having a negative mixing study and lupus anticoagulant or antiphospholipid antibodies. Further, platelet mapping with thromboelastography (TEG) was of particular clinical benefit to assist us in guiding the choice of antiplatelet medications and efficacy. The TEG results with R-time of 12.2 min, K-time of 1.5 min and a-angle of 69.0 for our patient are shown, which showed sufficiency with decreasing clot burden while on ticagrelor.

While there is an inherent risk for vascular events due to testosterone use, this association needs to be further elucidated with additional studies [8]. With the rise of exogenous testosterone use for performance enhancing reasons, particularly those that are not approved by the FDA, our case report demonstrates such potential risks and consequences, especially since the purity of the injected androgenic substance also could not be verified. Vigilance for testosterone as a potential risk factor for thrombogenicity is essential in patients with an unclear etiology as this can contribute to improved outcome in patients.

References

[1] D. Sagoe, "Methods used in a meta-analysis and meta-regression analysis of the global epidemiology of anabolic-androgenic steroid use," *Annals of Epidemiology*, vol. 24, no. 5, pp. 383–398, 2014.

[2] H. G. Pope, R. I. Wood, A. Rogol, F. Nyberg, L. Bowers, and S. Bhasin, "Adverse health consequences of performance-enhancing drugs: an endocrine society scientific statement," *Endocrine Reviews*, vol. 35, no. 3, pp. 341–375, 2013.

[3] D. E. Houghton, M. Alsawas, P. Barrioneuvo et al., "Testosterone therapy and venous thromboembolism: a systematic review and meta-analysis," *Thrombosis Research*, vol. 172, pp. 94–103, 2018.

[4] A. A. L. Ajayi, R. Mathur, and P. V. Halushka, "Testosterone increases human platelet thromboxane A 2 receptor density and aggregation responses," *Circulation*, vol. 91, no. 11, pp. 2742–2747, 1995.

[5] E. Bachman, T. G. Travison, S. Basaria et al., "Testosterone induces erythrocytosis via increased erythropoietin and suppressed hepcidin: evidence for a new erythropoietin/hemoglobin set point," *The Journals of Gerontology Series A: Biological Sciences and Medical Sciences*, vol. 69, no. 6, pp. 725–735, 2014.

[6] S. M. Nguyen, N. K. Ko, A. S. Sattar, E. G. Ipek, and S. Ali, "Pulmonary embolism secondary to testosterone-enhancing herbal supplement use," *Cureus*, 2017.

[7] A. D. Seftel, "Re: association between testosterone replacement therapy and the incidence of deep vein thrombosis and pulmonary embolism: a retrospective cohort study of the veterans administration database," *Journal of Urology*, vol. 196, no. 6, pp. 1723–1723, 2016.

[8] C. Martinez, S. Suissa, S. Rietbrock et al., "Testosterone treatment and risk of venous thromboembolism: population based case-control study," *BMJ*, p. i5968, 2016.

17

Transient Complete Unilateral Oculomotor Nerve Palsy following Clipping of Ruptured Anterior Communicating Artery Aneurysm: An Abstruse Phenomenon

Joe M. Das[1] **Rashmi Sapkota**[2] **and Manish Mishra**[3]

[1] *Consultant Neurosurgeon, Department of Neurosurgery, College of Medical Sciences–Teaching Hospital, Bharatpur-10, Chitwan, Nepal*
[2] *Sister-in-Charge, Department of Neurosurgery, College of Medical Sciences–Teaching Hospital, Bharatpur-10, Chitwan, Nepal*
[3] *Medical Officer, Department of Neurosurgery, College of Medical Sciences–Teaching Hospital, Bharatpur-10, Chitwan, Nepal*

Correspondence should be addressed to Joe M. Das; drjoemdas@gmail.com

Academic Editor: Nilda Espinola-Zavaleta

Background. Aneurysmal subarachnoid hemorrhage may be associated with different cranial nerve palsies, with oculomotor nerve palsy (ONP) being the most common. ONP is especially associated with posterior communicating artery aneurysms, due to the anatomical proximity of the nerve to the aneurysmal wall. Anterior communicating artery (Acom) aneurysms are very unlikely to produce ONP due to the widely separated anatomical locations of Acom and oculomotor nerve. *Case Description.* Here we describe the case of a 60-year-old nondiabetic lady who presented with Acom aneurysmal subarachnoid hemorrhage having a World Federation of Neurosurgical Societies (WFNS) grade I. She underwent an uneventful right pterional craniotomy and clipping of the aneurysm, except for a short period of controlled rupture of the aneurysm. Postoperatively she developed complete ONP on the right side, though her sensorium was preserved. Computed Tomogram and Magnetic Resonance Imaging scans of the brain did not yield any useful information regarding its etiology. She was conservatively managed and kept on regular follow-up. She had a gradual recovery of ONP in the following order: pupillary reaction, ocular movements, and finally ptosis. On postoperative day 61, she had complete recovery from ONP. *Conclusion.* We describe a very unusual case of complete ONP following Acom aneurysm clipping and its management by masterly inactivity.

1. Introduction

"Perhaps the most important evidence of aneurysm is the sudden repeated sharp pains in the eye or in the frontal or temporal region, frequently followed by ptosis of the upper lid and extraocular palsies on the same side. These manifestations are almost pathognomonic of carotid or nearby aneurysms." (Dandy WE, 1944) [1].

This holds true even now. In any patient presenting with spontaneous painful oculomotor nerve palsy (ONP), intracranial aneurysm has to be suspected, especially that located in the posterior communicating, cavernous internal carotid, basilar, posterior cerebral, anterior choroidal, or superior cerebellar arteries [2]. In these situations, it is easy to explain the presence of ONP due to the close proximity of oculomotor nerve to the above-said aneurysms. The aneurysm, once it enlarges, can compress on the nerve producing pain and palsy. The other causes of ONP in patients with aneurysmal subarachnoid hemorrhage (aSAH) are transtentorial herniation, iatrogenic injury, or associated diabetes mellitus. We encountered a patient who developed a painful ophthalmoplegia, following surgical clipping of ruptured anterior communicating artery (Acom) aneurysm. Though rarely reported to produce both abducens and trochlear nerve palsies [3], Acom aneurysm is very unlikely to produce ONP (with only 11 such cases reported till date in the literature) due to the anatomically remote locations of the two structures.

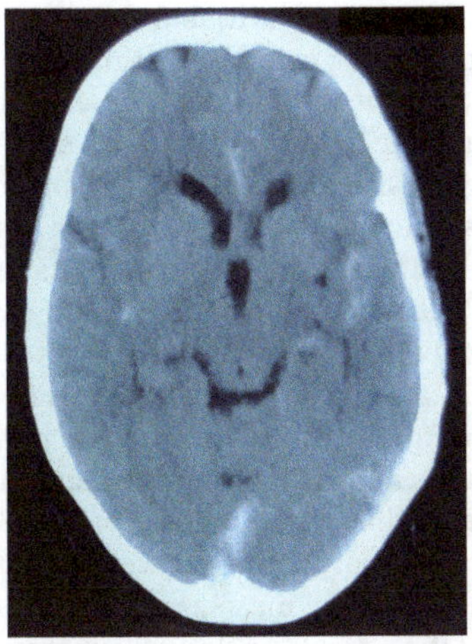

FIGURE 1: Preoperative plain Computed Tomogram scan of the brain showing subarachnoid hemorrhage.

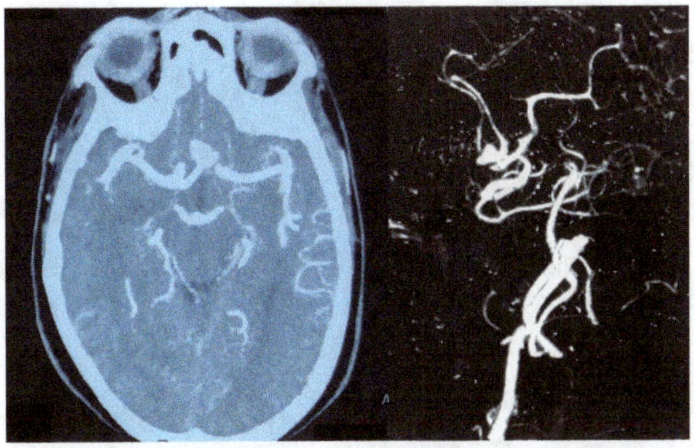

FIGURE 2: Computed Tomogram Angiography films showing the anterior communicating artery aneurysm.

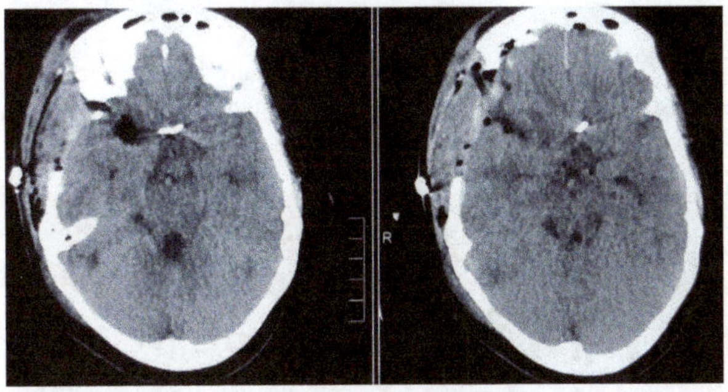

FIGURE 3: Postoperative plain Computed Tomogram scan of the brain showing the absence of hematoma or infarct.

2. Case Report

A 60-year-old lady, who was a hypertensive patient under irregular medication, presented with mild-to-moderately-severe headache episodes for four days for which she did not seek medical attention. This was followed by sudden onset severe headache for one day prior to presentation in our emergency room (ER). Headache was holocranial and associated with vomiting. There was no history of trauma, fever, seizures, weakness of limbs, or loss of consciousness. She was not a diabetic and did not have any addictions.

When she presented to our ER, her Glasgow Coma Scale score was 15 and did not have any neurological deficits (World Federation of Neurosurgical Societies grade I). She underwent plain Computed Tomogram (CT) scan of the brain, which showed subarachnoid hemorrhage (SAH) in the left sylvian fissure and interhemispheric fissure (Modified Fisher grade 1) (Figure 1). Suspecting an aneurysmal SAH, she was admitted in neurosurgery intensive care unit and was started on antiedema measures, anticonvulsant, analgesic, and Nimodipine.

The next day, she underwent CT cerebral angiogram, which revealed a bilobed anterior communicating artery aneurysm, projecting anterosuperiorly and measuring 8 × 7 × 5 mm in size (Figure 2). There was no evidence of any other aneurysms or vascular malformations. On the fourth day of ictus, she underwent right pterional craniotomy and clipping of aneurysm.

Intraoperatively, the sphenoid drilling and craniotomy were uneventful. After exposure of the aneurysm, there was controlled rupture during permanent clipping with a blood loss of around 20 ml and temporary clipping was not required. Papaverine was not instilled. Since the brain was slightly full at the end of surgery, the bone flap was not replaced. She was extubated postoperatively on table and was fully conscious.

Three hours after the surgery, she started developing right sided ptosis, which progressed into complete right sided oculomotor nerve paralysis with dilated and nonreacting pupil. An emergency CT scan of the brain was taken which revealed only postoperative changes (Figure 3). There was no hematoma in the basal cisterns or infarct. But her oculomotor nerve palsy persisted and was painful (Figure 4). Her further postoperative period was uneventful, pupillary reaction to light started to appear, and pain started to disappear by day 7. But pupillary size remained the same (Figure 5). She was discharged on the eighth postoperative day. On follow-up after one week, a Magnetic Resonance Imaging scan of the brain with venogram was done to rule out any infarct or thrombosis of the cavernous sinus. But it turned out to be normal. She was kept under regular follow-up in our outpatient department. Nimodipine was continued for a total of 21 days following the ictus. On review at the end of one month, her ocular movements were normal except for impaired adduction and pupils were normal in size and reaction, but complete ptosis was persisting. On the 61st postoperative day, her ptosis suddenly disappeared on waking up and when she came for follow-up in outpatient department, her ONP had fully recovered (Figure 6).

3. Discussion

Oculomotor nerve is the most common cranial nerve affected in patients with aneurysmal subarachnoid hemorrhage [11]. Depending on the series, 15% to 50% of oculomotor nerve palsies (ONP) are caused by an intracranial aneurysm [10]

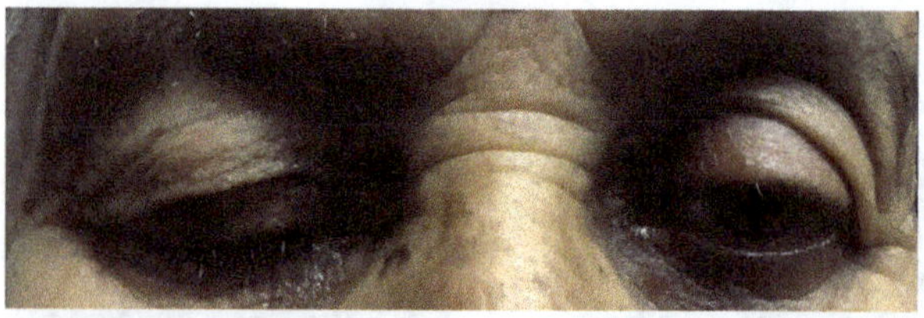

FIGURE 4: Photograph showing the right sided ptosis due to oculomotor nerve palsy.

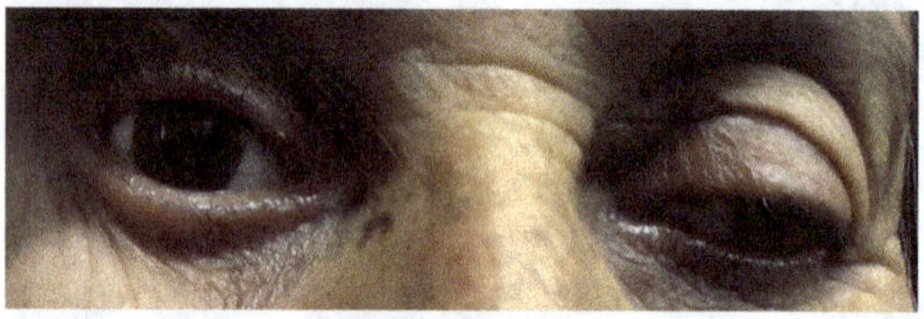

FIGURE 5: Photograph showing the manually lifted right eye lid demonstrating mydriasis and impaired adduction of right eye.

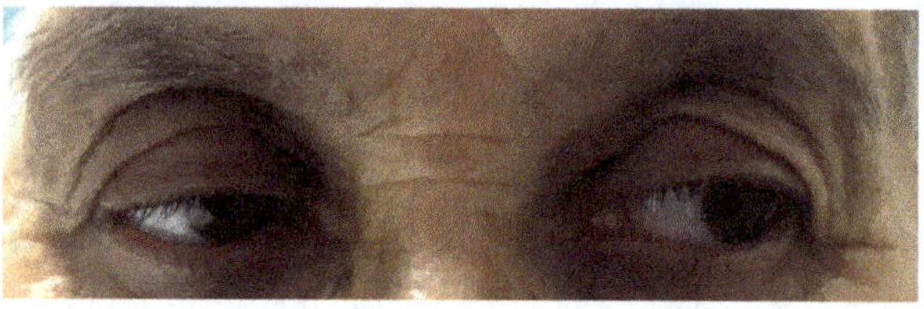

FIGURE 6: Photograph showing the resolved oculomotor palsy with full adduction of right eye.

and paresis of oculomotor nerve is associated with ruptured aneurysms in 30% of patients [12]. Aneurysmal ONP typically presents with pain, mid-dilated pupil with poor or absent light reaction, and complete or partial external paresis including ptosis with supra-, infra-, and adduction deficits [13].

Compressive lesions of oculomotor nerve usually affect both the central somatomotor fibers and the peripheral superomedial pupil fibers, while ischemic lesions spare the latter. This anatomy is the basis for the "rule of the pupil," which states that a complete motor third-nerve palsy (complete external paresis) with a normal pupil is most probably ischemic in origin and not compressive [14].

When the peripheral oculomotor nerve is involved by an aneurysm, usually the pupilloconstrictor fibers are involved first, followed by palsy of the levator palpebrae, superior rectus, and medial rectus, in order [8]. In general, after both surgery and coiling, functional recovery is usually noted first in the levator palpebrae muscle, followed by the medial rectus muscle, superior rectus muscle, constrictor muscles of the iris, and ciliary muscle. Patients with incomplete recovery often had residual diplopia in upward gaze and pupillary dysfunction [15].

But in our case, the patient had reversal of ptosis occurring last in the order of recovery. In a large study on the prognosis of ocular motor nerve palsies conducted by Richards BW et al., it was concluded that the mean recovery time from ONP was 5.4 months and the range was from less than one month to 48 months. The median tended to be earlier, about 2.6 months. As might be expected, the more benign the cause, the more rapid the recovery [16]. In a study on cranial nerve lesions following aSAH, oculomotor nerve lesions regressed in 39.2% of cases within a period of six months; the remaining lesions were permanent [11]. But our patient had a relatively early recovery in two months.

There are only 12 properly reported cases of ONP associated with Acom artery complex aneurysms in the literature till date, including our case (Table 1). The initial reports of this rare phenomenon date back to as early as 1974, when ocular motor disturbances occurring as false localizing signs in ruptured intracranial aneurysms were reported by Suzuki J and Iwabuchi T [3]. The mean age of the patients was 58.7 and majority of the patients, including our case, were females (5:1). Most of them had a Fisher grade of 3 and Glasgow Coma Scale score of 15 at the time of admission. Six patients were hypertensive. Only three patients had partial ONP, whereas all others had complete ONP. The right side oculomotor nerve was affected in five patients and left side in another five, and bilateral oculomotor nerves were paralyzed in two patients. Even though 10 patients had Acom aneurysm, one patient had A1 aneurysm [3] and another one had ACA-A2 aneurysm [9]. Two patients had some other vascular anomaly [3, 5] and one had developed a pontine infarct [8]. Though average number of days to recovery from ONP was slightly higher (98.1 days), the median duration was 60.5 days. Among the reported cases, fastest complete recovery occurred in 24 days.

The probable causes by which ONP can occur postoperatively following surgical clipping of an aneurysm are

(1) damage to the nerve during drilling of lesser wing of sphenoid [17];

(2) uncal herniation due to brain edema or hematoma;

(3) direct injury to the nerve or pressure effect;

(4) aneurysm clip accidentally incorporating or applying pressure over the nerve;

(5) the presence of an unrecognized aneurysm in the vicinity of third nerve, which was missed in angiogram;

(6) instillation of papaverine over the surrounding blood vessels, as a preventive attempt against vasospasm [18];

(7) development of cavernous sinus thrombosis;

(8) brainstem infarction or hemorrhage.

Our case is unique in that this is the only case in which ONP occurred postoperatively following clipping of a ruptured Acom aneurysm, without any evidence of cisternal clot and direct or indirect injury to the nerve by any of the mechanisms described above. The hypothetical explanations to the development of ONP in our patient are as follows:

(1) Direct injury to the nerve produced neurapraxia by the jet of blood during intraoperative rupture of aneurysm.

(2) As a part of cerebral vasospasm, which may have affected the vasa nervorum of oculomotor nerve. Ipsilateral

TABLE 1: Cases of oculomotor nerve palsy associated with subarachnoid hemorrhage from aneurysms at anterior communicating artery complex.

Sr No.	Author (Year)	Age/Sex*	Fisher grade	GCS†	Day of appearance	Complete/ Partial	Side affected	Aneurysm size and projection	Day of recovery	Comments	Possible explanation
1	Suzuki J et al. (1974) [3]	59 / F	NA‡	NA	0	Partial	Right	Right A1§ 15 × 10 × 10 mm	24	Megadolichobasilar anomaly	Raised ICP II / Vascular malformation
2	Suzuki J et al. (1974) [3]	48 / M	NA	15 (EVD)¶	2 (EVD)	Complete	Bilateral	3 mm (on autopsy)	Expired	None	Tentorial herniation
3	Coyne TJ et al. (1994) [4]	59 / F	3	14	0	Complete	Bilateral	NA	120	HTN#	Clot in cistern / raised ICP
4	Aiba et al. (2003) [5]	61 / F	3	15	0	Complete	Left	NA	30	Inverted left PCA and SCA**	Unusual anatomy
5	Aiba et al. (2003) [5]	70 / F	3	Confused Delirious	0	Complete	Right	NA	60	None	Clot in cistern / raised ICP
6	Satyarthee et al. (2004) [6]	65 / F	3	15	0	Complete	Right	NA	180	HTN	Medial temporal haematoma
7	White JB et al. (2007) [7]	46 / M	3	15	0	Complete	Left	10 mm × 9 mm × 7 mm	NA	HTN	Clot / blood products
8	Kang SD et al. (2007) [8]	68 / F	3	Semicomatose	0	Complete	Left	NA	Partial – 1 year	Lacunar infarct of pons	Clot, herniation / vasospasm
9	Fairbanks C et al. (2011) [9]	? / F	3	15	0	Partial	Left	Superiorly and anteriorly measured 1×2×1 mm	30	ACA-A2*** aneurysm HTN	Mass effect, hemotoxicity and ischemia
10	Balossier A et al. (2012) [10]	55 / F	3	15	1 (Emb) ****	Complete	Right	NA	90	HTN	interpeduncular cistern haematoma
11	Srinivasan A et al. (2015) [2]	55 / F	3	9	0	Partial	Left	Antero-superior	Partial - 21	HTN	Perfusion deficits, hemorrhagic dissection of the nerve
12	Our case	60 / F	2	15	2 (PO)*****	Complete	Right	Antero-superior 8 mm × 7 mm ×5 mm	61	HTN	Neurapraxia by jet of blood or vasospasm

* M: Male, F: Female; †: Glasgow Coma Scale score; ‡: details not available; §: A1 segment of anterior cerebral artery; II: intracranial pressure; ¶: following external ventricular drainage; #: systemic hypertension; ** PCA: posterior cerebral artery; SCA: superior cerebellar artery; ***ACA: anterior cerebral artery; A2: A2 segment of anterior cerebral artery; ****: following embolization; *****: postoperative.

periorbital pain, as occurred in this patient following ONP, stands more in favor of vasospasm, as it can involve the sensory ganglia located within the nerve. But our patient had a Modified Fisher grade 1, which is reported to cause vasospasm only in 21.6% of cases [19].

(3) A right posterior communicating artery aneurysm, which was not able to be diagnosed with CT angiogram and postoperative Magnetic Resonance Angiogram, is a very rare possibility. Digital Subtraction Angiogram could not be done due to economic constrains. But the spontaneous resolution of ONP and of the pain associated with it stands against such a possibility. Also the order of recovery of ONP also is against it, since in our patient ptosis was the last to resolve, whereas it is the first to resolve in aneurysmal ONP [14].

4. Conclusion

ONP can very rarely occur following aSAH, even from aneurysms located away from the oculomotor nerve. If there are no features of raised intracranial pressure, there is not much to panic. Usual natural history is one of gradual recovery over a period of time, usually within a year.

Acknowledgments

We would like to thank the Department of Radiodiagnosis for providing us with the angiogram images.

References

[1] W. E. Dandy, *Intracranial Arterial Aneurysms in The Carotid Canal*, Comstock, Ithaca, NY, USA, 1942.

[2] A. Srinivasan, S. Dhandapani, and A. Kumar, "Pupil sparing oculomotor nerve paresis after anterior communicating artery aneurysm rupture: False localizing sign or acute microvascular ischemia?" *Surgical Neurology International*, vol. 6, no. 1, p. 46, 2015.

[3] J. Suzuki and T. Iwabuchi, "Ocular motor disturbances occurring as false localizing signs in ruptured intracranial aneurysms," *Acta Neurochirurgica*, vol. 30, no. 1-2, pp. 119–128, 1974.

[4] T. J. Coyne and M. C. Wallace, "Bilateral third cranial nerve palsies in association with a ruptured anterior communicating artery aneurysm," *World Neurosurgery*, vol. 42, no. 1, pp. 52–56, 1994.

[5] T. Aiba and M. Fukuda, "Unilateral oculomotor nerve paresis associated with anterior communicating artery aneurysm rupture - two case reports," *Neurologia medico-chirurgica*, vol. 43, no. 10, pp. 484–487, 2003.

[6] G. D. Satyarthee and A. K. Mahapatra, "Unusual neuro-ophthalmic presentation of anterior communicating artery aneurysm with third nerve paresis," *Journal of Clinical Neuroscience*, vol. 11, no. 7, pp. 776–778, 2004.

[7] J. B. White, K. F. Layton, and H. J. Cloft, "Isolated third nerve palsy associated with a ruptured anterior communicating artery aneurysm," *Neurocritical Care*, vol. 7, no. 3, pp. 260–262, 2007.

[8] S. D. Kang, "Ruptured anterior communicating artery aneurysm causing bilateral oculomotor nerve palsy: a case report," *Journal of Korean Medical Science*, vol. 22, no. 1, pp. 173–176, 2007.

[9] C. Fairbanks and J. B. White, "Oculomotor nerve palsy in the setting of an anterior cerebral A2 segment aneurysm," *Journal of NeuroInterventional Surgery*, vol. 3, no. 1, pp. 74–76, 2011.

[10] A. Balossier, A. Postelnicu, S. Khouri, E. Emery, and J. M. Derlon, "Third nerve palsy induced by a ruptured anterior communicating artery aneurysm," *British Journal of Neurosurgery*, vol. 26, no. 5, pp. 770–772, 2012.

[11] A. Laun and J. C. Tonn, "Cranial nerve lesions following subarachnoid hemorrhage and aneurysm of the circle of willis," *Neurosurgical Review*, vol. 11, no. 2, pp. 137–141, 1988.

[12] J. Hamer, "Prognosis of oculomotor palsy in patients with aneurysms of the posterior communicating artery," *Acta Neurochirurgica*, vol. 66, no. 3-4, pp. 173–185, 1982.

[13] J. T. Kissel, R. M. Burde, T. G. Klingele, and H. E. Zeiger, "Pupil-sparing oculomotor palsies with internal carotid—posterior communicating artery aneurysms," *Annals of Neurology*, vol. 13, no. 2, pp. 149–154, 1983.

[14] J. Lemos and E. Eggenberger, "Neuro-Ophthalmological Emergencies," *The Neurohospitalist*, vol. 5, no. 4, pp. 223–233, 2015.

[15] M. C. Hanse, M. C. Gerrits, W. J. van Rooij, M. P. Houben, P. C. Nijssen, and M. Sluzewski, "Recovery of posterior communicating artery aneurysm-induced oculomotor palsy after coiling," *American Journal of Neuroradiology*, vol. 29, no. 5, pp. 988–990, 2008.

[16] B. W. Richards, F. R. Jones Jr, and B. R. Younge, "Causes and prognosis in 4,278 cases of paralysis of the oculomotor, trochlear, and abducens cranial nerves," *American Journal of Ophthalmology*, vol. 113, no. 5, pp. 489–496, 1992.

[17] S. Spektor, S. Dotan, and C. J. Mizrahi, "Safety of drilling for clinoidectomy and optic canal unroofing in anterior skull base surgery," *Acta Neurochirurgica*, vol. 155, no. 6, pp. 1017–1024, 2013.

[18] G. Menon, S. S. Baldawa, and S. Nair, "Transient oculomotor nerve palsy after topical administration of intracisternal papaverine," *Acta Neurochirurgica*, vol. 153, no. 6, pp. 1357-1358, 2011.

[19] J. A. Frontera, J. Claassen, J. M. Schmidt et al., "Prediction of symptomatic vasospasm after subarachnoid hemorrhage: The modified fisher scale," *Neurosurgery*, vol. 59, no. 1, pp. 21–26, 2006.

18

Laparoscopic Release for Median Arcuate Ligament Compression Syndrome Associated with a Celiac-Mesenteric Trunk

Shamir O. Cawich, Dave Harnanan, and Lemuel Pran

Department of Surgery, University of the West Indies, St. Augustine Campus, Trinidad and Tobago West Indies

Correspondence should be addressed to Shamir O. Cawich; socawich@hotmail.com

Academic Editor: Konstantinos A. Filis

The median arcuate ligament compression syndrome is a rare entity that occurs in 2 per 100,000 unselected individuals. We present a case where the median arcuate ligament compression syndrome was associated with an equally uncommon anatomic variation—a celiac-mesenteric trunk, which occurs in 0.42-2.7% of unselected individuals. We could find no prior report of a celiac-mesenteric trunk being associated with the median arcuate ligament compression syndrome. This report also adds to the literature to show that a laparoscopic approach to median arcuate ligament release is feasible.

1. Introduction

Compression of the celiac trunk (CT) by the median arcuate ligament (MAL) may produce symptoms such as postprandial abdominal pain, weight loss, nausea, and vomiting [1]. This symptom complex is known by several names including Harjola-Marable syndrome, Dunbar syndrome, celiac artery compression syndrome, and median arcuate ligament syndrome [2].

The symptoms can become quite distressing and may require operative division of the MAL. Most authors recommend that this should be achieved using an open approach because it requires dissection of the aorta and its ventral branches, from which bleeding can be catastrophic. However, there are increasing numbers of reports, suggesting that the laparoscopic approach is becoming increasingly accepted for this procedure [2–4]. We report our experience with laparoscopic MAL release in a patient with a rare anatomic anomaly—the celiac-mesenteric trunk—thus adding to the existing literature to show that a minimally invasive approach is feasible even in the case of anatomic anomalies.

2. Report of a Case

A 44-year-old woman with no comorbidities presented to our facility with abdominal pain. There was no history of trauma, viral illnesses, or COVID vaccinations within the preceding 8 weeks. She complained of a six-month history of incapacitating epigastric pain, nausea, and vomiting that occurred within minutes of her meals. The symptoms were so severe that she developed anxiety before meals. In addition, she experienced unintentional loss of 25 pounds.

Persistent symptoms prompted computer tomographic mesenteric angiography. This revealed a variant celiac-mesenteric trunk (CMT) with evidence of celiac trunk/SMA compression and intraluminal thrombus in the SMA (Figure 1). Investigations did not reveal any other causes of thrombosis, including negative COVID swabs, normal blood coagulation studies, normal echocardiogram, and normal thoraco-aortograms.

Since this patient presented relatively late to the surgical team, it was thought that embolectomy would be difficult as we expected that the thrombus would be solidified. In addition, she had tolerated the luminal thrombus for six months without developing frank bowel necrosis. Therefore, a decision was made to commence therapeutic anticoagulation. Despite anticoagulation for four weeks, her symptoms persisted and prompted repeat angiography at six weeks. At this point, the thrombus was no longer present, but there was now perijejunal fat stranding, oral contrast hold-up, and mural thickening, suggestive of an ischemic jejunal stricture.

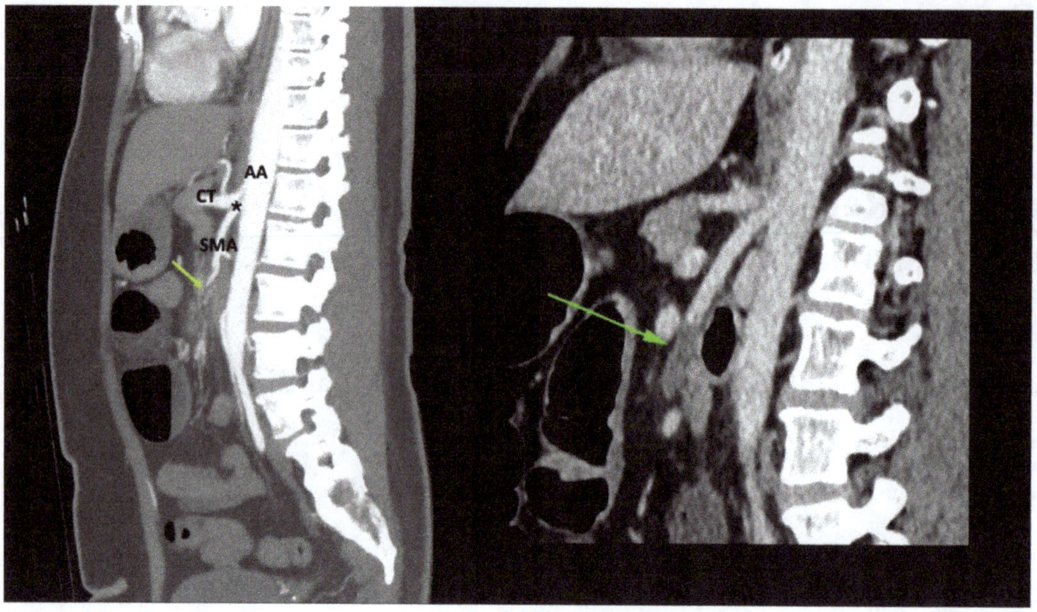

Figure 1: Sagittal view of a CT mesenteric angiogram showing a short celiac-mesenteric trunk (asterisk) arising from the abdominal aorta. The trunk further branches into the celiac trunk (CT) and superior mesenteric artery (SMA). Inset: an intraluminal thrombus can be seen within the SMA appearing as a filling defect (green arrow) and causing flow cessation in the lumen.

A Doppler ultrasound was performed, and this revealed cyclic angulation and compression of the celiac trunk on forced expiration, with expiratory dilatation (Figure 2). A maximum expiratory peak systolic velocity of 374 cm/sec was recorded within the celiac axis and secured our diagnosis of MAL syndrome.

This patient was offered a laparoscopic release of the MAL with resection of the jejunal stricture and primary anastomosis. The patient was prepared for anaesthesia, and a 12 mmHg pneumoperitoneum was created. The operation commenced by interrupting the hepato-gastric ligament to enter the lesser sac. The left gastric artery was identified and traced retrograde to the CMT trunk (Figure 3).

We carefully and patiently dissected at the superior aspect of the CMT using blunt instruments in order to avoid arterial injury. For this, we used combinations of a peanut gauze swab and a 5 mm LigaSure™ Maryland dissector (Medtronic, Minneapolis, USA), taking care to remain in the avascular adventitial plane. This allowed us to expose the ventral part of the aorta. Once the CMT and the aorta were clearly identified and separated from the MAL, the release was performed using the LigaSure TM (Medtronic, Minneapolis, USA). An immediate and audible release resulted from MAL division. The MAL was divided until the ventral surface of the aorta was exposed for 5-6 cm (Figure 4).

The jejunal stricture was then identified and resected, with primary intracorporeal anastomosis. In order to confirm viability and perfusion of the anastomotic ends, we used fluorescence angiography with intravenous indocyanine green (Figure 5). Once mesenteric flow and viability of the resected bowel ends were confirmed, a primary stapled anastomosis was completed and the specimen removed. The operation was completed in 120 minutes without a recorded complication.

Eight months after her operation, there has been complete resolution of symptoms and thirty-one pounds of weight gain. A follow-up CT scan revealed complete resolution of the thrombus (Figure 6) and resolution of intra-abdominal findings, such as fat stranding and mural thickening.

3. Discussion

The patient in this report had a CMT—an anatomic variation first described by Lipshutz [5]. He coined the term "*truncus celiaco-mesenterica*" to describe 2 cadavers with a variant where the SMA and CT took a common origin from the aorta. Published data suggest that the CMT occurs in 0.42% [6] to 2.7% [7] of unselected persons across the globe. In the Caribbean population, it occurs in 0.45% of autopsies [8] and is commoner in males. According to the classification proposed by Wang et al. [9], this was a short trunk (<15 mm from aortic origin), type I variant (all 3 coeliac trunk branches having a common origin with superior mesenteric artery). The anatomic variant detected here is uncommon and has only been reported in association with the MAL syndrome in one prior report by Chaiwatcharayut et al. [10].

In traditional anatomic descriptions, the aorta passes behind the MAL of the diaphragm into the abdomen at the twelfth thoracic vertebral level [5]. Approximately 1 cm distal to the MAL, the celiac trunk arises as the first ventral branch of the abdominal aorta [5]. However, in approximately 10-20% of persons, the MAL is located caudally and compresses the celiac artery and adjacent sympathetic ganglia [5, 11, 12]. The clinical syndrome was first described in 1963 by Harjola, a Finnish surgeon who also described the first recorded MAL release [11]. Later in 1965, Dunbar et al.

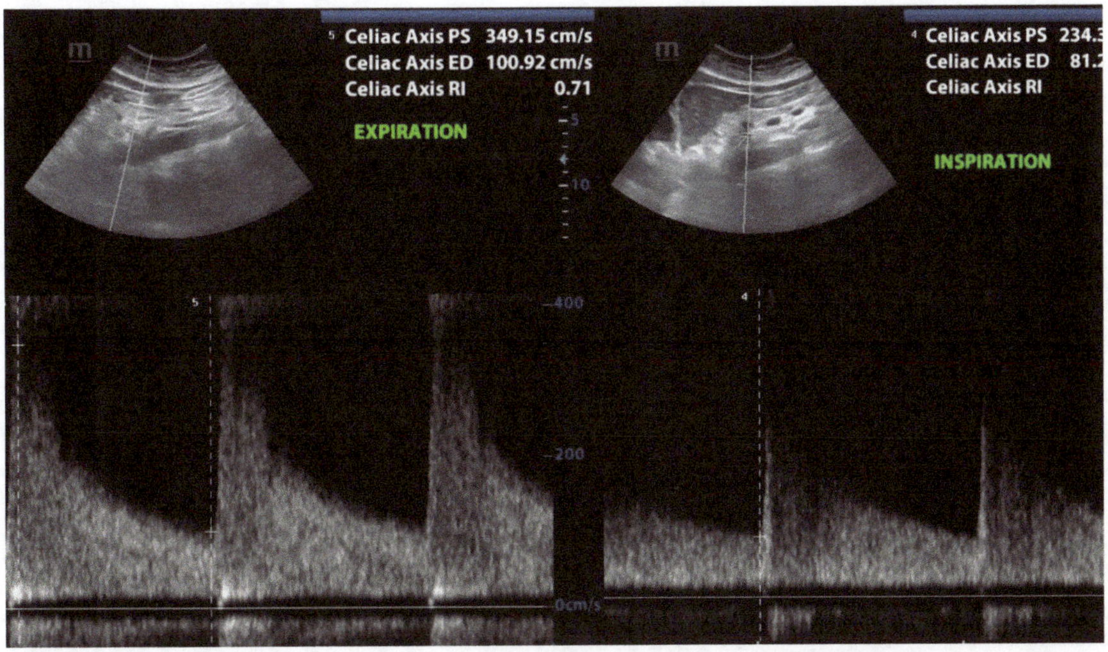

FIGURE 2: Duplex Doppler ultrasound images demonstrating narrowing of the CMT during forced expiration and dilation in the inspiratory phase. A maximum expiratory peak systolic velocity of 374 cm/sec was recorded within the coeliac axis.

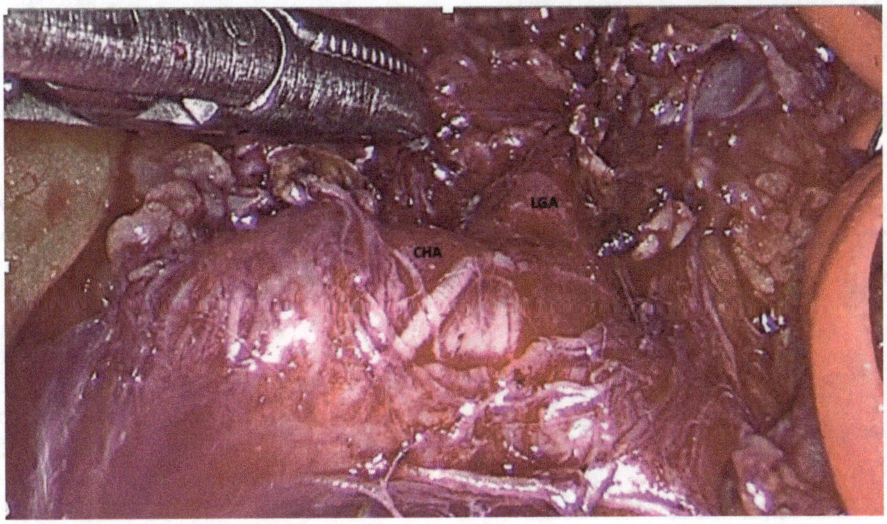

FIGURE 3: Intraoperative view showing that the left gastric artery (LGA) and common hepatic artery (CHA) have been dissected. The vessel will be encircled with loops and followed retrograde to the celiaco-mesenteric trunk.

[12], radiologists, published a series of 15 cases. Both names have been eponymously attached to this syndrome.

The MAL syndrome is also a rare phenomenon in which the celiac trunk is compressed as it passes behind the diaphragm [1]. It is reported to occur in 2 per 100,000 persons and is approximately four times more common in women, especially those between the ages of 30 and 50 years of age [13]. While most persons with a CMT are asymptomatic [7, 8], we can only surmise that the presence of a CMT may have predisposed this patient to the MAL syndrome. There has only been one prior report of this association between the CMT and MAL syndrome described previously in the medical literature [10].

There is controversy about the pathophysiology producing this syndrome. One theory is that compression becomes more marked as the diaphragm is depressed during inspiration, producing ischaemia in the organs supplied by branches of the celiac trunk [1]. An alternative theory is that compression of the sympathetic ganglion in the celiac trunk produces neuropathic pain [1, 13] and hyperstimulation of the celiac ganglion produces splanchnic vasoconstriction [1, 13]. The prevailing theory is that both mechanisms may be involved to produce the characteristic triad of vomiting, postprandial pain, and weight loss [1, 3].

Because the symptoms are nonspecific and pathophysiology is poorly understood, there has been no consensus

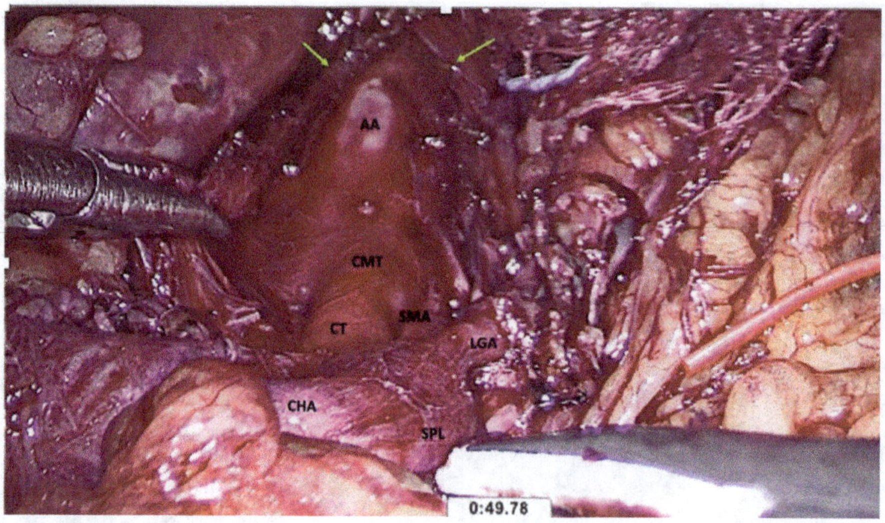

FIGURE 4: Completed dissection reveals a 5 cm segment of the ventral abdominal aorta (AA). The short celiaco-mesenteric trunk (CMT) can be seen branching into the superior mesenteric artery (SMA) and celiac trunk (CT). The three branches of the celiac trunk can be traced: common hepatic artery (CHA), splenic artery (SPL), and left gastric artery (LGA). The fibers of the divided median arcuate ligament are also visible (arrows).

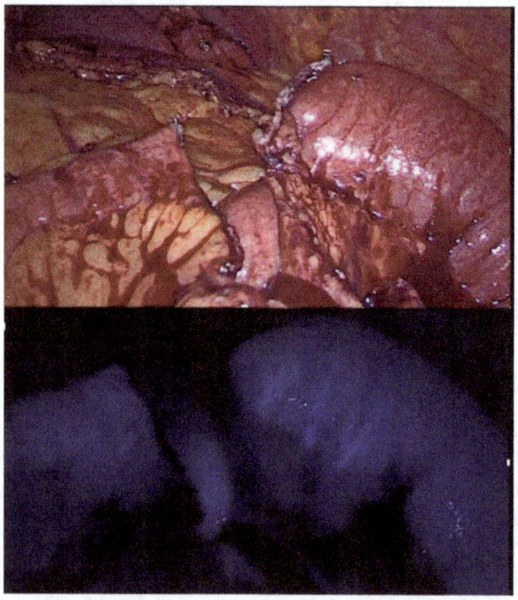

FIGURE 5: Intraoperative view of the laparoscopic feed. The strictured jejunal segment has been resected using an endo-GIA stapler (a). In order to confirm perfusion of the jejunal ends, ICG has been injected intravenously (b), and perfusion was confirmed.

on the criteria for diagnosis. Therefore, the diagnosis is largely made by excluding alternative diagnosis that may explain the patient's symptoms [2, 3, 14]. Often, a Doppler ultrasound is the initial diagnostic test. This may demonstrate the stenotic vessel and dynamic flow variations [3]. It is a readily available, inexpensive investigation that avoids exposure to radiation [3, 14].

The point of compression can be identified by digital subtraction angiography, computer tomographic angiography, or magnetic resonance angiography [4, 15]. CT/MR offers the advantage of being noninvasive, able to identify concurrent intra-abdominal pathology and exclude differential diagnoses. In our case, CT angiography and DSA were performed and supported the diagnosis. The features on angiography that most authors consider diagnostic are (1) demonstrating the area of compression, (2) cephalad movement of the celiac axis during inspiration, and (3) poststenotic dilation upon expiration [16, 17]. All three features were present in our case.

Once the diagnosis is made, operative decompression is required. This involves division of the MAL and dissection of periaortic tissues to interrupt neural tissue that may be responsible for neuropathic pain [14]. This operation was traditionally performed using the open approach because the dissection required exposure of the abdominal aorta and the celiac trunk, with the potential for catastrophic bleeding in the event of an injury. However, in the past decade, there have been increasing reports of laparoscopic celiac decompression [14].

The benefits of a laparoscopic approach are similar to those for other major open operations and include reduced postoperative pain, wound complications, respiratory sequelae, gastrointestinal disfunction, and hospitalization [1]. We acknowledge the concern that catastrophic bleeding may occur if there is iatrogenic injury to the aorta during dissection. However, we found that the periarterial adventitial plane provided an avascular plane for dissection. Therefore, we advocate patient dissection with blunt instruments and care to stay in the adventitial plane. We found the use of a laparoscopic peanut gauze and the LigaSure™ Maryland dissector useful to expose the correct dissection plane.

Operative decompression of the MAL is considered to be the gold standard treatment. The largest contemporary series reported that 75% of patients remained symptom-free after MAL release with mean follow-up of nine years [17]. Endovascular techniques such as angioplasty and stenting have been attempted, but they have been largely

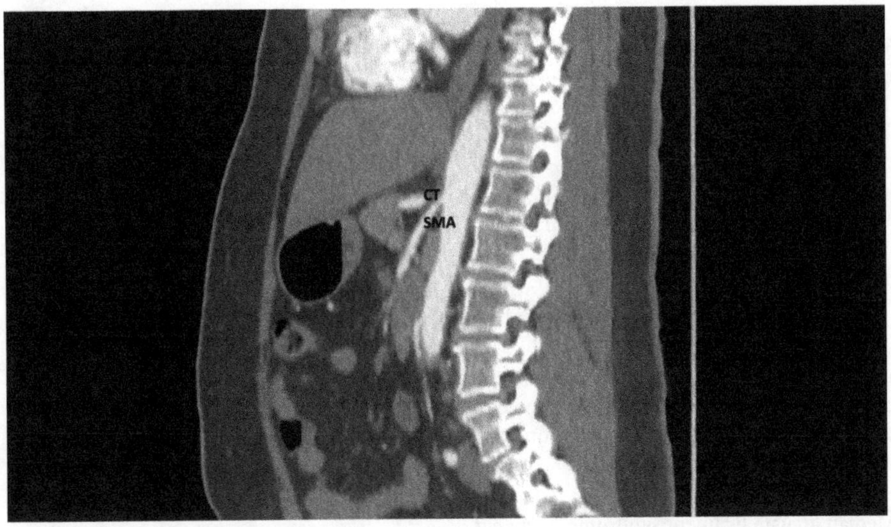

Figure 6: Follow-up CT scan at 8 months showing resolution of the thrombus in the superior mesenteric artery.

ineffective as a therapeutic maneuver as they do not effectively address the extrinsic compression of the celiac trunk [3, 14, 16].

In order to confirm complete decompression, intraoperative Doppler assessment and/or angiography may be considered. In our case, we used fluorescence angiography with intravenous indocyanine green to confirm mesenteric perfusion and small bowel viability. Fluorescence angiography with intravenous indocyanine green is a relatively new technique that allows the surgeon to evaluate perfusion in transected viscera in real time. Recently, it has gained application in laparoscopic colorectal and foregut surgery as well as bariatric procedures to reduce the incidence of anastomotic leaks. We have not encountered reports of this application in patients with MAL syndrome and suggest that it may be useful as an alternative to intraoperative Doppler evaluation. In the event of persistent stenosis after decompression, the other therapeutic options are aorto-celiac bypass or celiac artery angioplasty [1].

4. Conclusion

Although there are increasing reports of the MAL syndrome in medical literature, this case was unique because it is the second recorded case in which there has been an association between the presence of a celiac-mesenteric trunk, an uncommon anatomic anomaly. It is likely that the anatomic anomaly in this patient contributed to the symptomatology from the MAL syndrome.

In addition to noting this association, we also add to the literature by suggesting that fluorescence angiography with intravenous indocyanine green may be used to confirm mesenteric perfusion following operative decompression. Finally, we also add to the growing body of literature that a laparoscopic approach is feasible for MAL decompression.

References

[1] M. Kotarać, N. Radovanović, N. Lekić et al., "Surgical treatment of median arcuate ligament syndrome: case report and review of literature," *Srpski Arhiv za Celokupno Lekarstvo*, vol. 143, no. 1-2, pp. 74–78, 2015.

[2] M. Rubinkiewicz, P. K. Ramakrishnan, B. M. Henry, J. Roy, and A. Budzynski, "Laparoscopic decompression as treatment for median arcuate ligament syndrome," *Annals of the Royal College of Surgeons of England*, vol. 97, no. 6, pp. e96–e99, 2015.

[3] P. Baccari, E. Civilini, L. Dordoni, G. Melissano, R. Nicoletti, and R. Chiesa, "Celiac artery compression syndrome managed by laparoscopy," *Journal of Vascular Surgery*, vol. 50, no. 1, pp. 134–139, 2009.

[4] Z. Sun, D. Zhang, G. Xu, and N. Zhang, "Laparoscopic treatment of median arcuate ligament syndrome," *Intractable & Rare Diseases Research*, vol. 8, no. 2, pp. 108–112, 2019.

[5] B. Lipshutz, "A composite study of the celiac axis artery," *Annals of Surgery*, vol. 65, no. 2, pp. 159–169, 1917.

[6] N. Ognjanović, D. Jeremić, I. Živanović-Mačužić et al., "MDCT angiography of anatomical variations of the celiac trunk and superior mesenteric artery," *Archives of Biological Sciences*, vol. 66, no. 1, pp. 233–240, 2014.

[7] S. Y. Song, J. W. Chung, Y. H. Yin et al., "Celiac axis and common hepatic artery variations in 5002 patients: systematic analysis with spiral CT and DSA," *Radiology*, vol. 255, no. 1, pp. 278–288, 2010.

[8] M. T. Gardner, S. O. Cawich, M. T. Gardner et al., "Rare anatomic variant: celiac-mesenteric trunk in an Afro-Caribbean population," *National Journal of Clinical Anatomy*, vol. 10, no. 3, p. 112, 2021.

[9] Y. Wang, C. Cheng, L. Wang, R. Li, J. H. Chen, and S. G. Gong, "Anatomical variations in the origins of the celiac axis and the superior mesenteric artery: MDCT angiographic findings and their probable embryological mechanisms," *European Radiology*, vol. 24, no. 8, pp. 1777–1784, 2014.

[10] P. T. Harjola, "A rare obstruction of the celiac artery," *Annales Chirurgiae et Gynaecologiae*, vol. 52, pp. 547–550, 1963.

[11] W. Chaiwatcharayut, A. Lekah, and A. Kurklinsky, "Celiacomesenteric trunk as a cause of median arcuate ligament syndrome," *Journal of Medical Ultrasound*, vol. 21, no. 1, pp. 39–42, 2013.

[12] J. D. Dunbar, W. Molnar, F. F. Beman, and S. A. Marable, "Compression of the celiac trunk and abdominal angina,"

The American Journal of Roentgenology, Radium Therapy, and Nuclear Medicine, vol. 95, no. 3, pp. 731–744, 1965.

[13] E. N. Kim, K. Lamb, D. Relles, N. Moudgill, P. J. DiMuzio, and J. A. Eisenberg, "Median arcuate ligament syndrome-review of this rare disease," *JAMA Surgery*, vol. 151, no. 5, pp. 471–477, 2016.

[14] R. Goodall, B. Langridge, S. Onida, M. Ellis, T. Lane, and A. H. Davies, "Median arcuate ligament syndrome," *Journal of Vascular Surgery*, vol. 71, no. 6, pp. 2170–2176, 2020.

[15] K. M. Horton, M. A. Talamini, and E. K. Fishman, "Median arcuate ligament syndrome: evaluation with CT angiography," *Radiographics*, vol. 25, no. 5, pp. 1177–1182, 2005.

[16] M. Chaum, D. Shouhed, S. Kim, A. E. Walts, and A. M. Marchevsky, "Clinico-pathologic findings in patients with median arcuate ligament syndrome (celiac artery compression syndrome)," *Annals of Diagnostic Pathology*, vol. 52, article 151732, 2021.

[17] A. A. Duncan, "Median arcuate ligament syndrome," *Current Treatment Options in Cardiovascular Medicine*, vol. 10, no. 2, pp. 112–116, 2008.

Superior Mesenteric Artery Syndrome: A Community Hospital Case Series

Brian Welch,[1] Alex Schaal,[1] Thomas F. O'Shea,[2] and Roberto Cantu[1]

[1]*Flushing Hospital Medical Center, 4500 Parsons Blvd., Flushing, NY 11355, USA*
[2]*Boston University School of Medicine, 72 E Concord St., Boston, MA 02118, USA*

Correspondence should be addressed to Alex Schaal; aschaal.fhmc@jhmc.org

Academic Editor: Nilda Espinola-Zavaleta

Superior mesenteric artery syndrome is an obstruction of the small bowel between the aorta and the superior mesenteric artery. Patients with this disease are initially managed medically and those patients who fail medical treatment require surgery. A retrospective case series of thirteen patients diagnosed with SMAS at Flushing Hospital, Flushing, NY, from 2011 to 2020 was performed. Descriptive statistics were used to summarize the characteristics of the entire cohort, and comparative statistics were used to compare the patients who failed medical treatment and required surgery to those who were successfully managed medically. Nine patients were managed conservatively and four patients required operative intervention. BMI was significantly lower in patients requiring operation compared to those who were successfully managed medically. This retrospective community hospital case series adds to the literature on SMAS and provides evidence of BMI as a potential predictor of requiring surgery in SMAS.

1. Introduction

Superior mesenteric artery syndrome (SMAS) is a rare gastrointestinal disorder that results from the compression of the third part of the duodenum between the angle of the aorta and superior mesenteric artery (SMA) [1]. SMAS was originally identified in 1842 by Carl von Rokitansky, and later extensively described in a comprehensive case series by David Wilkie in 1927, leading to the name "Wilkie's syndrome" [2, 3]. The normal SMA-aorta angle is from 38 to 65°, with an aortomesenteric distance (AMD) of 10-28 mm [4]. Narrowing of the angle to less than 25° with a distance less than 10 mm can cause compression of the third part of the duodenum and may cause obstructive symptoms [5, 6]. This narrowing of the SMA-aorta angle has been correlated with decreasing BMI, believed to be due to a decrease in size of the mesenteric fat pad [7]. As such, SMAS has been associated with patients that have experienced substantial weight loss, such as those with eating disorders, malignancy, AIDS, recent gastric bypass surgery, and malabsorption syndromes [8–12]. Clinically, SMAS presents with acute symptoms of postprandial epigastric abdominal pain, nausea, vomiting, fullness, and acid reflux with electrolyte imbalance [1, 2]. These symptoms overlap with many other upper GI pathologies, and therefore, SMAS is often a diagnosis of exclusion that is coupled with imaging studies to confirm the narrowing of the SMA-aorta angle [13]. SMAS is incredibly rare, with an estimated incidence of 0.013%-0.03% and therefore is often low on many clinician's differential diagnosis for these common constellation of symptoms leading to a delay in necessary treatment [14, 15]. Although this disease is often initially treated conservatively, surgical management may be warranted via a duodenojejunostomy or a Ligament of Treitz release procedure (Strong procedure) if conservative management fails to resolve symptoms [16, 17]. This case series is aimed at describing the characteristics of our patients and our surgical experience with this disease in a community hospital setting in order to add to the body of knowledge about this pathology and help identify characteristics of patients that fail conservative management.

2. Methods

A retrospective case series of thirteen patients diagnosed with SMAS at Flushing Hospital, Flushing, NY, from 2011 to 2020 was performed. Patient data including BMI, symptoms type/duration, associated comorbidities, SMA angle, AMD, and patient management were reviewed via our EPIC database. For the purpose of this study, patients were split into two groups: those who were managed conservatively and those who underwent either duodenojejunostomy or Strong procedure after failing conservative management. Conservative management protocols included left lateral decubitus position or knee-chest positioning, Hayes maneuver, multiple small feedings, passing of nasoenteric tube past the point of the obstruction, and intravenous fluid resuscitation. Descriptive statistics were used to summarize the data for the entire cohort; results are reported as medians and interquartile ranges or means and standard deviations, as appropriate. Categorical variables were represented as counts with percentages. Comparative statistics were used to examine differences between the conservative and operative treatment groups with unpaired two-tailed t-tests used to compare continuous variables and chi-square tests used to compare categorical variables.

3. Results

3.1. Demographics and Characteristics of Patients. Thirteen total patients diagnosed with SMAS were included in this study. The demographic and characteristic information for the entire cohort is shown in Table 1. The median age (IQR) at diagnosis for this cohort was 29 (24-43) years. Four patients were male, and nine were female. Median duration of symptoms (IQR) was 4 (2-180) days. The mean SMA-aorta angle was 23.75 (±10.0) degrees, the mean (±SD) AMD was 5.4 (±1.9) mm, and the mean (±SD) BMI was 21.7 (±3.1) kg/m^2. Nine were managed conservatively (69.9%) and four patients required operative intervention (30.1%, three duodeno-jejunostomies 75% and one Strong's procedure 25%). The demographic and characteristic information for each of the two treatment modalities, along with comparative statistics, are shown in Table 2. The mean (±SD) BMI of those patients who failed conservative management and required surgery was significantly lower than those that were successfully managed with conservative therapy (18.9 ± 2.6 vs. 23.2 ± 2.3, $P = 0.02$). There was no significant difference between the two patient groups in sex, age at diagnosis, symptoms duration until diagnosis, SMA-aorta angle, and AMD.

3.2. Clinical Courses. The decision of which procedure to perform on the patients who failed conservative management was largely based on surgeon preference. Of note, the patient who underwent Strong's procedure had a diagnosis with Marfan's syndrome (with concurrent aortic root dilatation, severe pectus excavatum, scoliosis, and vitreous degeneration). Follow-ups were obtained from all patients. Of those operated on, 1 patient who had a duodenojejunostomy continued to have several emergency department visits (eleven times since surgery) for epigastric pain and emesis, once requiring a cholecystectomy. Several interval abdominal CT scans failed to yield a diagnosis. Eventually, she underwent an EGD which revealed duodenitis and gastritis, was treated conservatively, and has since been lost to follow up. Another patient who received a duodenojejunostomy was asymptomatic until 4 years postop when she presented with a small bowel obstruction which was treated conservatively. The other two surgically managed patients have had no issues since surgery. Of those treated conservatively, seven of them were either asymptomatic after initial management or lost to follow-up. One patient had persistently worsening reflux symptoms and was treated conservatively. One patient had undergone laparoscopic jejuno-jejunum reduction for intussusception prior to diagnosis of SMAS which was managed conservatively. She has since had two ED visits for epigastric pain/emesis—neither time surgery was consulted nor has she followed up with a general surgeon.

Table 1: Characteristics of patients with SMAS.

Characteristic	Patients ($N = 13$)
Patient age at diagnosis (years), median (IQR)	29 (24-43)
Patient sex, N (%)	
(i) Male	4 (30.1%)
(ii) Female	9 (69.9%)
Symptoms duration (days), median (IQR)	4 (2-180)
BMI, mean (SD)	21.7 (3.1)
SMA-aorta angle (degrees), mean (SD)	23.8 (10.0)
Aortic mesenteric distance (millimeter), mean (SD)	5.4 (1.9)
Treatment, N (%)	
(i) Conservative treatment	9 (69.9%)
(ii) Operative treatment	4 (30.1%)
(1) Duodenojejunostomy	3 (75%)
(2) Strong procedure	1 (25%)

4. Discussion

SMAS is a rare condition that is well described in the literature; however, it is often misdiagnosed resulting in delay of appropriate treatment [14, 15]. This retrospective community hospital case series describes thirteen patients with imaging confirmed diagnoses of SMAS with symptomatic presentations that were treated with either conservatively or operatively. This series is aimed at adding to the literature on SMAS, specifically in the community hospital setting, aiding in syndrome's accurate diagnosis, and providing insight into potential characteristics of patients that fail conservative management.

Radiological criteria used in the diagnosis of patients with SMAS include dilatation of the first and second parts of the duodenum, sudden vertical compression of the mucosal fold, flow of the barium against the peristaltic flow in the area proximal to the obstruction, delay of 4-6 hours in the gastroduodenal region, or relief of the obstruction when the patient was repositioned in the left lateral decubitus/knee-chest positions [13, 17]. The most sensitive finding for SMAS on imaging, however, is a SMA-aorta angle of <25 degrees with an AMD of <8 mm [4, 5]. In our cohort,

TABLE 2: Characteristics of conservatively treated vs. operatively treated patients.

Characteristics	Conservative Tx ($N = 9$)	Operative Tx ($N = 4$)	P value
Patient sex, N (%)			
(i) Male	4 (44.4%)	0 (0.0%)	0.11
(ii) Female	5 (66.6%)	4 (100%)	
Patient age at diagnosis (years), mean (SD)	31.4 (12.9)	33.25 (20.7)	0.85
Symptom duration until diagnosis (days), mean (SD)	274.89 (594.17)	185.25 (363.17)	0.78
BMI, mean (SD)	23.2 (2.3)	18.9 (2.6)	**0.02**
SMA-aorta angle (degrees), mean (SD)	(32.1-35)	34 (32.6-34.5)	0.97
Aortic mesenteric distance (mm), mean (SD)	5.7 (2.0)	4.8 (1.5)	0.43

the mean SMA-aorta angle was 23.75 (±10.0) degrees, and the mean (±SD) AMD was 5.4 (±1.9) mm in patients presenting with symptoms of SMAS (Table 1) matching the recommended diagnostic guidelines. However, there were still three patients who presented symptomatically with SMA – aorta angles > 25 degrees; therefore, our data suggest that SMA-aorta angle is not a completely sensitive test for SMAS, and it should still be considered as a potential cause of obstructive symptoms even in the presence of a larger SMA-aorta angle with a less than 8 mm AMD.

Our cohort had a median age at diagnosis of 29 with IQR 24-43, and more female patients were diagnosed than male patients. Our patients exhibited a wide range of symptom duration before diagnosis of SMAS, with some experiencing symptoms for as long as 5 years and some as little as 2 days before diagnosis. Most common symptoms reported were epigastric pain, nausea, vomiting, and fullness. There was no significant difference in the duration of symptoms before diagnosis between patients that were managed conservatively compared to those with surgery.

Management of SMAS can vary depending on the severity of the symptoms. A nonoperative approach is typically the first line of treatment [16]. The three most common operative treatments are gastrojejunostomy, duodenojejunostomy, and Strong's operation (mobilization of the right colon then sectioning of the ligament of Treitz with mobilization of the transverse and ascending duodenum) [13]. Nine of our patients were successfully managed with strategies including left lateral decubitus position or knee-chest positioning, Hayes maneuver, multiple small feedings, passing of nasoenteric tube past the point of the obstruction, and intravenous fluid resuscitation. Four of our patients failed this conservative management regiment and required operative intervention. The BMI of the patients who failed conservative treatment was found to be significantly lower than those that were managed successfully with conservative treatment. In this cohort, there was no other significant differences between the treatment groups. This finding is consistent with previous data that demonstrate a correlation between decreased BMI and decreased SMA aorta angle [7]. This suggests a role for BMI as a predictor of which patients will require surgical management; however, due to the low power nature of this case series, further larger scale studies are warranted. But given the rarity of this disease, it may be hard to establish.

There are several limitations of this study. First, this case series has a very low sample size of 13 patients. Part of this is inherent in studying SMAS due to its low incidence; thus, multicenter studies should be conducted to provide further significant data. Second, our postdiagnosis data is underwhelming due to many patients in both treatment cohorts who were lost to follow-up; however, the patients that were managed conservatively and surgically seemed to have unique posttreatment complications and courses. Finally, it is important to note that the decision to perform surgery, and which specific operation was performed, was at the preference of the attending surgeons.

SMAS is a disease that requires consideration for any patient with obstructive GI symptoms, especially ones with lower BMI or other predisposing conditions. This retrospective community hospital case series adds to the literature on SMAS, specifically in the community hospital setting, and provides evidence of BMI as a potential predictor for failure of conservative management that requires further investigation.

References

[1] M. T. Mandarry, L. Zhao, C. Zhang, and Z. Q. Wei, "A comprehensive review of superior mesenteric artery syndrome," *European Surgery*, vol. 42, no. 5, pp. 229–236, 2010.

[2] T. Welsch, M. W. Büchler, and P. Kienle, "Recalling superior mesenteric artery syndrome," *Digestive Surgery*, vol. 24, no. 3, pp. 149–156, 2007, Epub 2007 Apr 27.

[3] D. P. D. Wilkie, "Chronic duodenal ileus," *The American Journal of the Medical Sciences*, vol. 173, no. 5, pp. 643–648, 1927.

[4] J. R. Derrick and H. A. Fadhli, "Surgical anatomy of the superior mesenteric artery," *The American Surgeon*, vol. 31, pp. 545–547, 1965.

[5] B. Unal, A. Aktaş, G. Kemal et al., "Superior mesenteric artery syndrome: CT and ultrasonography findings," *Diagnostic and Interventional Radiology*, vol. 11, no. 2, pp. 90–95, 2005.

[6] S. Neri, S. S. Signorelli, E. Mondati et al., "Ultrasound imaging in diagnosis of superior mesenteric artery syndrome," *Journal of Internal Medicine*, vol. 257, no. 4, pp. 346–351, 2005.

[7] H. Ozkurt, M. M. Cenker, N. Bas, S. M. Erturk, and M. Basak, "Measurement of the distance and angle between the aorta and superior mesenteric artery: normal values in different BMI categories," *Surgical and Radiologic Anatomy*, vol. 29, no. 7, pp. 595–599, 2007.

[8] A. Haider, M. Sharma, and A. Siddiqa, "Superior mesenteric artery syndrome: a forgotten cause of duodenal obstruction," *Cureus*, vol. 12, no. 9, 2020.

[9] D. E. Adson, J. E. Mitchell, and S. W. Trenkner, "The superior mesenteric artery syndrome and acute gastric dilatation in eating disorders: a report of two cases and a review of the literature," *The International Journal of Eating Disorders*, vol. 21, no. 2, pp. 103–114, 1997.

[10] B. Clapp and B. Applebaum, "Superior mesenteric artery syndrome after Roux-en-y gastric bypass," *JSLS*, vol. 14, no. 1, pp. 143–146, 2010.

[11] M. T. Baker, M. D. Lara, and S. N. Kothari, "Superior mesenteric artery syndrome after laparoscopic Roux-en-Y gastric bypass," *Surgery for Obesity and Related Diseases*, vol. 2, no. 6, p. 667, 2006.

[12] T. Agarwal, T. A. Rockall, A. R. Wright, and S. W. Gould, "Superior mesenteric artery syndrome in a patient with HIV," *Journal of the Royal Society of Medicine*, vol. 96, no. 7, pp. 350-351, 2003.

[13] J. Hines, "Superior mesenteric artery syndrome: diagnostic criteria and therapeutic approaches," *The American Journal of Surgery*, vol. 148, no. 5, pp. 630–632, 1984.

[14] V. Zaraket and L. Deeb, "Wilkie's syndrome or superior mesenteric artery syndrome: fact or fantasy," *Case Reports in Gastroenterology*, vol. 9, no. 2, pp. 194–199, 2015.

[15] N. Van Horne and J. P. Jackson, "Superior Mesenteric Artery Syndrome. [Updated 2020 Jul 21]," in *StatPearls*, StatPearls Publishing, Treasure Island (FL), 2021.

[16] B. J. Pottorf, F. A. Husain, H. W. Hollis, and E. Lin, "Laparoscopic management of duodenal obstruction resulting from superior mesenteric artery syndrome," *JAMA Surgery*, vol. 149, no. 12, pp. 1319–1322, 2014.

[17] P. Gaikwad, N. Ambrose, and S. Sharma, "Management of superior mesenteric artery syndrome: two paths to go by," *Current Medical Issues*, vol. 17, no. 4, pp. 140–143, 2019.

20

Fourteen-Year Patency of an Anterior Tibial Artery-Saphenous Vein Fistula in an Ambulatory Patient

Zerrin Pulathan and Gökalp Altun

Cardiovascular Surgery Department, Karadeniz Technical University Faculty of Medicine, Trabzon, Turkey

Correspondence should be addressed to Zerrin Pulathan; zerrin.pulathan@gmail.com

Academic Editor: Hiroyuki Nakajima

Background. Ankle arteriovenous fistulas are the rarest vascular access type among lower extremity fistulas for hemodialysis patients with end-stage renal disease. Here, we present a case of a tibial-saphenous fistula that remained open for a long time despite a recurrent anastomotic aneurysm. *Case Presentation.* A 43-year-old female patient who had been undergoing hemodialysis via a right femoral tunnel catheter for six months was referred for recurrent catheter infection and a 4 cm pulsatile mass in the anterior aspect of the ankle. While she had been undergoing hemodialysis through a right tibial-saphenous fistula for fourteen years, hemodialysis continued after the fistula's closure due to total occlusion of the great saphenous vein through the tunneled catheter. After balloon angioplasty to the right subclavian vein, we performed right upper extremity basilic vein transposition. Later, after starting adequate dialysis from the basilic vein fistula and removing the femoral catheter, we performed a resection of the anastomotic aneurysm in the right ankle and repaired the anterior tibial artery. Because this is the only ambulatory patient and the one with the longest patency of ankle arteriovenous fistulas in the literature and the only case in which the anterior tibial artery was used, the case is presented and discussed in light of the literature. *Conclusion.* Despite many complications and low patency rates reported in the literature, ankle vessels should be considered for autogenous vascular access in selected patients.

1. Introduction

Upper extremity autogenous arteriovenous fistulas (AVF) are the best options for hemodialysis (HD). The most common indications for vascular access in the lower extremities are inadequate vascular structures in the upper extremities or bilateral central vein occlusion. Creating an autogenous arteriovenous fistula for the lower extremities is extremely rare, and usually, a saphenofemoral AV fistula is used [1]. Interventions below the knee are rare due to maturation problems related to inadequate dilatation of the great saphenous vein, frequent stenosis due to intimal hyperplasia, and ischemic complications due to diabetes and peripheral arterial disease [2, 3]. Typically, the posterior tibial artery is used in this body region. In our case, the fistula was formed between the anterior tibial artery and the saphenous vein.

2. Case Presentation

A nephrologist referred a 43-year-old female due to pulsatile swelling at the anterior part of the right ankle, pain, and recurrent infection of the femoral tunneled catheter. The patient was on hemodialysis for seventeen years, and hemodialysis had been performed through left radiocephalic, left brachiocephalic, right radiocephalic, right forearm prosthetic loop, and right brachiocephalic fistulas created in the upper extremities for three years. Then, the tibial-saphenous fistula was created fourteen years ago on the right ankle after the initial fistulas had become unusable. Hemodialysis was started on the below-knee saphenous vein two months after the creating that fistula. However, an ankle aneurysm developed three years later, and an aneurysmoplasty was performed in the fifth year after creating this fistula. After that, hemodialysis was effectively performed for

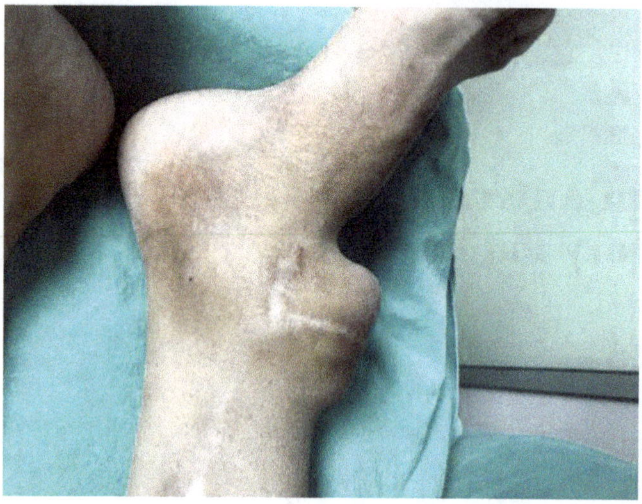

(a)

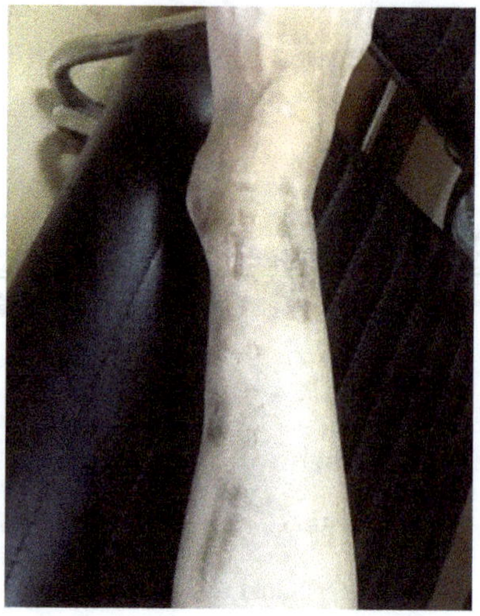

(b)

FIGURE 1: (a) Aneurysm and surgical incisions on right ankle (transverse scar is due to aneurysmoplasty operation performed nine years ago). (b) Image of the right ankle at the 3rd year postoperatively.

another nine years (fourteen years in total). Although the swelling at the ankle worsened, the fistula was used without further intervention, as long as it was functional. When the great saphenous vein was occluded while the patient was being followed in another center six months ago, a tunneled catheter was placed in the right femoral vein, and hemodialysis was continued without any invasive or surgical procedure to render the fistula functional. Physical examination revealed a pulsatile mass on the anterior aspect of the right ankle, transverse and longitudinal surgical incision scars on the aneurysm sac and medial malleolus, pigmentation secondary to cannulation of the great saphenous vein, an increase in calf circumference of 1 cm, fibrotic thickening, and thrombosed aneurysmal dilatation on the great saphenous vein (Figure 1). There was no palpable thrill over the pulsatile aneurysm sac. The posterior tibial pulse was strong; the anterior tibial pulse was weak, and there were no findings suggestive of ischemia. Lower extremity arterial Doppler's ultrasonography revealed a 41×45 mm nonthrombosed aneurysm sac at ankle level in the right anterior tibial artery and a biphasic flow pattern in the distal artery. In venous Doppler's ultrasound, the deep venous system was patent; the saphenous vein was occluded entirely at the level below the knee, and the diameter of the proximal saphenous vein at the level above the knee was 3.4 mm. An aneurysmatic segment with a diameter of 45 mm was detected in computed tomography angiography (CTA) examination of the right ankle (Figure 2). Physical examination and upper extremity Doppler's ultrasonography revealed that only the right basilic vein was open with an appropriate diameter (3.5 mm) to create a new AVF. Upper extremity venography performed due to dilated collateral veins around the shoulder showed stenosis of the short segment of the brachiocephalic vein, and complete patency was obtained by balloon angioplasty. A functional AVF was obtained after right basilic vein transposition (BVT), and HD was initiated 34 days later. The tunneled catheter in the right femoral vein was removed, and surgical repair of the ankle aneurysm was performed one week later. A 4 cm incision was made on the anterior tibial artery trace in the ankle. After vascular control was achieved, the aneurysm sac was excised, and the artery was repaired with 7/0 Prolene sutures laterally. Anterior tibial pulse was palpable after the surgery. Hemodialysis has continued for three years via the right BVT, thanks to balloon angioplasty repeated twice in the right brachiocephalic vein. The patient is still on the transplant list and waiting for a donor.

3. Discussion

Creation of a lower extremity saphenous arteriovenous fistula is quite rare and is usually performed above-knee level. The ankle region is rarely chosen due to the tendency towards trauma, arterial calcifications frequently seen in patients with kidney disease, and possible intolerance of the distal vascular bed due to diabetic angiopathy or peripheral artery disease. In addition, the wall structure of the saphenous vein and compression of the surrounding fascia may cause insufficient dilatation and maturation as well as increased neointimal hyperplasia. Kahraman et al. reported that they could initiate hemodialysis in only three (27.3%) of eleven tibial saphenous fistula cases in which they applied balloon dilation to the saphenous vein and its fascia while creating the ankle fistula [2]. Also, lower extremity edema, which may be caused due to volume burden or impaired venous circulation due to fistula, may lead to difficult cannulation. In the long-term, complications such as infection, steal syndrome, thrombosis, and aneurysm caused by the fistula cause a greater risk of extremity loss in this region than in other areas. No complications other than an aneurysm developed in the long-term were observed in this patient, which may be due to the patient's age and the absence of other comorbidities such as obesity, diabetes, hypertension, and peripheral arterial disease [1, 3]. If indicated, fistula

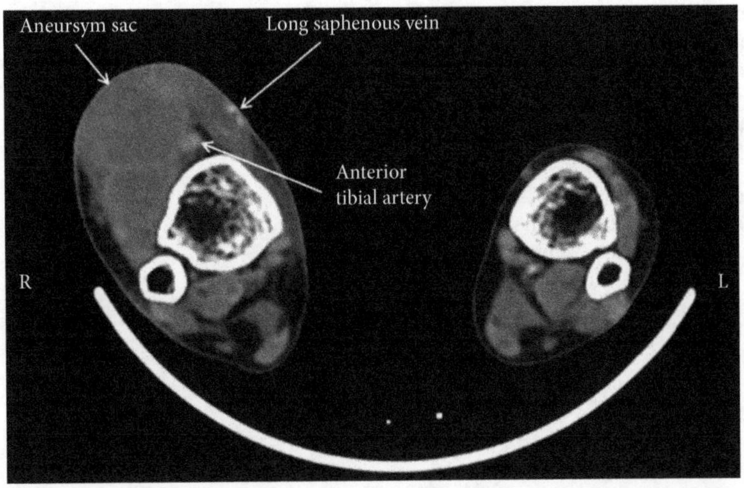

FIGURE 2: Computed tomography of the patient's right ankle aneurysm shows calcification in the saphenous vein and an intact aneurysm.

functionality can be prolonged with interventions such as aneurysmorrhaphy, aneurysmoplasty, and remodeling in aneurysmatic fistulas. Although primary and secondary patency rates, infection rate, and incidence of critical ischemia for autogenous fistulas of the femoral region for one year were 83%, 93%, 1.6%, and 21%, respectively, literature data for patency and complication rates of ankle fistulas is quite limited [1]. Flora et al. reported that thrombosis developed in one of the three cases with tibial-saphenous AV fistula in the fourth month [4]. In the other two patients, AV fistulas remained functional after a mean follow up of twelve months. Goh et al. reported that they formed a posterior tibia-saphenous AVF in a 50-year-old female patient with central vein occlusion, and cannulation was performed with a flow of 300 ml/min at the twelfth week. It was stated that anastomotic thrombosis developed in this patient five months later, the AVF was moved more proximal and remained functional for six months [5]. The longest patency in the literature was reported as 24 years in a 63-year-old paraplegic patient. Rim et al. reported no complications related to the fistula in this paraplegic patient, but they did not recommend this method because of the risk of trauma in outpatients [6]. Hara et al. reported the second-longest patency [7]. In this case, the posterior tibial artery-saphenous vein fistula remained open for fifteen months until kidney transplantation. Our case is a female patient who could perform daily routine activities for fourteen years until the fistula occluded. She is the first mobile patient with the longest duration of patency. Most of the cases in the literature are posterior tibial artery-saphenous vein fistulas. Our case is the only anterior tibial artery-saphenous vein fistula case in the literature to the best of our knowledge. In our case, 14-year fistula patency can be attributed to the aneurysmorraphy intervention performed nine years ago and presented by Günday [8]. Inston et al. reported that the one-year patency rate of fistulas whose aneurysms were treated was over 80% [9]. A basilic vein transposition is a good option for vascular access due to high maturation and patency rates in patients with insufficient superficial veins [10]. The rarity of imaging and intervention methods in previous years may explain why BVT fistula had not been tried in this patient earlier. Imaging central veins and performing angioplasty in patients with shoulder venous collaterals may allow upper extremity AVF patency and create more complex fistulas like BVT.

4. Conclusion

Despite the limited case series in the literature and uncertain long-term patency rates, ankle AVFs should be considered as an alternative autogenous vascular access route in selected patients.

References

[1] G. A. Antoniou, M. K. Lazarides, G. S. Georgiadis, G. S. Sfyroeras, E. S. Nikolopoulos, and A. D. Giannoukas, "Lower-extremity arteriovenous access for haemodialysis: a systematic review," *Europian Journal of Vascular and Endovascular Surgery*, vol. 38, no. 3, pp. 365–372, 2009.

[2] D. Kahraman, U. Şener, T. Olgaç, M. Moda, and B. Yoğurtçuoğlu, "Preliminary balloon dilation of both saphenous fascia and the saphenous vein increases the below-knee fistula patency, but not maturation," *The Journal of Vascular Access*, vol. 22, no. 2, pp. 266–272, 2021.

[3] E. Elamurugan and R. Hemachandar, "Ankle arteriovenous fistula – a rare site of choice for hemodialysis," *The Journal of Vascular Access*, vol. 17, no. 3, pp. 291-292, 2016.

[4] H. S. Flora, E. J. Chaloner, C. Day, and S. G. Barker, "The ankle arterio-venous fistula: an approach to gaining vascular access for renal haemodialysis," *Europian Journal of Vascular and Endovascular Surgery*, vol. 22, no. 4, pp. 376–378, 2001.

[5] M. A. Goh, J. M. Ali, R. Lagaac, and G. J. Pettigrew, "Ankle fistula as the last resort for vascular access: case report and literature review," *The Journal of Vascular Access*, vol. 16, no. 1, pp. 68–71, 2015.

[6] H. Rim, H. S. Shin, and Y. S. Jung, "Arteriovenous fistula between the posterior tibial artery and great saphenous vein," *Kidney International*, vol. 81, no. 9, p. 925, 2012.

[7] T. Hara, T. Sofue, and M. Kohno, "Hemodialysis arteriovenous fistula created from the posterior tibial artery and a saphenous vein branch," *American Journal of Kidney Disease*, vol. 62, no. 6, pp. 1222-1223, 2013.

[8] M. Günday, "Aneurysm of the tibial-saphenous fistula in hemodialysis patient: the results of surgical treatment," *Vascular Health and Risk Management*, vol. 7, pp. 657–660, 2011.

[9] N. Inston, H. Mistry, J. Gilbert et al., "Aneurysms in vascular access: state of the art and future developments," *The Journal of Vascular Access*, vol. 18, no. 6, pp. 464–472, 2017.

[10] S. Wang, M. S. Wang, and W. C. Jennings, "Basilic elevation transposition may improve the clinical outcomes for superficialization of basilic arteriovenous fistula veins," *The Journal Vascular of Surgery*, vol. 65, no. 4, pp. 1104–1112, 2017.

Balloon-Assisted Percutaneous Thrombin Injection for Treatment of Iatrogenic Left Subclavian Artery Pseudoaneurysm in a Critically Ill COVID-19 Patient

Hassan Al-Thani,[1] Ahmed Hussein,[1] Ahmed Sadek,[1] Ali Barah,[2] and Ayman El-Menyar[3,4]

[1]*Vascular Surgery Section, Department of Surgery, Hamad General Hospital (HGH), Doha, Qatar*
[2]*Radiology Department, HGH, Doha, Qatar*
[3]*Clinical Research, Trauma and Vascular Surgery Section, HGH, Doha, Qatar*
[4]*Clinical Medicine, Weill Cornell Medical College, Doha, Qatar*

Correspondence should be addressed to Ayman El-Menyar; aymanco65@yahoo.com

Academic Editor: Hiroyuki Nakajima

Background. Central venous catheter represents an important tool in the management of critically ill patient. In this report, we described a COVID-19-positive case who had COVID-related complications and iatrogenic left subclavian artery pseudoaneurysm after central venous catheter insertion. *Case Presentation.* A 58-year-old male patient presented with a high-grade fever, myalgia, and shortness of breath due to COVID-19 infection. He required mechanical ventilation support and hemodialysis. He also developed uneventful deep vein thrombosis and myocardial infarction. As a complication of central line insertion, the patient developed pseudoaneurysm that originated from the subclavian artery with significant bleeding and large hematoma. Balloon-assisted percutaneous thrombin injection was done under ultrasound guidance. The patient was extubated 2 days later with no evidence of flow in the pseudoaneurysm. However, he lost movement in the left arm secondary to the compression of the brachial plexus from the pseudoaneurysm/hematoma, and therefore, 1.5 litres of the hematoma was evacuated in the operating room through a lateral left chest wall incision along the anterior axillary line to relieve the compression over the brachial plexus. The patient declined surgical reconstruction of the brachial plexus, and the flaccid paralysis of the arm did not recover during the follow-up. *Conclusion.* This is a case of unusual complications of COVID infection and iatrogenic left subclavian artery pseudoaneurysm postcentral vein cannulation. Balloon-assisted percutaneous thrombin injection for treatment of left subclavian artery pseudoaneurysm is feasible; however, delayed diagnosis could be associated with long-term or permanent disability.

1. Introduction

Central venous catheter represents an important tool in the management of critically ill patients [1]. During the peak of the COVID pandemic, more critically ill patients required admission into intensive care unit with increased number of central venous catheter insertion with possible increase in the rate of complications [2] including the rare ones as subclavian artery pseudoaneurysm. In this report, we described a case of COVID-related complications and iatrogenic left subclavian artery pseudoaneurysm after central venous catheter insertion in a patient with severe COVID-19 infection.

2. Case Report

A 58-year-old male patient presented with high-grade fever, myalgia, and shortness of breath and proved to be COVID-19 positive on the 16th of May 2020. The patient's clinical condition rapidly deteriorated on the second day of admission due to severe pneumonia that required mechanical ventilation support after failure of the conventional support including prone position. He was started on azithromycin 500 mg intravenous, tocilizumab 600 mg intravenous single dose, hydroxychloroquine 400 mg tablets once a day, and methylprednisolone 40 mg twice daily (for five days for all). He developed acute kidney injury requiring renal replacement therapy in the form of sustained low-efficiency dialysis (SLED) through a right femoral vein central line due to hemodynamic instability on the 19th of May. The patient developed deep vein thrombosis on the same side of the hemodialysis catheter despite the prophylaxis with low molecular heparin. A second central line using the left internal jugular was placed under ultrasound guidance on the 24th of May. When the patient was connected to the hemodialysis machine, the venous pressure was high which indicates possible arterial flow. Another line was inserted on the 25th of May on the right internal jugular using ultrasound guidance, and at this time, it worked well (Figure 1(a)). The left internal jugular catheter was removed, and pressure dressing was applied (Figure 1(b)).

The patient developed left upper arm and supraclavicular swelling, and his hemoglobin dropped by 4-5 to 5 g from the initial 9.5 g. The patient was stabilized by fluid resuscitation and blood transfusion. No melena or any sign of active bleeding was identified. The patient was extubated on the 1st of June, breathing well with retrosternal chest pain with elevated troponin level which was diagnosed as myocardial infarction type II that was treated conservatively. He also had left shoulder pain and was unable to move his left arm; orthopedic consultation was requested and the plan for conservative management as no obvious radiological orthopedic insult.

A CT scan of the abdomen and upper chest was done to rule out the source of bleeding on the 2nd of June. CT scan confirmed evidence of large intramuscular and extramuscular hematoma involving the muscle of the left side of the chest wall extending to the lateral aspect of the abdominal wall, and there was no intra-abdominal free fluid or collection. The CT scan was limited to the upper chest and abdomen but did not cover the neck and the supraclavicular area. There was a plan for another CT scan of the neck and upper chest, but because of acute kidney injury and risk of more nephrotoxicity, the CT scan was postponed until the 9th of June when his kidney function improved and his last hemodialysis was on the 7th of June. CT angiogram for the head, neck, and chest revealed a large homogenously hyperdense sac-like structure with a tongue projecting superiorly noted posterior to the left clavicle and in close proximity to the anterior wall of the proximal part of the left subclavian artery possibly arising from it with narrow neck, measuring 2.1 × 3.5 × 4.5 cm (Figure 2). It was seen associated and surrounded with large mixed density area extending from the left lower neck opposite the level of epiglottis towards the left axilla, subscapular region, lateral chest wall, and the left upper abdominal quadrant approximately more than 25 cm in craniocaudal dimension and 8 cm in maximum transverse dimension in the lateral chest wall with more heterogeneous density inferiorly. The rest of the left subclavian artery appeared stretched by the hematoma but otherwise patent. The left internal jugular vein was significantly attenuated and could not be seen in the lower neck. Ultrasound showed pseudoaneurysm originating from the subclavian artery (Figures 2(b) and 3(c)).

Vascular surgery consultation was done on the 12th of June regarding the large hematoma extending from the neck to the left side of the chest. Attempt to evacuate the pseudoaneurysm was postponed because of the fear of rupturing the pseudoaneurysm. The left arm was flaccid with no movement; however, pulses over the brachial and radial arteries were palpable with no sign of ischemia.

The patient was transferred from the COVID facility to the tertiary hospital for management of the pseudoaneurysm on the 13th of June with full infection control precautions taken, as the patient's COVID test remained positive for 6 weeks. Due to his general condition and extent of the hematoma, the plan was to use ultrasound-guided thrombin injection of the pseudoaneurysm. This was done under general anaesthesia to reduce the risk of coronavirus transmission in case of the need to proceed with open surgical repair for the pseudoaneurysm. On the 15th of June, under ultrasound guidance with complete aseptic technique and local anaesthesia, micropuncture set was used to puncture the left brachial artery. Using Seldinger technique, access of the aortic arch with a 6-French sheath was obtained. Flush aortic angiogram was done using a 4-French pigtail catheter; it showed pseudoaneurysm arising from the proximal part of left subclavian artery distal to the origin of left vertebral artery and left internal mammary artery (Figures 3 and 3(b)). Mapping of the neck of pseudoaneurysm was done, and an 8 mm × 3 cm balloon was used to cover the pseudoaneurysm neck. Bedside ultrasound documented the absence of the flow within the pseudoaneurysm by inflating the balloon (Figure 3(c)). After inflation of the balloon, injection of 2000 U of thrombin was done under ultrasound guidance (Figure 3(c)). Follow-up left subclavian angiogram showed good opacification of the left vertebral artery and internal mammary artery with nonopacification of the pseudoaneurysm (Figure 3(d)). The sheath was removed, and manual compression for 10 minutes was applied at the puncture site. Postcompression ultrasound of the left brachial artery showed good flow distally with no hematoma. Radial and ulnar pulses were intact.

The patient was extubated 2 days after the procedure; however, he had no movement in the left arm which was considered secondary to the compression of the brachial plexuses from the hematoma which was confirmed by electromyography (EMG) and nerve conduction studies (Figure 4). On the 24th of June, the patient was taken to the operating theatre for evacuation of 1.5 litres of hematoma through a lateral left chest wall incision along the anterior axillary line to relieve the compression over the brachial plexus. The patient was offered surgical reconstructions for the brachial plexus (grafting and transfer) but he declined. Despite that, the patient's flaccid paralysis did not recover during the three months of follow-up.

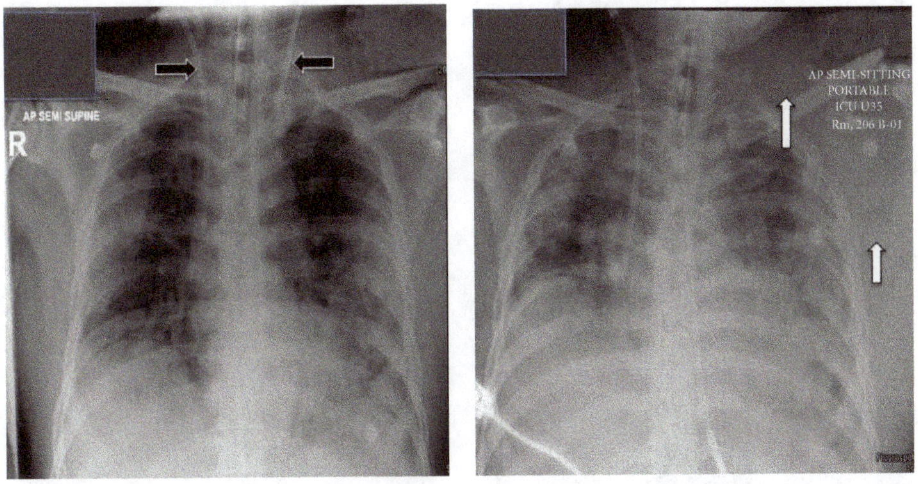

(a) (b)

Figure 1: (a) Chest X-ray showing two double lumen hemodialysis central vascular access. (b) Chest X-ray after the removal of the one on the left side with significant soft tissue swelling around the left shoulder associated with left lateral displacement of the scapula.

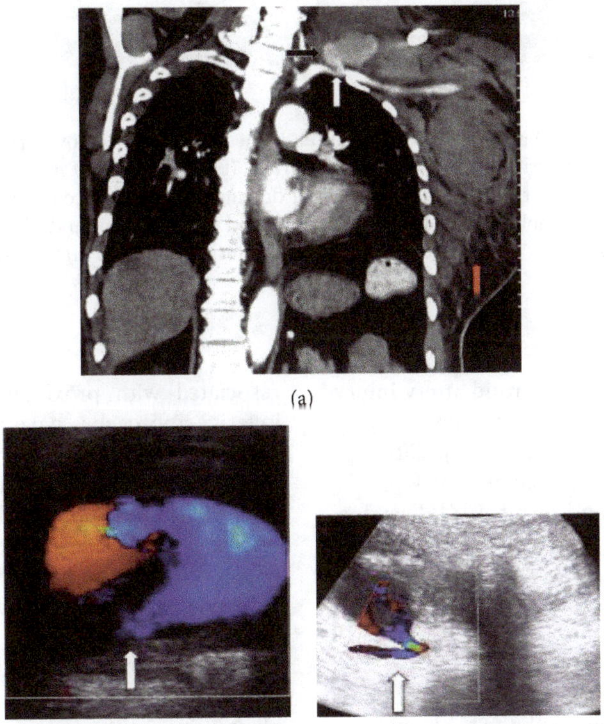

(a)

(b) (c)

Figure 2: (a) CT coronal section showing the left subclavian artery (white arrow) with pseudoaneurysm (black arrow) and large intra- and extramuscular chest wall and left side hematoma (red arrow). (b, c) Ultrasonography showing a pseudoaneurysm originating from the subclavian artery (white arrow).

3. Discussion

The present COVID-positive case developed many complications related to the COVID infection such as reversible organ failure (lung and kidney) and arterial and venous thromboembolism (myocardial infarction and deep vein thrombosis) as well as iatrogenic complication (subclavian pseudoaneurysm and nerve injury). For faster detection of such iatrogenic injuries in an intubated patient, the healthcare giver should follow proper physical examination, bedside imaging, and CTA imaging with little contrast when renal failure is present, in addition to adherence to the precautionary measures during pandemic. Cannulation of the central veins can have various complications (4-35%)

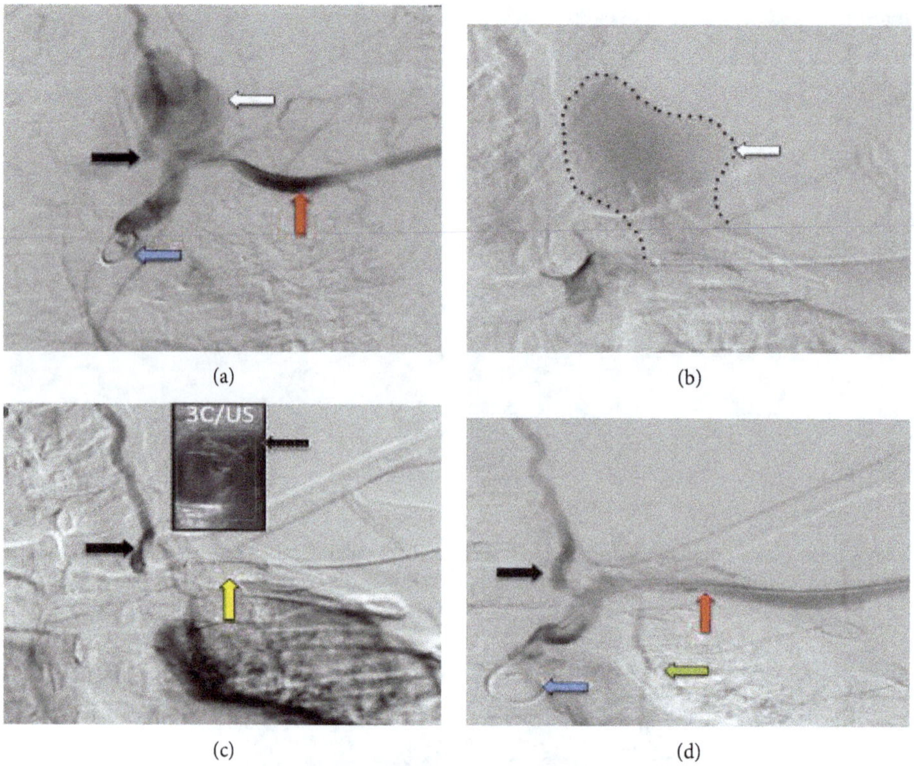

Figure 3: (a, b) Pigtail catheter (blue arrow) arteriogram showed pseudoaneurysm (white arrow) arising from the proximal part of the left subclavian artery (red arrow) distal to the origin of the left vertebral artery (black arrow). (c) Angioplasty balloon-tipped catheter (yellow arrow) covering the neck of the pseudoaneurysm. Bedside ultrasound documents the absence of the flow within the pseudoaneurysm by inflating the balloon, and injection of thrombin was done under ultrasound guidance ((c) and US). (d) Arteriogram after the thrombin injection shows no pseudoaneurysm, and it shows the left subclavian artery (red arrow), left vertebral artery (black arrow), and left internal mammary artery (green arrow).

including pneumothorax, chylothorax, carotid artery injury, stroke, arteriovenous fistula, pseudoaneurysm, nerve injury, cardiac perforation, and cardiac tamponade [3]. Although some of these complications are rare, it can be fatal if not discovered and treated successfully and on time [4]. Pseudoaneurysm formation is diagnosed based on clinical findings of pulsatile mass, palpable thrill, or pressure and ischemic manifestations although it might be asymptomatic. Imaging modalities include ultrasonography, CT angiography, MR angiography, and conventional angiography [5].

In our case, the investigations were focused on finding the cause of dropping of hemoglobin with the big hematoma in the chest wall extending into the upper abdomen which caused delay in the diagnosis and treatment of the left subclavian pseudoaneurysm. The conventional CT and CT angiogram offered valuable information regarding the anatomy and morphology of the pseudoaneurysm and helped in planning the treatment options. Symptomatic pseudoaneurysm should be treated; traditionally, it was treated by surgical repair which carries significantly higher morbidities and mortality rates.

The management of the subclavian artery pseudoaneurysm evolved over the years. Although open surgical repair had been the primary method in its management, due to the difficult surgical exposure and the difficulties associated with proximal and distal control, other less-invasive approaches have been utilized, including endovascular option. Endovascular approach is aimed at excluding the pseudoaneurysm from the circulation by covered stent or by embolization. On the other hand, percutaneous approach usually utilizes ultrasound or CT-guided thrombin injection. Direct compression of the pseudoaneurysm using ultrasound guidance is another noninvasive management. This needs a cycle of 10-20 minutes or up to 1 hour with operator and patient discomfort. There are limitations for its use including location and depth and the outcome affected using anticoagulants, size, configuration, and diameter of the neck of the pseudoaneurysm. The treatment options should be tailored to the site, rupture risk, clinical situation, and patient comorbidities [6].

In our case, the suitable size of the covered stent was not available. Our choice was to proceed for thrombin injection to induce thrombosis of the pseudoaneurysm and exclude it from the circulation. This technique was developed initially for the treatment of the femoral pseudoaneurysm after catheterization and extended to other vessels [7].

Few case reports described thethrombin injection technique for the treatment of the subclavian artery pseudoaneurysm [4, 7–16]. The success rate is around 82% and can be used as a salvage procedure of failed endovascular

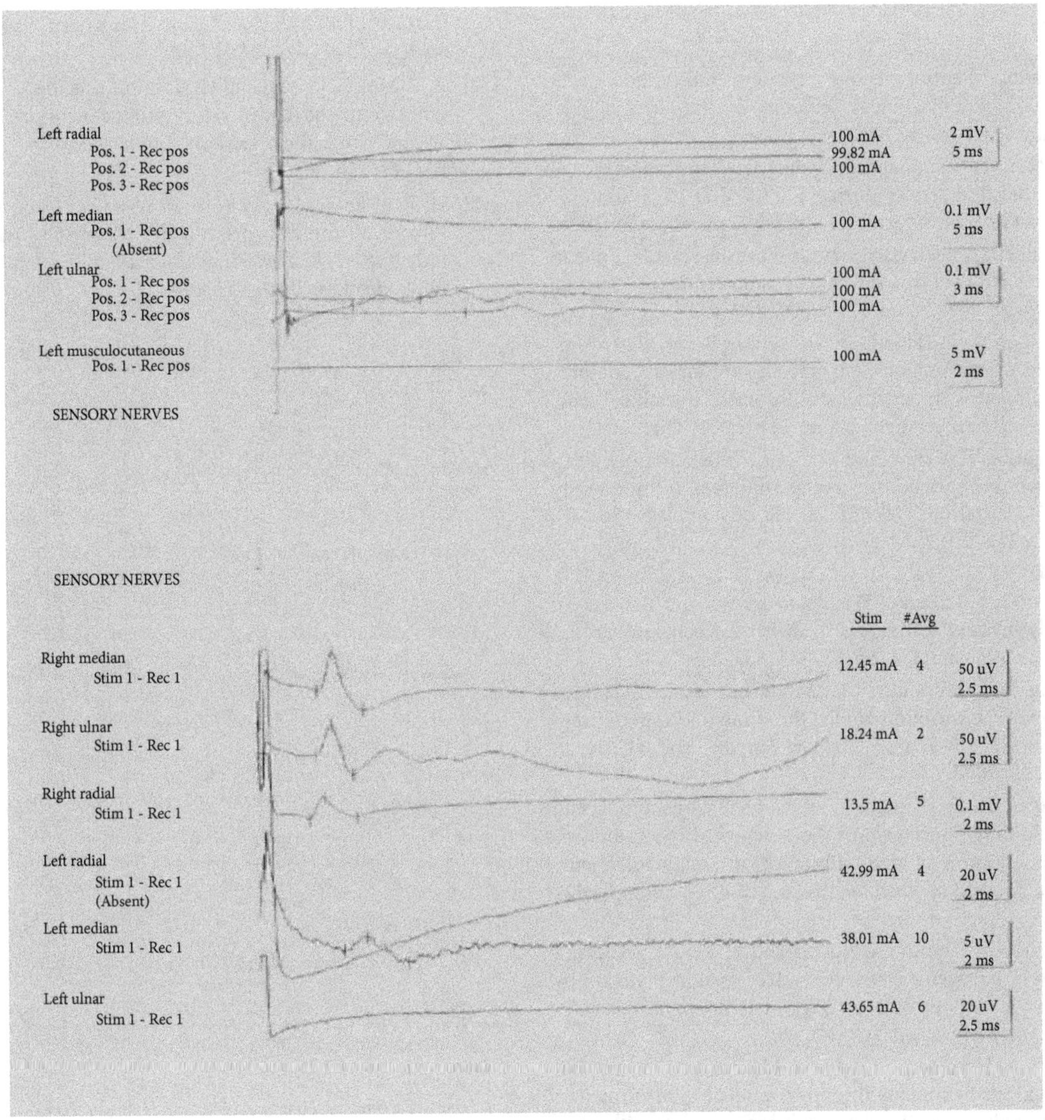

FIGURE 4: Nerve conduction studies of the upper limbs.

stenting with low complication rate. In our case, we successfully used the balloon-assisted percutaneous injection of thrombin for the treatment of left subclavian artery pseudoaneurysm in the critically ill COVID-19 patient.

Lastly, the fear of direct contact and lack of proper daily physical examination of patients with severe COVID infection could lead to serious outcomes because of missing important signs particularly in intubated patients who had invasive procedure such as center line insertion. There are few case reports in the literature describing the subclavian aneurysm causing brachial plexus injury even after removal of the subclavian central line with a partial recovery [3]. Also, subclavian artery pseudoaneurysm has been reported to cause brachial plexus injury [17, 18]. The authors stated that early surgical intervention of compressive hematoma within the first 2 days showed improvement in all patients; however, late intervention > 2 days could lead to improvement in only 50% of cases [17].

4. Conclusion

These are unusual complications in a COVID ill patient. Iatrogenic subclavian artery injury and pseudoaneurysm secondary to central vein cannulation are not common but could be associated with serious morbidity. Balloon-assisted percutaneous thrombin injection without stenting for treatment of left subclavian artery pseudoaneurysm is feasible; however, delayed diagnosis and evacuation of the subsequent hematoma could be associated with long-term or permanent disability.

Consent

No written consent has been obtained from the patient as there is no patient identifiable data included in this case report.

References

[1] R. Jamshidi, "Central venous catheters: indications, techniques, and complications," *Seminars in Pediatric Surgery*, vol. 28, no. 1, pp. 26–32, 2019.

[2] N. Ilonzo, A. Rao, K. Soundararajan et al., "The importance of a centralized line service during the COVID-19 pandemic," *Journal of Vascular Surgery*, vol. 72, no. 2, pp. 403-404, 2020.

[3] F. M. Walden, "Subclavian aneurysm causing brachial plexus injury after removal of a subclavian catheter," *British Journal of Anaesthesia*, vol. 79, no. 6, pp. 807–809, 1997.

[4] R. Jeganathan, D. W. Harkin, P. Lowry, and B. Lee, "Iatrogenic subclavian artery pseudoaneurysm causing airway compromise: treatment with percutaneous thrombin injection," *Journal of Vascular Surgery*, vol. 40, no. 2, pp. 371–374, 2004.

[5] O. Sarioglu, A. E. Capar, and U. Belet, "Interventional treatment options in pseudoaneurysms: different techniques in different localizations," *Polish Journal of Radiology*, vol. 84, pp. e319–e327, 2019.

[6] N. E. Saad, W. E. Saad, M. G. Davies, D. L. Waldman, P. J. Fultz, and D. J. Rubens, "Pseudoaneurysms and the role of minimally invasive techniques in their management," *Radiographics*, vol. 25, suppl_1, pp. S173–S189, 2005.

[7] S. S. Kang, N. Labropoulos, M. A. Mansour et al., "Expanded indications for ultrasound-guided thrombin injection of pseudoaneurysms," *Journal of Vascular Surgery*, vol. 31, no. 2, pp. 289–298, 2000.

[8] A. D. Brown, D. H. Hirpara, A. Jaberi, G. D. Oreopoulos, and M. E. Simons, "Successful balloon assisted percutaneous thrombin injection of right subclavian artery pseudoaneurysm," *The Journal of Vascular Access*, vol. 18, no. 5, pp. e62–e65, 2017.

[9] Y. Yamashita, S. Kimura, K. Kurisu, and Y. Ueno, "Successful treatment of iatrogenic subclavian artery pseudoaneurysm by ultrasound-guided thrombin injection," *Annals of Vascular Diseases*, vol. 9, no. 2, pp. 108–110, 2016.

[10] E. Lorenz, J. Herold, A. Udelnow, M. Pech, M. Pech, and Z. Halloul, "Percutaneous thrombin embolisation of an iatrogenic pseudoaneurysm of the subclavian artery with neuroprotection in a critically ill patient," *VASA*, vol. 44, no. 5, pp. 391–394, 2015.

[11] M. Kim, E. S. Kang, H. W. Kim et al., "Delayed presentation of catheter-related subclavian artery pseudoaneurysm," *JNMA; Journal of the Nepal Medical Association*, vol. 53, no. 198, pp. 130–133, 2015 Apr-Jun.

[12] G. S. Lee, J. Brawley, and R. Hung, "Complex subclavian artery pseudoaneurysm causing failure of endovascular stent repair with salvage by percutaneous thrombin injection," *Journal of Vascular Surgery*, vol. 52, no. 4, pp. 1058–1060, 2010.

[13] P. I. McConnell, J. Rehm, D. L. Oltman, T. G. Lynch, and B. T. Baxter, "Thrombin injection for treating a subclavian artery pseudoaneurysm," *Surgery*, vol. 127, no. 6, pp. 716–718, 2000.

[14] B. Shaygi, D. Kinsella, and A. F. Watkinson, "Amplatzer vascular plug 4 insertion for the treatment of a left subclavian artery pseudoaneurysm," *Annals of Vascular Surgery*, vol. 43, pp. 311.e5–311.e7, 2017.

[15] W. Woźniak, R. K. Mlosek, G. Górski, P. Myrcha, and P. Ciostek, "Thrombin obliteration of subclavian artery aneurysm with intravascular balloon protection," *Kardiochir Torakochirurgia Pol*, vol. 2, no. 2, pp. 202–204, 2014.

[16] A. Derom, S. Ottenheim, H. Raat, and J. van Kleef, "Endovascular treatment of acute subclavian pseudo-aneurysm after fracture of the clavicle," *Acta Chirurgica Belgica*, vol. 108, no. 4, pp. 441–443, 2008.

[17] T. N. Mol, A. Gupta, and U. Narain, "Brachial plexus compression due to subclavian artery pseudoaneurysm from internal jugular vein catheterization," *Indian J Nephrol.*, vol. 27, no. 2, pp. 148–150, 2017.

[18] M. R. O'Leary, "Subclavian artery false aneurysm associated with brachial plexus palsy: a complication of parenteral drug addiction," *The American Journal of Emergency Medicine*, vol. 8, no. 2, pp. 129–133, 1990.

22

Cyclist Endofibrosis (Exercise-Induced Arterial Endofibrosis) Treated by Drug-Coated Balloon Angioplasty

Ahmed S. Zugail,[1,2] **Hossam I. Shaabi**,[3,4] **Slimane Idir**,[1] **and Jean-Pierre Becquemin**[1]

[1]*East Paris Vascular Institute (IVPE), Paul d'Égine Private Hospital (Ramsay Santé), Champigny-sur-Marne, France*
[2]*Department of Surgery, Faculty of Medicine in Rabigh, King Abdulaziz University, Jeddah, Saudi Arabia*
[3]*Department of Vascular and Endoluminal Surgery, Nancy Regional and University Hospital Center (CHRU), Nancy, France*
[4]*Department of Surgery, Faculty of Medicine, Jazan University, Jazan, Saudi Arabia*

Correspondence should be addressed to Ahmed S. Zugail; zugail2@hotmail.com

Academic Editor: Muzaffer Sindel

Exercise-induced arterial endofibrosis is an uncommon entity that is most frequently identified in high-performance athletes, especially cyclists. We present this disease in a male professional cyclist of 22 years of age. The course of his condition, clinical manifestations, modalities of investigation, and a nonprecedent treatment plan are demonstrated.

1. Introduction

Arterial diseases are rare in young people, but they could appear in the form of endofibrosis in special circumstances. Initially witnessed in highly skilled male cyclists, it has been found in many other endurance athletes of both genders. Exercise-induced arterial endofibrosis (EIAE) was first described in competitive cyclists in 1985 [1]. Sometimes, it is very challenging to diagnose this disease, and failure to do so could have grave consequences both socially and career-wise. Therefore, we believe that medical and paramedical health workers such as orthopedists, neurologists, rheumatologists, and physiotherapists should be aware of this rare condition that could imitate musculoskeletal disorders. Two distinctive characteristics remain for this ailment; it affects high-level endurance athletes, and the histopathological studies show endofibrosis [2]. To this day, the pathophysiology of this disease is unknown. We would like to add that the patient agreed to the publishing of his case details and radiological images.

2. Case Presentation

We report a professional athletic male cyclist—more than 25,000 kilometers (km) per year—of 22 years of age with no past medical, surgical, or traumatic history who was referred by his family doctor to the vascular surgery outpatient clinic for left thigh claudication on maximal effort. The patient's symptom had already been explored with a Duplex scan and a computed tomographic angiography (CTA). The Duplex scan showed a posterior intraluminal nonatheromatous fibrous thickening at the junction of the left common and external iliac arteries of about 20 millimeters (mm) of length. At rest, no hemodynamic changes were found compared to a velocity increase at the level of the stenosis and a slight drop of the ankle-brachial index after performing 50 squats. On the CTA, an endofibrotic plaque of the left external artery (LEA) was seen Figures 1 and 2. The patient was labelled with an exercise-induced arterial endofibrosis (EIAE) or more commonly known as a "Cyclist Endofibrosis." The patient was proposed four management plans given in the following order. The first was to withhold cycling which was refused by the patient. The second was surgery consisting of endofibrosectomy angioplasty with shortening of the LEA. The third was intervention by balloon angioplasty and self-expandable stent. The fourth was a balloon angioplasty using a drug-coated balloon (DCB). All the pros and cons of each treatment were discussed with the patient. He opted for the latter treatment although no scientific data

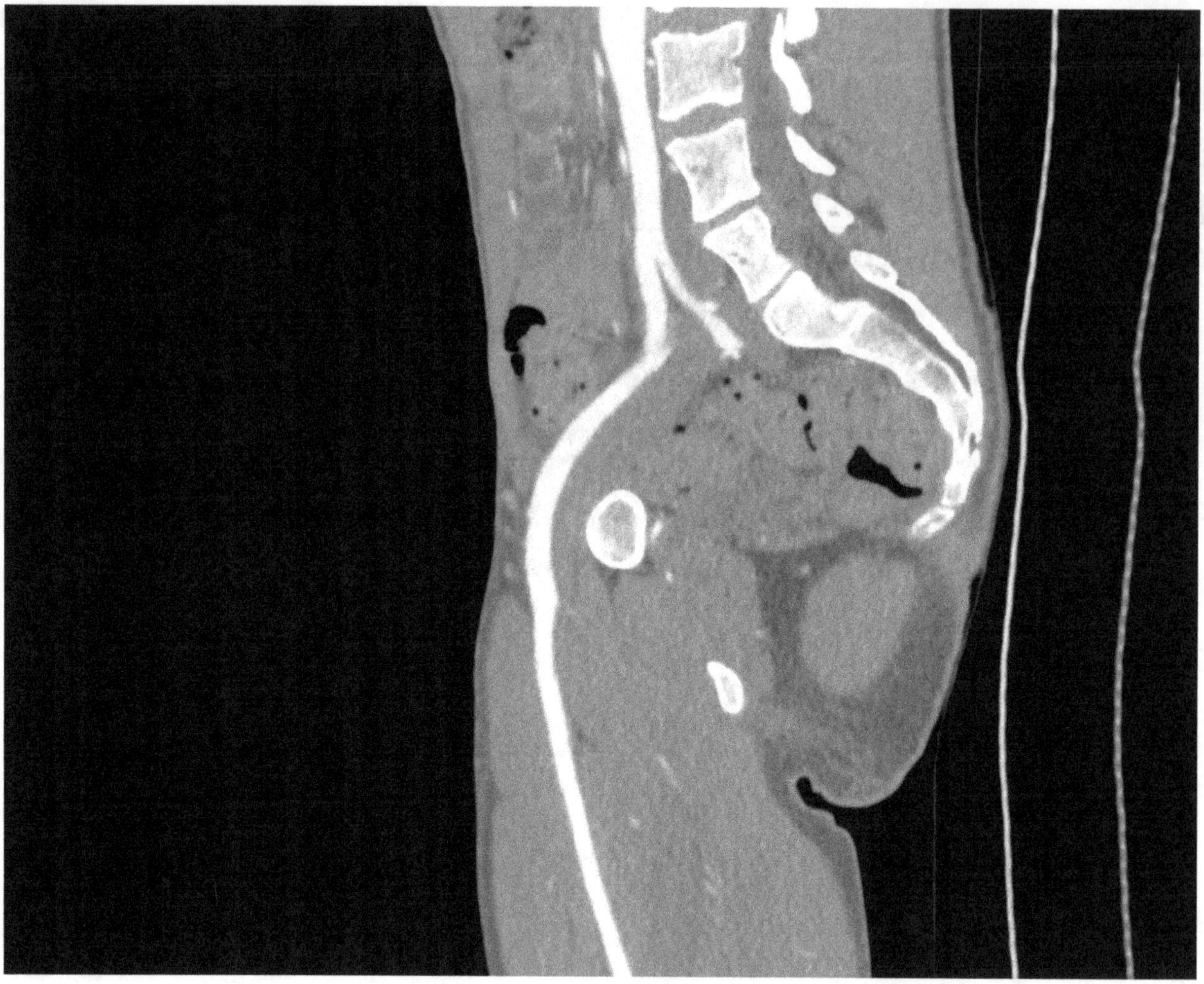

FIGURE 1: A reconstructed sagittal computed tomographic angiogram of the abdominal aorta and the left iliac arteries using the stretch reformation technique, revealing a stenosis and kink in the proximal half of the left external iliac artery (an endofibrotic plaque). Poststenotic dilation is noted. (The patient agreed to the publishing of his radiological images.)

supports it. The patient was admitted to the outpatient surgical department and was discharged home on the same day. After the patient's consent and under general anesthesia, an endovascular intervention was done in a hybrid operating room. An 8 mm × 60 mm LUTONIX® 035 DCB from BARD Medical, C. R. BARD, Inc. was placed over the lesion. Upon discharge, he was prescribed 75 milligrams of acetylsalicylic acid and clopidogrel once daily for one month and recommended a one-week rest before competing in a race. At the one-month clinical follow-up appointment, the patient declared no recurrence of claudication upon resuming previous cycling activity and was able to compete successfully in several races. Six months after the intervention, the patient came back with a relapse of symptoms.

3. Discussion

EIAE was previously known as "external iliac artery endofibrosis" as it was affected in 90% of the cases. The term was changed later since other locations were affected such as the common iliac artery, the common femoral artery, the profunda femoris, and quadricipital artery [3]. EIAE is most commonly described in cyclists; however, it has also been recognized in speed skaters, race walkers, endurance runners, triathletes, rowers, rugby players, soccer players, cross-country skiers, and body-builders [4]. EIAE is predominantly found in male endurance cyclists who are younger than 40 years of age [4, 5] and who have practiced a minimum of 45,000 to 50,000 km in more than 5 years [6]. At the onset of symptoms, these athletes will have cycled an average of 120,000 km completing between 14,500 km and 20,000 km per year [7]. Cyclists who undergo surgical treatment would have cycled a mean of 14 years and a total of 210,000 km [3, 8]. The symptoms of vascular disease in endurance athletes are seldom defined as typical claudication; they usually complain of an unexplained progressive decrease in performance and thigh discomfort in one leg or rarely both legs in 15% of cases. Sometimes, the patient describes a sensation of a swollen limb or complains of deep vague pain. Other symptoms include hardening of the thigh, cramps, and/or paralysis. Symptoms occur more commonly on the left side [9]. In 1995, Beck studied 164 cases of arterial endofibrosis

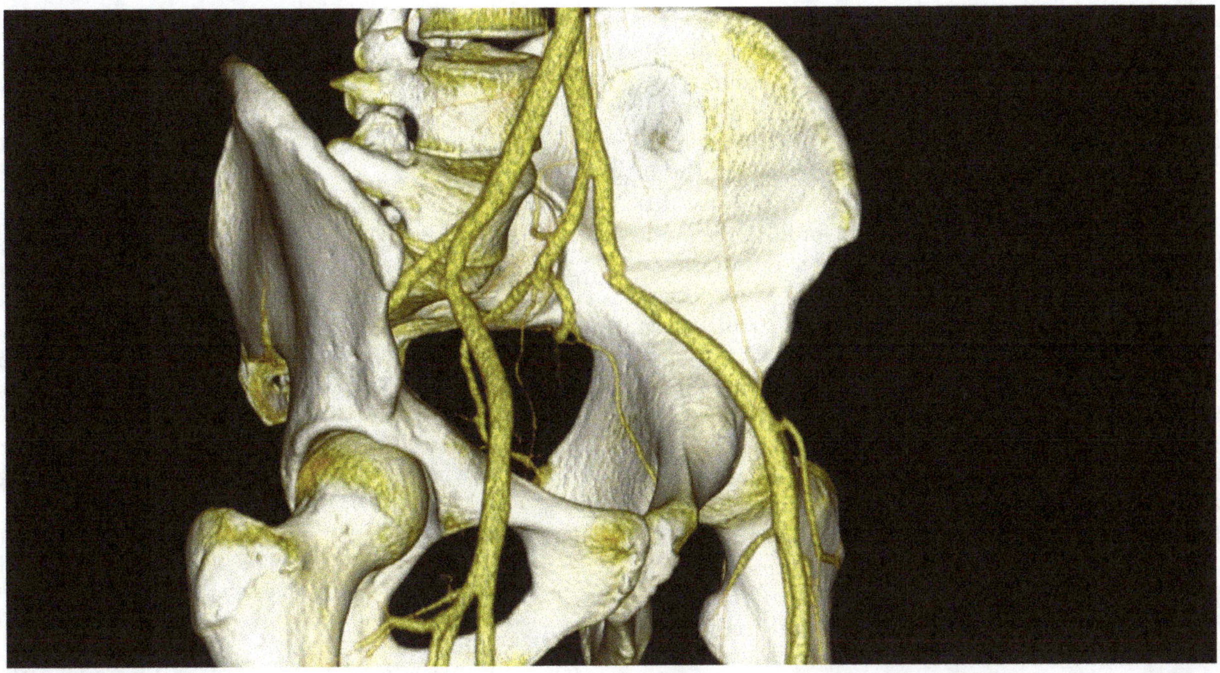

FIGURE 2: A 3-dimensional reconstruction of the patient's computed tomographic angiogram of the abdominal aorta and common iliac arteries, revealing the stenosis and kink in the proximal half of the left external iliac artery (LEA). We can observe two atypical branches of the LEA; one climbing towards the ilium and the other passing anterior to the left femoral head. Poststenotic dilation is noted. (The patient agreed to the publishing of his radiological images.)

and found that 50% of these patients complained of a paralyzing pain, a swollen thigh in 23%, both previous manifestations in 17%, typical claudication in 9%, and 1% had critical ischemia [10]. On the other hand, Feugier and Chevalier reported claudication of the lower limb at supramaximal exercise in 350 patients diagnosed with arterial endofibrosis [3]. All authors agree that these clinical manifestations appear during maximal effort and disappear at rest. A typical acute arterial claudication is rarely found and usually suggests a complication such as an occlusion [11] or a dissection [12]. Complications of endofibrosis include thrombosis, dissection, and secondary atheroma [3]. Direct trauma or familial history of vascular disease must be explored to exclude direct arterial damage or early atherosclerosis. Clinical examination is usually normal, but patients could present with an arterial systolic bruit at the groin at or with the thigh flexed. This sign is commonly found in highly trained athletes due to low resting heart rate and could be found in normal subjects, thus, not specific for endofibrosis. Differential diagnosis of EIAE includes atherosclerosis of familial origin, any musculotendinous lesion that can mimic claudication, fibromuscular dysplasia, compartment syndrome affecting the thigh, adductor canal syndrome, kinking of the femoral or iliac arteries, atypical sciatica with truncated symptoms, abnormal muscle metabolism that could be responsible for cramps during exercise, and femoral stress fractures. Different factors have been suggested that could explain the pathophysiology of endofibrosis; the aerodynamic posture and repetitive limb flexion during exercise may cause repeated stretching and lengthening of the artery that could lead to arterial kinking, and the presence of atypical arterial branches to the hypertrophied psoas muscle may displace, limit the mobility, or produce kinking of the artery and/or hereditary and metabolic factors [3, 4, 13]. The presence of a large sciatic artery acting like a pin around the affected artery has also been proposed [14], but this does not explain cases of femoral or quadricipital artery involvement. The increased blood flow and shear forces may cause stress injuries to the arterial wall with intense exercises. Contrariwise, these minor arterial lesions can lead to a significant flow impairment upon heavy load exercises where high blood flow is demanded due to an inverse relationship between the pressure drop and both the percentage of the stenosis and blood flow through these lesions [15]. Moreover, the significant increase in homocysteine in the blood and urine after methionine loading could suggest a metabolic predisposition as a minor dysfunction of the methionine cycle [3]. This abnormality increases the exercise diastolic blood pressure response and causes endothelial dysfunction [16]. Histologically, the lesion consists of an asymmetric intimal thickening with normal-appearing endothelium. The subendothelial layer shows coarse fibrous tissue with few cells that are mostly myofibroblasts in a milieu rich in collagen but poor in elastic fibers. The richly cellular intima with myofibroblasts suggests medialization. A neointimal elastic membrane in proximity to the arterial lumen is shown occasionally. The internal elastic membrane, media, and adventitia are usually normal, but the elastic membrane could be duplicated [14]. These histopathological features cause stenosis of the artery thus restricting the blood flow to muscles and produce the symptoms during maximal effort [2]. Numerous methods are used to diagnose EIAE, exercise testing with the Doppler velocimetry or ultrasound imaging, which will confirm the acceleration of blood flow with low frequencies on the spectral analysis due to turbulence [17]. Typical ultrasound imaging features include parietal thickening, enhanced echogenicity of the arterial wall, straightness of the abnormal arterial segment, and mild narrowing of the arterial diameter of the proximal or medial segment by using the B-mode that has 78% sensitivity and an 80% specificity for EIAE diagnosis [18]. In most cases, the Doppler velocimetry or ultrasound imaging at rest shows normal profiles. Furthermore, postexercise ankle-brachial systolic pressure index (ABI) is an important diagnostic tool; at rest ABI is normal. ABI measurements taken in the supine position that are less than 0.5 after completing a one-minute exercise can identify 80% of cases with 100% specificity for EIAE [4]. Little is known about computerized tomographic scans and magnetic resonance imaging of EIAE; as a result, most patients have been studied with arteriography. With the widespread of CTA and magnetic resonance angiography (MRA), arteriography with the Seldinger technique preoperatively is becoming obsolete. Sensitivity and specificity of CTA in detecting 50% aortoiliac stenosis, for example, are 96% (95% CI: 91–99) and 98% (95% CI: 95–99) [19]. The role of MRA is limited to those patients without identified endovascular lesions and whose symptoms may be due to arterial kinking [20]. Angioscopy (endovascular ultrasound) has been performed in a large number of patients showing a large eccentric white regular plaque and defining its extensions [10]. This modality needs to be broadly studied since it is certainly a promising technique although it is rarely used nowadays. The two most commonly used methods to repair EIAE are endofibrosectomy with patch angioplasty or interposition grafting with recalibrated saphenous vein grafts providing long-term satisfactory results [3]. Polytetrafluoroethylene (PTFE) prosthetic grafts should not be used in treating EIAE because almost all prostheses have occluded in the experience of Chevalier et al. and Beck [10, 14]. Percutaneous balloon angioplasty may be used when temporary relief is needed, but patients generally have recurring symptoms within 8 weeks of treatment [21]. We believe that this is the first case of EIAE treated primarily with a drug-coated balloon (DCB) angioplasty after reviewing both the English and the French literature. We believe that this method should be suggested for these patients because it is minimally invasive, relatively safe, and easily reproducible and has in the current case an excellent immediate outcome, but further studies are indispensable to confirm its long-term efficacy. In conclusion, EIAE is an uncommon ailment and is typically diagnosed in high-performance athletes, especially cyclists. The condition should be considered early in athletes who experience reproducible symptoms with exercise. Failure to diagnose and treat EIAE in young athletes has both career and social implications; a high index of suspicion for this condition is important. Ultrasound, the Doppler, and ABI studies should always be performed at rest and after exertion. CTA in appropriate patients, MRA, should be done systematically. No guidelines are available for the management of EIAE; thus, all treatment modalities should be discussed carefully with the patient including DCB angioplasty.

Acknowledgments

We acknowledge the role of Mrs. Christelle Villaumé for her technical assistance.

References

[1] J. Walder, F. Mosimann, G. Van Melle, and R. Mosimann, "Iliac endofibrosis in 2 cycling racers," *Helv Chir Acta*, vol. 51, no. 6, pp. 793–795, 1985.

[2] M. C. Rousselet, J. P. Saint-Andre, P. L'Hoste, B. Enon, A. Megret, and J. M. Chevalier, "Stenotic intimal thickening of the external iliac artery in competition cyclists," *Human Pathology*, vol. 21, no. 5, pp. 524–529, 1990.

[3] P. Feugier and J. M. Chevalier, "Endofibrosis of the iliac arteries: an underestimated problem," *Acta Chirurgica Belgica*, vol. 104, no. 6, pp. 635–640, 2016.

[4] G. Peach, G. Schep, R. Palfreeman, J. D. Beard, M. M. Thompson, and R. J. Hinchliffe, "Endofibrosis and kinking of the iliac arteries in athletes: a systematic review," *European Journal of Vascular and Endovascular Surgery*, vol. 43, no. 2, pp. 208–217, 2012.

[5] G. Schep, M. H. Bender, G. van de Tempel, P. F. Wijn, W. R. de Vries, and B. C. Eikelboom, "Detection and treatment of claudication due to functional iliac obstruction in top endurance athletes: a prospective study," *Lancet*, vol. 359, no. 9305, pp. 466–473, 2002.

[6] J. M. Chevalier, P. L'Hoste Ph, E. Bouvat, A. Megret, J. P. SaintAndre, and P. RuaultPh, "L'endofibrose artérielle du sportif de haut niveau: Formes inhabituelles," *J Traumatol Sport*, vol. 8, pp. 176–181, 1991.

[7] G. Schep, M. H. Bender, S. L. Schmikli et al., "Recognising vascular causes of leg complaints in endurance athletes. Part 2: the value of patient history, physical examination, cycling exercise test and echo-Doppler examination," *International Journal of Sports Medicine*, vol. 23, no. 5, pp. 322–328, 2002.

[8] M. H. M. Bender, G. Schep, S. W. Bouts, F. J. G. Backx, and F. L. Moll, "Endurance Athletes with Intermittent Claudication Caused by Iliac Artery Stenosis Treated by Endarterectomy with Vein Patch - Short- and Mid-term Results," *European Journal of Vascular and Endovascular Surgery*, vol. 43, no. 4, pp. 472–477, 2012.

[9] O. Rouvière, P. Feugier, J. P. Gutiérrez, and J. M. Chevalier, "Arterial endofibrosis in endurance athletes: angiographic features and classification," *Radiology*, vol. 273, no. 1, pp. 294–303, 2014.

[10] F. Beck, *L'endofibrose artérielle: formes typiques et atypiques (À propos de 164 cas)*, Doctoral dissertation, Université Claude-Bernard Lyon, France, 1995.

[11] C. R. R. Gallegos, J. G. N. Studley, and D. B. Hamer, "External iliac artery occlusion–Another complication of long distance running?," *European Journal of Vascular Surgery*, vol. 4, no. 2, pp. 195-196, 1990.

[12] P. S. Cook, L. S. Erdoes, P. M. Selzer, F. J. Rivera, and J. C. Palmaz, "Dissection of the external iliac artery in highly trained athletes," *Journal of Vascular Surgery*, vol. 22, no. 2, pp. 173–177, 1995.

[13] J. K. Clifft, F. A. Coleman, and C. B. Malone, "Vascular disorder in a competitive cyclist: a case report," *Physiotherapy Theory and Practice*, vol. 30, no. 7, pp. 517–520, 2014.

[14] J.-M. Chevalier, B. Enon, J. Walder et al., "Endofibrosis of the external iliac artery in bicycle racers: an unrecognized pathological state," *Annals of Vascular Surgery*, vol. 1, no. 3, pp. 297–303, 1986.

[15] G. Weber, A. L. Strauss, H. Rieger, A. Scheffler, and J. Eisenhoffer, "Validation of Doppler measurement of pressure gradients across peripheral model arterial stenosis," *Journal of Vascular Surgery*, vol. 16, no. 1, pp. 10–16, 1992.

[16] S. E. Brett, B. Y. Jiang, C. Turner, J. M. Ritter, and P. J. Chowienczyk, "Elevation of plasma homocysteine by methionine loading increases the diastolic blood pressure response to exercise," *Journal of Hypertension*, vol. 24, no. 10, pp. 1985–1989, 2006.

[17] P. Abraham, J. L. Saumet, and J. M. Chevalier, "External iliac artery endofibrosis in athletes," *Sports Medicine*, vol. 24, no. 4, pp. 221–226, 1997.

[18] P. Abraham, G. Leftheriotis, Y. Bourre, J. M. Chevalier, and J. L. Saumet, "Echography of external iliac artery endofibrosis in cyclists," *The American Journal of Sports Medicine*, vol. 21, no. 6, pp. 861–863, 2016.

[19] R. Met, S. Bipat, D. A. Legemate, J. A. Reekers, and M. J. W. Koelemay, "Diagnostic performance of computed tomography angiography in peripheral arterial Disease," *JAMA*, vol. 301, no. 4, pp. 415–424, 2009.

[20] M. H. M. Bender, G. Schep, W. R. de Vries, A. R. Hoogeveen, and P. F. F. Wijn, "Sports-related flow limitations in the iliac arteries in endurance athletes: aetiology, diagnosis, treatment and future developments," *Sports Medicine*, vol. 34, no. 7, pp. 427–442, 2004.

[21] L. D. Wijesinghe, P. A. Coughlin, I. Robertson, D. Kessel, P. J. Kent, and R. C. Kester, "Cyclist's iliac syndrome: temporary relief by balloon angioplasty," *British Journal of Sports Medicine*, vol. 35, no. 1, pp. 70-71, 2001.

23

Spontaneous Renal Artery Dissection in a Man with Previous Spontaneous Superior Mesenteric Artery Dissection

Yujiro Yokoyama[1] and Masato Nakajima[2]

[1]*General Surgery Department, Easton Hospital, 18042, USA*
[2]*Cardiovascular Surgery Department, Yamanashi Prefectural Central Hospital, 400-8506, Japan*

Correspondence should be addressed to Yujiro Yokoyama; yujiyoko429@gmail.com

Academic Editor: Nilda Espinola-Zavaleta

Both spontaneous superior mesenteric artery dissection (SMAD) and spontaneous renal artery dissection (SRAD) are very rare conditions. Their etiologies and natural histories are not precisely defined, but they are thought to be associated with underlying conditions. In this report, we describe an extremely rare case of SRAD in a man who had a history of spontaneous SMAD. We successfully treated SRAD with endovascular intervention. Isolated spontaneous SMAD and SRAD are both rare conditions. Their optimal treatment has not been established due to their rare entities, but endovascular treatment is a good option because it can prevent both advancement of infarction and renovascular hypertension, and it has become safer as device technology has improved. Patients with isolated visceral artery dissection should be carefully followed up.

1. Introduction

Both spontaneous superior mesenteric artery dissection (SMAD) and spontaneous renal artery dissection (SRAD) are very rare conditions. Their etiologies and natural histories are not precisely defined, but they are thought to be associated with underlying conditions. In this report, we describe an extremely rare case of SRAD in a man who had a history of spontaneous SMAD.

2. Case Report

A 41-year-old man presented to our hospital with a history of abdominal pain for the last 3 days. He had no past medical history. He did not have hypertension, hyperlipidemia, diabetes, or any collagen vascular disease. Contrast-enhanced computerized tomography (CT) showed SMAD without bowel ischemia (Figure 1). The patient was admitted and received 1 week of anticoagulant therapy. He was discharged from the hospital without complications and started taking 100 mg aspirin daily.

He was followed up once in 3 months, but 2 years later he was brought to our hospital with right-sided flank pain. His blood pressure was 142/96 mmHg, and his heart rate was 66 bpm. His abdomen was soft but not tender. Contrast-enhanced CT revealed right renal artery dissection with right renal infarction of the upper one-third portion (Figure 2). His serum creatinine level was not elevated. Renal angiography revealed two focal aneurysms and narrowing of the upper branch due to dissection (Figure 3). Two stents (Palmatz genesis 6.0 mm * 18 mm × 2) were deployed and the aneurysms were embolized by coiling (Target Detachable coils) in order to dilate the narrowing and obliterate the blood flow into aneurysms. We confirmed that the narrowing was diminished, that no blood flow entered the false lumens, and that no other branches were occluded (Figure 4).

Antiplatelet therapy with 100 mg aspirin daily was continued postoperatively and is to be continued indefinitely considering for his high risk for recurrence. His renal function did not decline, and contrast-enhanced CT performed 2 weeks after the intervention showed no advancement of renal infarction. He was discharged without complications.

He was followed up without symptom, and contrast-enhanced CT performed 6 months after discharge showed no advancement of both renal infarction and renal artery

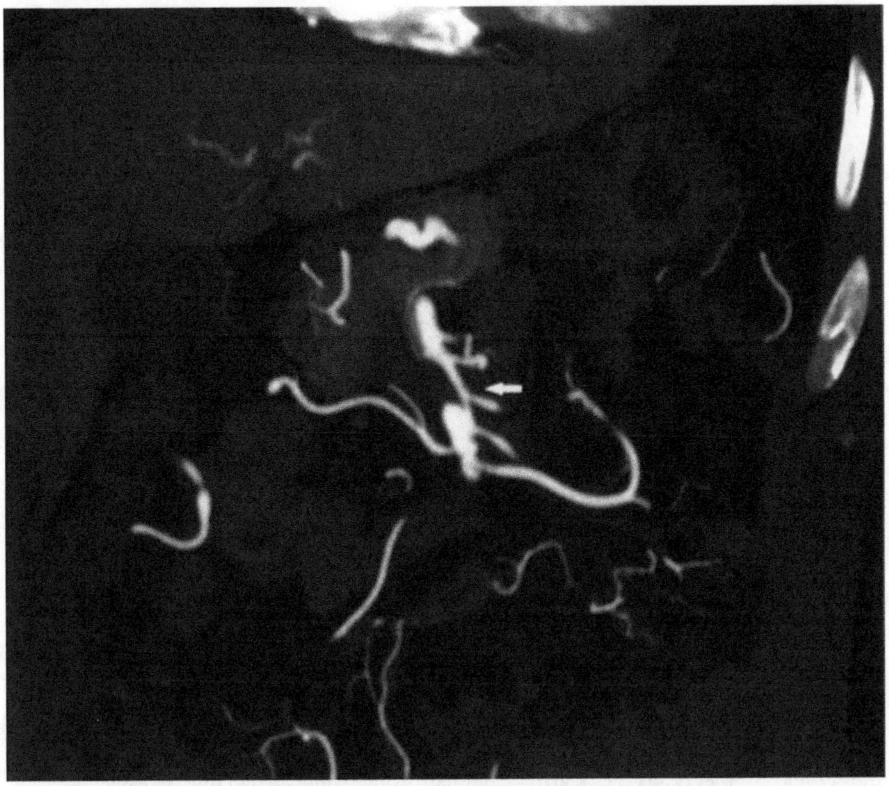

Figure 1: Dissection of the superior mesenteric artery (arrow).

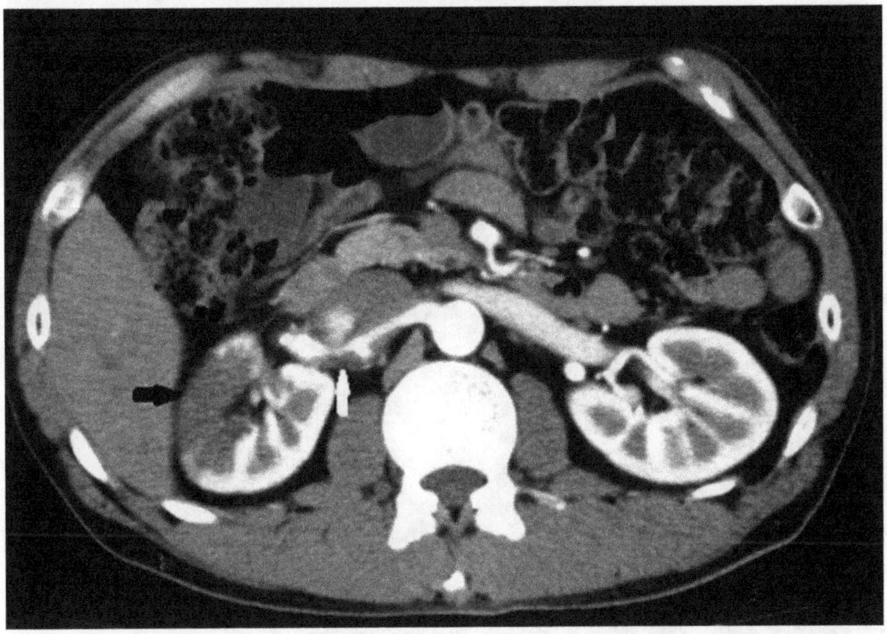

Figure 2: Right renal artery dissection (white arrow) and renal infarction (black arrow).

dissection. Genetic testing was performed but we could not find any abnormalities.

3. Discussion

SMAD is commonly associated with aortic dissection. Isolated spontaneous SMAD is a rare condition. Causes of spontaneous SMAD include atherosclerosis, fibromuscular dysplasia, segmental arterial mediolysis, connective tissue disorder, vasculitis like giant cell arteritis, Takayasu arteritis, and polyarteritis nodosa. It is accompanied by acute epigastric pain and may cause intestinal ischemia or intraabdominal rupture, but sometimes there are no symptoms [1]. There are three therapeutic

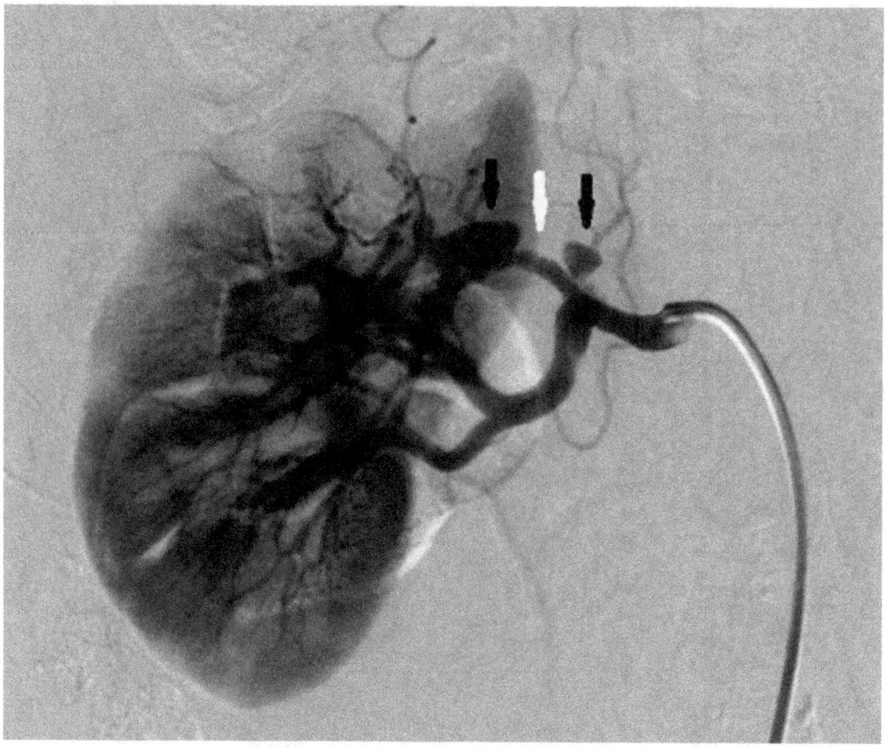

FIGURE 3: Aneurysms (black arrow) and narrowing (white arrow) due to dissection.

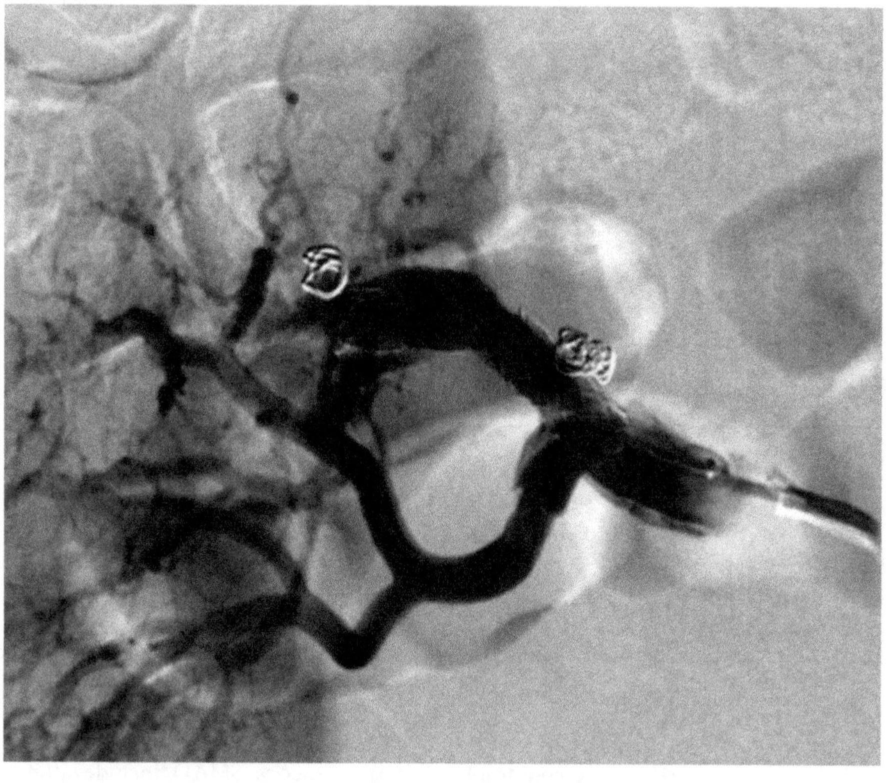

FIGURE 4: The false lumens are occluded by coiling, and the narrowing is diminished.

approaches: conservative management, endovascular therapy, and surgical revascularization. Conservative management includes anticoagulants, antiplatelet drugs, blood pressure control, and pain control, but there is no consensus on the optimal strategy for conservative management. Surgical revascularization is performed in cases with bowel necrosis, aneurysm rupture, or failure of endovascular repair.

SRAD is also rare, and the most common presenting symptom is sudden-onset flank pain; it may cause uncontrolled blood pressure, renal infarction, and renal failure [2]. It may be caused by fibromuscular dysplasia, segmental arterial mediolysis, connective tissue disorder, or vasculitis. SRAD is difficult to diagnose because of its nonspecific symptoms. Renal ultrasound and Doppler have poor diagnostic sensitivity, so contrast-enhanced CT is the gold standard for diagnosis [3]. The treatment for SRAD has not been established, so treatment should be based on the patient's clinical presentation and the anatomical features of the dissection. Treatment includes supportive medical treatment, endovascular intervention, and surgery. Supportive therapy including control of hypertension and systemic anticoagulation has shown good outcomes, but there is still a risk of acute infarction or renovascular hypertension. Endovascular treatment is a good option because it can prevent both advancement of infarction and renovascular hypertension, and it has become safer as device technology has improved [4]. The potential complications of endovascular treatment are puncture site hematoma, development of dissection, renal artery thrombosis, or perforation. Contraindications for endovascular treatment is unstable hemodynamics. The intravascular ultrasound may be helpful for the evaluation of etiology [5].

A combination of spontaneous SMAD and SRAD is extremely rare [6, 7]. We cannot identify the etiology of this patient, but he may have an underlying condition like segmental arterial mediolysis, so regular follow-up with contrast-enhanced CT will be needed for such a case. Furthermore, if the patients have another abdominal or back pain, prompt workup like contrast-enhanced CT will be needed and proper interventions should be done immediately if necessary to prevent severe consequences like organ ischemia or hemorrhage.

4. Conclusion

A combination of spontaneous SMA dissection and SRAD is a very rare condition. Patients with isolated visceral artery dissection should be carefully followed up.

Consent

The patient consented for publication.

References

[1] M. N. Tameo, M. J. Dougherty, and K. D. Calligaro, "Spontaneous dissection with rupture of the superior mesenteric artery from segmental arterial mediolysis," *Journal of Vascular Surgery*, vol. 53, no. 4, pp. 1107–1112, 2011.

[2] F. Afshinnia, B. Sundaram, P. Rao, J. Stanley, and M. Bitzer, "Evaluation of characteristics, associations and clinical course of isolated spontaneous renal artery dissection," *Nephrology, Dialysis, Transplantation*, vol. 28, no. 8, pp. 2089–2098, 2013.

[3] S. P. Gandhi, K. Patel, and B. C. Pal, "Isolated spontaneous renal artery dissection presented with flank pain," *Case Reports in Radiology*, vol. 2015, Article ID 896706, 5 pages, 2015.

[4] G. Tandon and R. Sukhija, "Isolated spontaneous renal artery dissection: a case report and review," *International Journal of Angiology*, vol. 21, no. 2, pp. 99–102, 2012.

[5] B. Peynircioğlu, S. Pişkinkaya, Ç. Özer, B. Cil, C. Yorgancioglu, and M. Arici, "Isolated spontaneous renal artery dissection: diagnosis and endovascular management," *Diagnostic and Interventional Radiology*, vol. 17, no. 1, pp. 101–104, 2009.

[6] K. G. Srinivasan, S. Srivdya, P. Ushanandhini, and S. Ramprabanath, "Spontaneous isolated superior mesenteric artery dissection - report of two cases," *Journal of Radiology Case Reports*, vol. 3, no. 9, pp. 6–13, 2009.

[7] T. Sugiura, K. Imoto, K. Uchida et al., "Fibromuscular dysplasia associated with simultaneous spontaneous dissection of four peripheral arteries in a 30-year-old man," *Annals of Vascular Surgery*, vol. 25, no. 6, pp. 838.e9–838.e11, 2011.

24

Endovascular Treatment of Venous Bypass Graft Pseudoaneurysm with the New Solaris Self-Expanding Covered Stent

Enrique M. San Norberto[1], **Liliana A. Fidalgo-Domingos**,[1] **Noelia Cenizo**,[1] **Álvaro Revilla**,[1] **James H. Taylor**,[2] **and Carlos Vaquero**[1]

[1]*Department of Vascular Surgery, Valladolid University Hospital, Valladolid, Spain*
[2]*Department of Cardiac Surgery, Valencia General University Hospital, Valencia, Spain*

Correspondence should be addressed to Enrique M. San Norberto; esannorberto@hotmail.com

Academic Editor: Muzaffer Sindel

Nonanastomotic pseudoaneurysm formation after vascular reconstruction is a rarely encountered problem. Covered stent graft constitutes a minimal approach. To our knowledge, the present study constitutes the first case of implantation of Solaris stent graft in Europe. A 69-year-old man with severe cardiac dysfunction presented a pseudoaneurysm of a popliteal to popliteal artery reversed saphenous vein bypass graft. The patient was successfully treated by the percutaneous placement of a Solaris self-expanding covered stent. The postimplantation arteriogram demonstrated exclusion of the pseudoaneurysm, complete apposition of the stent, and adequate runoff. No complications occurred, and the patient was discharged from the hospital one day later receiving 75 mg of clopidogrel. Endovascular exclusion by covered stent deployment offers a safe, rapid, and minimally invasive alternative to open surgical resection in patients with lower limb venous graft pseudoaneurysm. The Solaris covered stent provides a new catheter-based device with adequate navigability and exceptional accurate delivery system.

1. Introduction

Complications of procedures requiring saphenous vein grafts include stenosis, thrombosis, infection, and aneurysmal degeneration with or without late graft rupture [1]. Pseudoaneurysm formation is the result of an injury to the arterial wall that allows extravasation of blood, but that is contained by the adventitia or surrounding perivascular soft tissue. Nonanastomotic pseudoaneurysm formation after vascular reconstruction is a rarely encountered problem in the treatment of peripheral arterial disease. Pseudoaneurysms can, if left untreated, be complicated by thrombosis, rupture, or distal embolization [1, 2].

Although traditional treatment includes open surgical repair, minimally invasive methods such as thrombin injection, ultrasound-guided compression, embolization, and stent graft repair have been described. To our knowledge, the case described constitutes the first case of implantation of a Solaris stent graft in Europe. This Brazilian stent graft is more radiopaque than other conventional nitinol stents, and its unique delivery system prevents migration during its implantation.

2. Case Presentation

A 69-year-old man with severe cardiac dysfunction, hypertension, and hypercholesterolemia presented with bruising, tenderness, pain, and a palpable mass in the left knee. On physical examination, he had a large pulsatile mass on the posterior aspect of the knee; the popliteal, posterior tibial, and dorsalis pedis vessels had a palpable pulse, and Doppler signals were triphasic in all of them. Nine years ago, the patient was admitted to the Vascular Surgery Department for treatment of a popliteal aneurysm and a popliteal to popliteal artery with inverted saphenous vein bypass graft, and exclusion of the aneurysm was performed. A contrast-

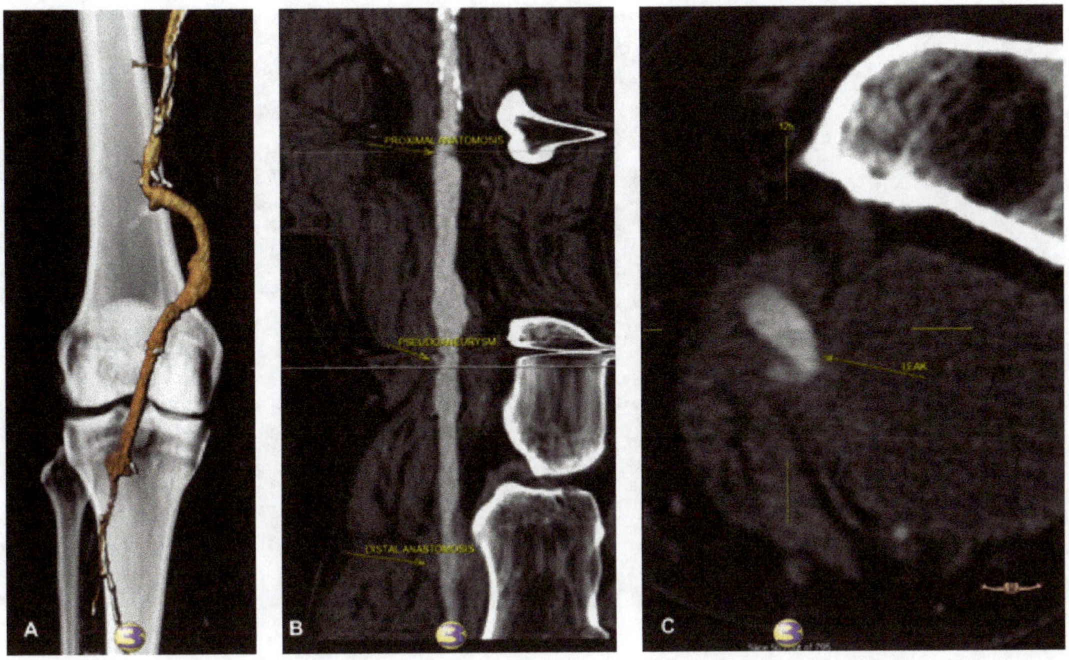

(a) (b) (c)

FIGURE 1: (a) 3D CT scan reconstruction showed a pseudoaneurysm of the popliteal-popliteal artery vein bypass graft. (b) Centre lumen line reconstruction for venous bypass graft pseudoaneurysm evaluation. (c) Pseudoaneurysm of the venous bypass graft with a 7.2 × 5 cm of maximum diameter.

enhanced computed tomography (angio-CT) demonstrated a pseudoaneurysm of the venous bypass graft (Figure 1) with a 7.2 × 5 cm of maximum diameter.

Through a right common femoral artery access with a 9 Fr contralateral sheath (Flexor, Cook Inc., Bloomington, USA), the selective catheterization of the popliteal to popliteal artery venous bypass graft was achieved using a 5 Fr catheter (TrailBlazer Support Catheter; Medtronic, Santa Rosa, USA) and a 0.035-inch angled hydrophilic wire (Radifocus M; Terumo, Leuven, Belgium). Angiography confirmed the presence of a pseudoaneurysm of the venous bypass graft adjacent to the knee joint and a large pseudoaneurysm in the distal left thigh (Figure 2). A second stiffer wire (Rosen, Cook Inc., Bloomington, USA) was exchanged through the catheter to facilitate the placement of an 8 × 80 mm self-expanding covered stent (Solaris, Scitech Medical, Brasil). The subsequent arteriogram demonstrated exclusion of the pseudoaneurysm, complete apposition of the stent, and adequate runoff. Pulse exam was comparable to preoperative examination with triphasic Doppler signals.

After the procedure, no complications occurred and the patient was discharged from the hospital one day later receiving 75 mg of clopidogrel. One-month duplex ultrasound follow-up confirmed persistent thrombosis of the pseudoaneurysm and stent patency.

3. Discussion

Pseudoaneurysm formation due to vein graft rupture is a rare complication described as a late complication of coronary and peripheral arterial bypass grafting [1, 2]. The clinical presentation of a popliteal pseudoaneurysm may vary from an asymptomatic pulsatile mass to acute or chronic limb ischemia, bleeding secondary to rupture or leg pain. The aetiology of this condition is uncertain, but it can occur owing to slippage from one of the tributaries of the saphenous veins, vein wall degeneration, or infection.

The treatment of cases of vein graft rupture should likely be surgical with preservation of distal flow [2]. Many infrainguinal bypass grafts are in a subcutaneous position, making surgical repair the most expeditious and desirable procedure. Other minimally invasive treatment options include ultrasound-guided compression, percutaneous thrombin injection, and endovascular treatment [3, 4]. In high-risk patients, an endovascular approach is a practical therapeutic method and offers an attractive option because it avoids the need for reoperation in a previously scarred area. Implantation of covered stents or glue embolization has been described. In our view, when faced with an especially large pseudoaneurysm, stent graft repair becomes the superior choice to other minimally invasive methods.

Covered stents can be either Dacron or polytetrafluoroethylene (PTFE), and they are used mainly for the treatment of traumatic arterial lesions, arteriovenous fistulas, aneurysms, and pseudoaneurysms or for the treatment of obstructive vascular disease of the aortoiliac and femoropopliteal sectors [5]. The covered stent Solaris (Scitech Medical, Brasil) is indicated in stenosis of AV fistulas, postangioplasty arterial dissection, in-stent restenosis, fenestrated prostheses, and vascular trauma [6, 7]. The Solaris system has been presented as a new covered stent with high flexibility designed for higher conformability, optimized radial force with a proximal and distal bare stent to minimize the migration risk, electrospinning PTFE ultrathin membrane

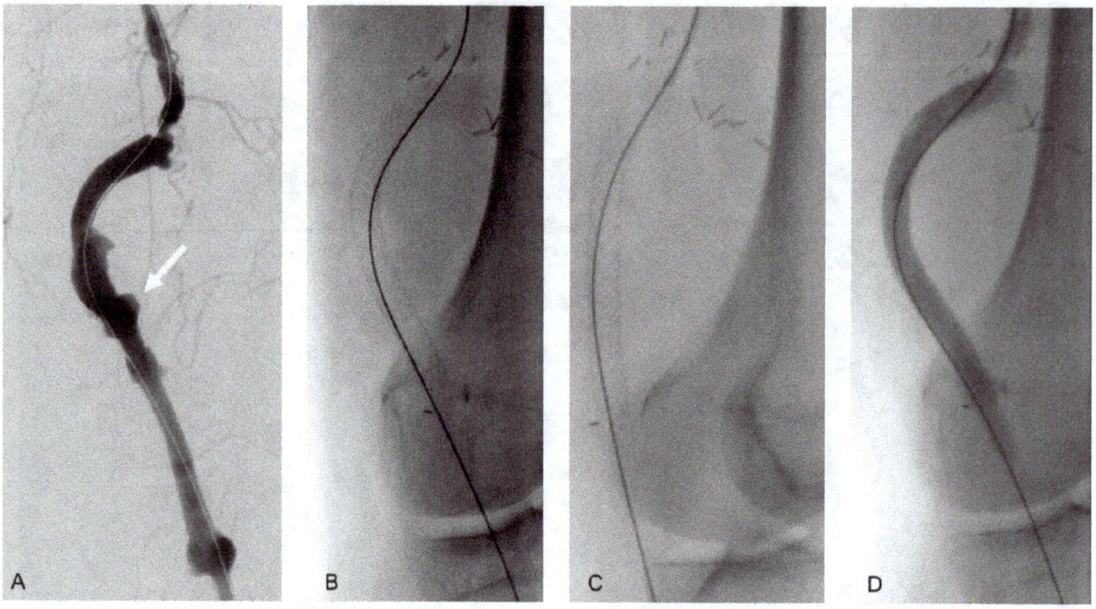

(a) (b) (c) (d)

Figure 2: Posteroanterior digital subtraction angiograms of the popliteal to popliteal artery vein bypass graft. (a) Pseudoaneurysm of the vein graft (white arrow). (b) Solaris covered stent deployed into the vein bypass graft, posteroanterior view. (c) Solaris covered stent deployed into the vein bypass graft, lateral view. (d) Control angiogram showing exclusion of the pseudoaneurysm.

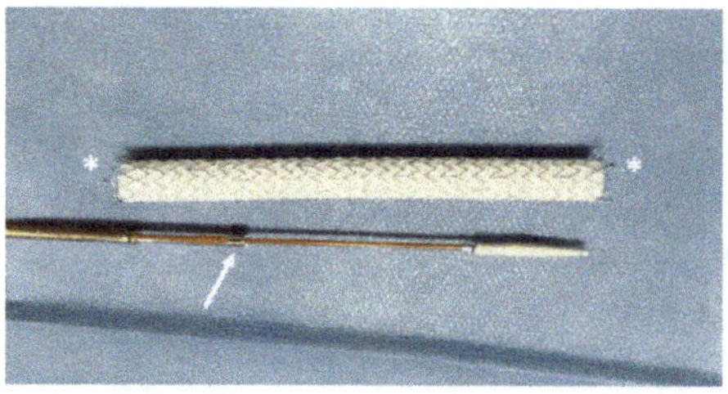

Figure 3: Solaris self-expanding covered stent. Arrow: antijumping system; asterisk: tantalum proximal and distal marker bands at uncovered stents at the ends.

encapsulating a nitinol stent structure with instantaneous sealing, and minimal shortening during deployment with an accurate delivery system (Figure 3). The pull-back hydrophilic delivery system provides superior navigability, and its antijumping system guarantees accurate deployment during the procedure. The Solaris device is configured in diameters of 6 to 9 mm and lengths of 40 to 100 mm. This stent graft has been used for the treatment of vascular trauma, aneurysmal disease, and occlusive peripheral disease.

Follow-up of this technique should be assessed by a duplex ultrasound or CT angiography surveillance program to detect late sequelae such as stent thrombosis, kinking, strut fracture, endoleak, or stent graft migration.

4. Conclusion

Endovascular exclusion with covered stent deployment offers a safe, rapid, and minimally invasive alternative to the open surgical resection in patients with lower limb venous graft pseudoaneurysms. The Solaris covered stent provides a new catheter-based minimally invasive device to the treatment of aneurysms, pseudoaneurysms, or stenotic vascular disease, with adequate navigability and an exceptional accurate delivery system.

Acknowledgments

The authors thank Raul Moro and Patricia Mesonero (superior technicians in image for diagnosis, Valladolid University Hospital) for their assistance during interventional procedures.

References

[1] L. E. Erdoes, "Spontaneous vein graft rupture after infrainguinal vascular reconstruction: report of three cases," *The American Surgeon*, vol. 74, no. 3, pp. 210–213, 2008.

[2] D. B. Davra, C. P. S Sravan, Vivekan et al., "Degenerative venous aneurysm of a reverse saphenous vein femoral artery to femoral artery cross over graft: case report and literature review of saphenous vein graft aneurysm," *Indian Journal of Vascular and Endovascular Surgery*, vol. 4, no. 4, pp. 169–172, 2017.

[3] A. Carollo, G. Gagliardo, P. M. DeVito, and M. Cicchillo, "Stent graft repair of anastomotic pseudoaneurysm of femoral–popliteal bypass graft following patch angioplasty," *Journal of Surgical Case Reports*, vol. 2016, no. 12, pp. 1–3, 2016.

[4] S. Garge, P. Vyas, K. Rathod, S. Jaggi, and I. Talwar, "Leaking pseudoaneurysm of lower limb saphenous vein graft: a rare complication and its successful treatment by endovascular embolization," *BJR|case reports*, vol. 3, no. 1, article 20150445, 2017.

[5] S. Hajibandeh, S. Hajibandeh, S. A. Antoniou, F. Torella, and G. A. Antoniou, "Covered vs uncovered stents for aortoiliac

and femoropopliteal arterial disease: a systematic review and meta-analysis," *Journal of Endovascular Therapy*, vol. 23, no. 3, pp. 442–452, 2016.

[6] M. Salvaji, M. Rajachandran, and K. Klym, "A quick fix: graft rescue for iatrogenic pseudoaneuysm," *The Journal of Invasive Cardiology*, vol. 19, pp. E19–E22, 2007.

[7] R. M. Ishii, C. H. Guillaux, R. Spósito, A. C. Silveira, H. L. Martinez Franco, and F. Folino, "Solaris stent angioplasty: an alternative to endovascular treatment in the femoropopliteal territory," *Vascular and Endovascular Surgery*, vol. 52, p. S12, 2018.

25

Carotid Thrombosis in a Crack Cocaine Smoker Woman

Mattia Cosenza, Luigi Panza, Anna Paola Califano, Carolina Defendini, Maria D'Andria, Roberto Romiti, Antonio Fabio Massimo Vainieri, and Sergio Morelli

Department of Internal Medicine and Atherosclerosis Prevention, University of Rome, La Sapienza, Italy

Correspondence should be addressed to Mattia Cosenza; mattia.cosenza@uniroma1.it

Academic Editor: Nilda Espinola-Zavaleta

Introduction. We report a case of stroke in a crack smoker with occlusion of the middle cerebral artery and a large thrombus in the carotid artery. *Case Presentation.* A 34-year-old female presented with left upper arm weakness, associated with paresthesia with onset of symptoms more than 24 hours before. Angio-RM sequences showed an area of ischemia, with occlusion of the M2 segment of the middle cerebral artery. Carotid ultrasound showed a soft plaque with distal end floating. Anticoagulant treatment was started, and seriated ultrasound evaluations showed its gradual dissolution. *Conclusions.* In atherothromboembolic stroke from carotid thrombosis, repeated ultrasound studies may be useful for either diagnosis and monitoring the efficacy of anticoagulant therapy.

1. Introduction

Cocaine use may be associated with stroke and carotid thrombosis. In the emergency setting, this abuse must be suspected in case of stroke of young adults. Accelerated atherosclerosis of carotid arteries can lead to thrombus formation. Whether the medical or surgical approach is to be preferred, it is unclear.

2. Case Presentation

A 34-years-old Caucasian female presented with left upper arm weakness associated with paresthesia. The symptoms had started about 24 hours before, on waking.

Physical examination revealed left hemiparesis, with diminished left upper (2/5) and lower (3/5) strength, and extensor plantar response on the left side. There were no cerebellar signs, and the cranial nerve examination was normal. The electrocardiogram showed normal sinus rhythm at 70 beats per minute, and blood pressure values were 160/90 mmHg. No other remarkable signs were present.

Cranial multimodal computed tomography (CT) imaging was performed, showing no sign of cerebral hemorrhage and hypodensity on cortical and subcortical right frontoparietal regions, compatible with ischemic stroke. Thrombolysis was not performed because of the remote onset of the symptoms. Cranial Magnetic Resonance Imaging (MRI) showed an area of ischemia in the acute/subacute phase, without hemorrhagic infarction, with occlusion of the M2 segment of the middle cerebral artery. She was given a loading dose of acetylsalicylic acid and transferred to our division.

Collecting a complete medical history, the patient revealed to be a habitual consumer of substances like heroine, methadone, cocaine, and alcohol; moreover, in the night before the episode, she had smoked crack cocaine. A toxicological screen resulted positive for cocaine and opioids. ECG and cardiac ultrasound were normal.

Carotid ultrasound (CU) showed a huge homogeneous soft plaque with an irregular surface, protrusive morphology, and circumferential blood flow at the distal end, inside the internal carotid artery (Figure 1).

Enoxaparin at the dosage of 100 U/kg twice/day was started, followed by warfarin therapy. Seriated CUs showed gradual dissolution of the thrombus (Figure 1). Her symptoms gradually improved during the next weeks, and she was discharged from the hospital in good general conditions. However, the patient continued drug abusing, and a new cerebral stroke occurred the year after.

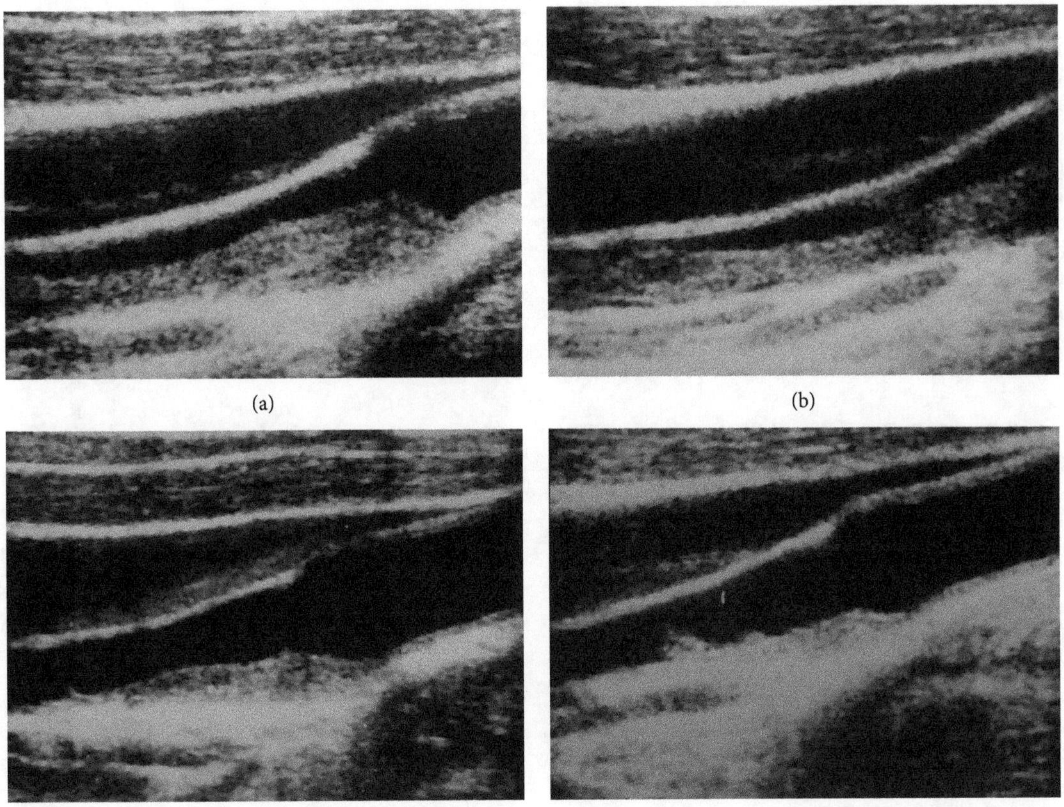

(a) (b) (c) (d)

Figure 1: (a, b) A huge homogeneous soft plaque with irregular surfaces and circumferential blood flow at the distal end along carotid bifurcation. (c) Image at 1 week after starting therapy. (d) Image at 2 weeks after anticoagulant.

3. Discussion

Stroke is a note complication of cocaine abuse [1]. The main peak in the description of cocaine-associated stroke happened in '80s-'90s, when crack use began. Crack cocaine has been associated with both ischemic and hemorrhagic stroke, whereas cocaine hydrochloride results more often in hemorrhagic events [2]. Recently, smoked cocaine intake was associated with stroke within 24 hours [3]. Ischemic infarctions usually affect the territories of midcerebral artery [4].

Many mechanisms may explain cocaine and crack cocaine neurotoxicity: vasospasm, endothelial damage, platelet dysfunction, and intracranial vasculitis [5]. When large vessels are involved, mechanisms include accelerated atherosclerosis with large lipid core [6]. Some authors suggest the possibility of vasospasm of large arteries and secondary intravascular thrombosis [7].

Free-floating thrombus is an uncommon condition, defined as an elongated thrombus attached to an arterial wall, with circumferential blood-flow at its distal end and cyclical motion relating to the cardiac cycle, with atherosclerosis as the most common etiology [8]. Both medical and surgical approaches were used, without clear evidence of the superiority of one over the other. In the last years, endovascular procedures were reported [9]. Nevertheless, medical therapy alone showed good results, and complete resolution of thrombosis was described [10–12].

To our knowledge, our case is the first that described the resolution of an intracarotid thrombus related to the assumption of crack-cocaine with medical therapy alone. The population of cocaine smokers is at high risk of stroke, and the management of these patients is complicated by low compliance and low adherence to therapy. The finding of a free-floating thrombus inside a supraaortic vessel is a hard clinical issue to face. The management of these patients is still uncertain, and more studies are required in this regard. Carotid ultrasound allowed to manage this patient-guiding therapy and follow-up.

References

[1] L. L. Cregler and H. Mark, "Medical complications of cocaine abuse," *The New England Journal of Medicine*, vol. 315, no. 23, pp. 1495–1500, 1986.

[2] S. R. Levine, J. C. Brust, N. Futrell et al., "Cerebrovascular complications of the use of the "crack" form of alkaloidal cocaine," *The New England Journal of Medicine*, vol. 323, no. 11, pp. 699–704, 1990.

[3] Y. C. Cheng, K. A. Ryan, S. A. Qadwai et al., "Cocaine use and risk of ischemic stroke in young adults," *Stroke*, vol. 47, no. 4, pp. 918–922, 2016, Epub 2016 Mar 10.

[4] S. Geibprasert, M. Gallucci, and T. Krings, "Addictive illegal drugs: structural neuroimaging," *AJNR. American Journal of Neuroradiology*, vol. 31, no. 5, pp. 803–808, 2010, Epub 2009 Oct 29.

[5] K. Bachi, V. Mani, D. Jeyachandran, Z. A. Fayad, R. Z. Goldstein, and N. Alia-Klein, "Vascular disease in cocaine addiction," *Atherosclerosis*, vol. 262, pp. 154–162, 2017, Epub 2017 Mar 14.

[6] J. Du, B. A. Wasserman, W. Tong et al., "Cholesterol is associated with the presence of a lipid core in carotid plaque of asymptomatic, young-to-middle-aged African Americans with and without HIV infection and cocaine use residing in inner-city Baltimore, Md., USA," *Cerebrovascular Diseases*, vol. 33, no. 3, pp. 295–301, 2012, Epub 2012 Feb 8.

[7] J. P. Konzen, S. R. Levine, and J. H. Garcia, "Vasospasm and thrombus formation as possible mechanisms of stroke related to alkaloidal cocaine," *Stroke*, vol. 26, no. 6, pp. 1114–1118, 1995.

[8] M. Roy, A. K. Roy, J. R. DeSanto, and M. Abdelsalam, "Free floating thrombus in carotid artery in a patient with recurrent strokes," *Case Reports in Medicine*, vol. 2017, Article ID 4932567, 4 pages, 2017, Epub 2017 Jan 10.

[9] N. Fitzpatrick, R. Motyer, B. Gibney et al., "Expanding the role of stent-retriever endovascular thrombectomy: a case series of free-floating thrombus," *Journal of NeuroInterventional Surgery*, vol. 10, no. 12, pp. 1164–1167, 2018, Epub 2018 Jun 20.

[10] A. K. Vellimana, Y. Kadkhodayan, K. M. Rich et al., "Symptomatic patients with intraluminal carotid artery thrombus: outcome with a strategy of initial anticoagulation," *Journal of Neurosurgery*, vol. 118, no. 1, pp. 34–41, 2013, Epub 2012 Oct 12.

[11] A. F. Bhatti, L. R. Leon Jr., N. Labropoulos et al., "Free-floating thrombus of the carotid artery: literature review and case reports," *Journal of Vascular Surgery*, vol. 45, no. 1, pp. 199–205, 2007.

[12] A. Gülcü, N. S. Gezer, S. Men, D. Öz, E. Yaka, and V. Öztürk, "Management of free-floating thrombus within the arcus aorta and supra-aortic arteries," *Clinical Neurology and Neurosurgery*, vol. 125, pp. 198–206, 2014, Epub 2014 Aug 15.

26

Acute Pulmonary Embolism Associated with Low-Dose Olanzapine in a Patient without Risk Factors for Venous Thromboembolism

Vu Hoang Vu,[1] Nguyen Duong Khang,[1] Mai Thanh Thao,[2] and Le Minh Khoi[1]

[1]*Cardiovascular Center, University Medical Center, University of Medicine and Pharmacy at Ho Chi Minh City, Vietnam*
[2]*Department of Radiology, University Medical Center, Ho Chi Minh City, Vietnam*

Correspondence should be addressed to Le Minh Khoi; khoi.lm@umc.edu.vn

Academic Editor: Muzaffer Sindel

Background. Olanzapine is a second-generation antipsychotic drug commonly prescribed for certain mental/mood conditions such as schizophrenia and bipolar disorders. This agent has been considered a precipitating factor for venous thromboembolism formation. Most of the cases previously reported were associated with high-dose olanzapine therapy or in patients with high-risk factors for the development of thromboembolism. *Case Presentation.* We report a patient who developed pulmonary embolism after a long course of low-dose olanzapine. A 66-year-old female patient suffering from insomnia had been prescribed olanzapine 2.5 mg and paroxetine 10 mg for two years. The patient suddenly developed a syncopal episode at home and was immediately brought to the hospital. The diagnosis of pulmonary embolism was made by chance during the computerized tomography of coronary arteries. The patient made a full recovery under conventional treatment and was discharged in stable condition. The thoracic computed tomography taken two months after discharge showed a completely normal pulmonary arterial tree. *Conclusion.* Olanzapine-associated pulmonary embolism is a rare entity and might be missed if the physician in charge is not vigilant and well informed. Even low-dose olanzapine can be associated with pulmonary embolism in patients with low classic risk factors if the treatment is prolonged. Pulmonary embolism should be sought in patients taking olanzapine even though the presenting manifestations are nonspecific.

1. Introduction

Venous thromboembolism is widely known as a common clinical entity with well-established classic risk factors, including but not limited to immobilization for more than three days, pregnancy, lower limb fracture, infection, cancer, and some medications. Olanzapine, a second-generation antipsychotic agent widely prescribed for patients with schizophrenia, has been recognized as a precipitating factor for venous thromboembolism [1, 2]. Most of the previous cases had been associated with high-dose olanzapine therapy or in patients with high-risk factors for the development of thromboembolism. We reported a patient without classic risk factors who developed symptomatic pulmonary embolism (PE) after being treated with low-dose olanzapine for insomnia.

2. Case Presentation

A 66-year-old female patient without a prior cardiovascular condition suddenly experienced a collapse for the first time and was reportedly unconscious for around 10 minutes. No abnormalities in facial expressions, limb weakness, drooling, or chest discomfort were noted during the crisis.

On admission to the emergency department, she was afebrile, alert, normotensive with a blood pressure of 135/82 mm Hg, a heart rate of 76 bpm, and nonobese with a BMI of 24.2 kg/m^2. Her oxygen saturation was 87% on room air. Physical examination showed no noticeable abnormalities. Complete blood cell count was in the normal range. Blood biochemistry, including blood urea nitrogen, creatinine, high-sensitive troponin T, and N-terminal pro-BNP, was all in the normal range. The non-ST elevated myocardial infarction was excluded. Due to the syncopal episode at home, a head computed tomography was then performed, showing an extradural hematoma due to the collapse, but no other cerebral malformation was noted. We decided to have a coronary computed tomography angiography performed that ruled out coronary artery disease but revealed a pulmonary embolism. Multiple emboli were noted, causing a subtotal occlusion of the distal segment of the right pulmonary artery (Figure 1). The left pulmonary artery was also partially occluded (Figure 2). A venous duplex scanning for proximal deep vein thrombosis was performed that revealed no venous clot. Due to the presence of PE, we proceeded to screen malignant diseases and autoimmune diseases and test the autoimmune antibodies and possible causes of hypercoagulopathy, which showed no abnormality. Retrospectively, we found that the patient had been taking olanzapine 2.5 mg daily for the previous two years for her insomnia. Olanzapine was then discontinued on the first day of hospitalization.

With the pulmonary embolism severity index (PESI) score of 66 points and the presence of an epidural hematoma, we decided to start continuous intravenous heparin for the first two days, followed by low molecular weight heparin for the next three days, and finally oral dabigatran 150 mg twice a day. The patient was discharged three weeks after the onset and has been regularly followed up at the outpatient clinic. During the follow-up period, she experienced no remarkable events. A computed tomographic pulmonary angiography ordered two months after her discharge showed complete resolution of the previously documented PE in the pulmonary arterial system (Figure 3). At the time of preparing this manuscript, the patient is still on oral Dabigatran.

3. Discussion

Olanzapine is a second-generation antipsychotic agent commonly prescribed for schizophrenia. Its typical side effects include weight gain, drowsiness, and other antimuscarinic effects. The association between antipsychotic agents and venous thromboembolism was first described in the 1950s [3]. Wagge and Gedde-Dahl [4] reported a clinical case of a 28-year-old male patient who developed after starting treatment with high-dose olanzapine. A case series also described the possible association between olanzapine and venous thromboembolism after a 2-week course of treatment in four patients. The doses of olanzapine in these patients ranged between 5 and 20 mg per day and lasted from seven weeks to 17 months [5, 6]. In clinical practice, if the physicians at the emergency department are not well informed, they may miss the early diagnosis of PE in patients taking olanzapine. Our emergency physician could not suspect the diagnosis of PE and did not proceed with the PE protocol by our institutional PE response team (PERT). The PE was incidentally

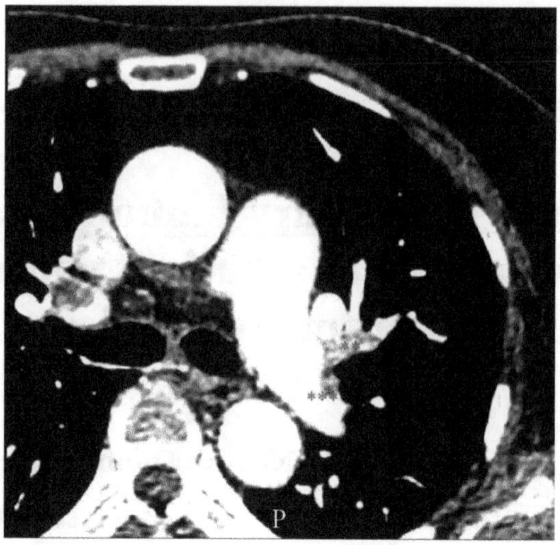

FIGURE 1: The spiral computed tomography angiogram obtained with highly concentrated contrast material and high flow technique showed multiple pulmonary emboli that subtotally occluded the right upper lobar pulmonary artery (*) and the left lingular artery (**). The left lower lobar pulmonary artery was also partially occluded (***).

established upon the thoracic CT to investigate the coronary artery system.

The mechanism by which olanzapine triggers or precipitates the thromboembolic conditions remains unknown. The olanzapine-induced metabolic changes such as dyslipidaemias, hyperleptinemia, hyperglycaemia, and hyperhomocysteinemia might, in part, account for a decreased thrombolysis but hardly responsible for the venous thromboembolism events [3]. Olanzapine is a 5-hydroxytryptamine receptor antagonist. Therefore, it may raise the blood serotonin leading to accelerated platelet aggregation and increased thromboembolic risk.

Our patient did not present any classic thrombotic risk factors (e.g., immobility, fracture, myocardial infarction, history of previous thromboembolism, malignant diseases, and hypercoagulable conditions). Thereby, we strongly suspected that it was associated with olanzapine. Of importance, the olanzapine dose in this patient was considerably low, only at 2.5 mg daily. Some case reports did recognize the thromboembolic events in patients taking olanzapine. However, the lowest dose reported in these observations was 5 mg per day. Like our case, these reports did not document any other thrombotic risk factors, except obesity in two patients. Our observation would emphasize the association between the oral olanzapine, even at a low dose, and thromboembolic events.

The management of olanzapine-associated venous thromboembolism consists of olanzapine discontinuation and guideline-based anticoagulation [7]. Our patient had a PESI score of 66 and an epidural hematoma secondary to falling at home; therefore, we decided to start continuous intravenous heparin but not thrombolytic therapy. This therapeutic approach proved effective: the patient became asymptomatic, and the pulmonary arterial tree was cleared of thrombus.

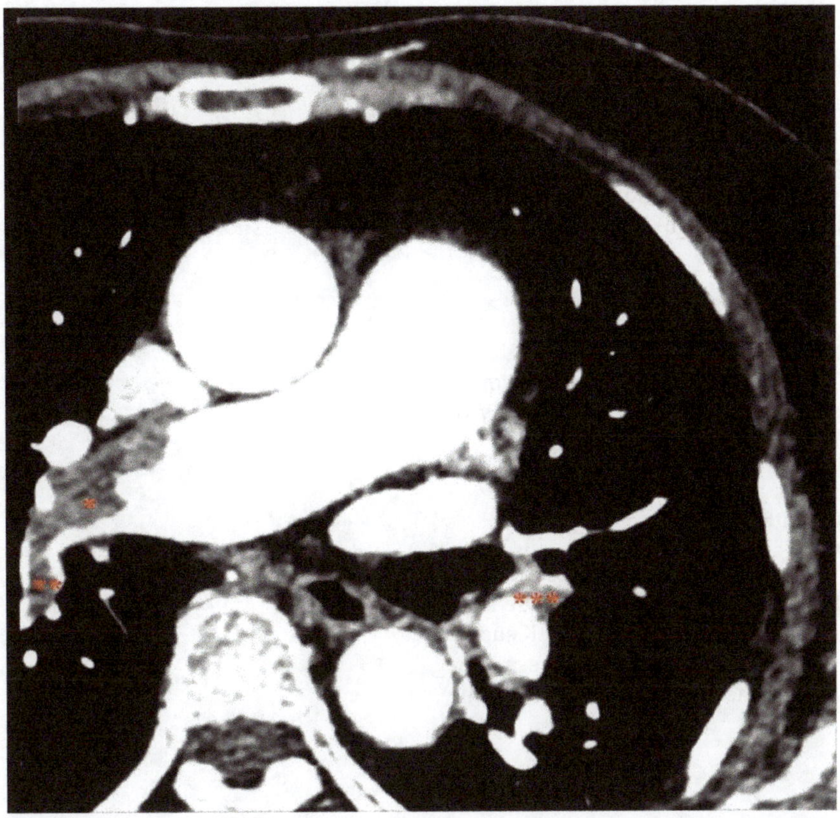

FIGURE 2: The spiral computed tomography angiogram obtained with highly concentrated contrast material and high flow technique showed multiple pulmonary emboli that partially occluded the right lower lobar pulmonary artery (*), the right lower lobar superior/apical segment (S6), and the left lower lobar anteromedial segment (S7-8) (***).

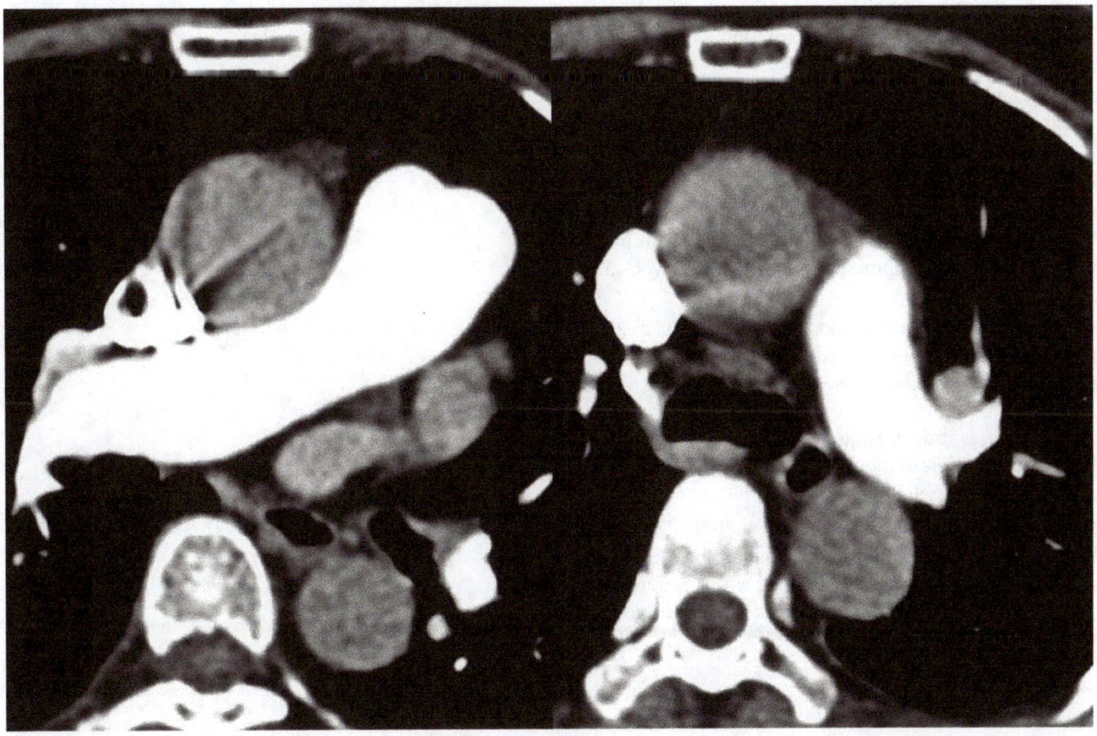

FIGURE 3: The spiral computed tomography angiogram obtained with highly concentrated contrast material and high flow technique showed that the contrast material filled the right pulmonary arterial system, and there was no embolus as previously documented in Figure 2.

4. Conclusion

Olanzapine-associated is a rare entity and might be missed if the physician in charge is not vigilant and well informed. Our report emphasized that even low-dose olanzapine can be associated with if the treatment is prolonged. Deep vein thrombosis and pulmonary embolism should be sought in patients taking olanzapine even though the presenting manifestations are atypical.

Disclosure

The current work was performed as part of the employment of the authors at University Medical Center, University of Medicine and Pharmacy at Ho Chi Minh City, Vietnam.

Authors' Contributions

V.H.V. conceived the presented idea. N.D.K. collected the data and drafted the first manuscript. M.P.T. analysed the computed tomographic pulmonary angiogram. L.M.K supervised the findings of this work and completed the manuscript. All authors discussed the results and approved the final manuscript.

References

[1] C. Barbui, V. Conti, and A. Cipriani, "Antipsychotic drug exposure and risk of venous thromboembolism: a systematic review and meta-analysis of observational studies," *Drug Safety*, vol. 37, no. 2, pp. 79–90, 2014.

[2] S. Hägg, A. Bate, M. Stahl, and O. Spigset, "Associations between venous thromboembolism and antipsychotics. A study of the WHO database of adverse drug reactions," *Drug Safety*, vol. 31, no. 8, pp. 685–694, 2008.

[3] R. Liperoti, C. Pedone, K. L. Lapane, V. Mor, R. Bernabei, and G. Gambassi, "Venous thromboembolism among elderly patients treated with atypical and conventional antipsychotic agents," *Archives of Internal Medicine*, vol. 165, no. 22, pp. 2677–2682, 2005.

[4] I. M. Waage and A. Gedde-Dahl, "Pulmonary embolism possibly associated with olanzapine treatment," *BMJ*, vol. 327, no. 7428, p. 1384, 2003.

[5] R. Maly, J. Masopust, L. Hosak, and A. Urban, "Four cases of venous thromboembolism associated with olanzapine," *Psychiatry and Clinical Neurosciences*, vol. 63, no. 1, pp. 116–118, 2009.

[6] T. Hägg, P. Tätting, and O. Spigset, "Olanzapine and venous thromboembolism," *International Clinical Psychopharmacology*, vol. 18, no. 5, pp. 299-300, 2003.

[7] S. V. Konstantinides, G. Meyer, C. Becattini et al., "2019 ESC Guidelines for the diagnosis and management of acute pulmonary embolism developed in collaboration with the European Respiratory Society (ERS)," *European Heart Journal*, vol. 41, no. 4, pp. 543–603, 2020.

27

Off-Label use of a Double-Layer Micromesh Carotid Stent for Hybrid Treatment of Popliteal Artery Aneurism Complicated by Chronic Distal Embolization

Sorin Barat[1] **and Dumitru Casian**[2]

[1]*Division of Vascular and Endovascular Surgery, Republican Clinical Hospital, 29 Nicolae Testemitanu Str., Chisinau, Moldova*
[2]*Department of General Surgery Nr.3, Vascular Surgery Clinic, Nicolae Testemitanu State University of Medicine and Pharmacy, 165 Stefan cel Mare si Sfant Bd., Chisinau, Moldova*

Correspondence should be addressed to Dumitru Casian; dumitru.casian@usmf.md

Academic Editor: Antonio Silvestro

We report our initial experience in off-label use of the double-layer micromesh (DLM) Roadsaver® stent for the hybrid treatment of a fusiform popliteal artery aneurism complicated by distal embolization and chronic limb threatening ischemia in a COVID-19-positive young male. A 36-year-old male patient was admitted with chronic limb threatening ischemia of the left lower limb. The duplex ultrasound and computer tomography angiography (CTA) demonstrated a fusiform popliteal artery aneurism with a maximal diameter of 14 mm and distal occlusion of peroneal and both tibial arteries. Urgent hybrid intervention was performed, starting with an open thrombectomy from the distal posterior tibial artery via a retromalleolar access followed by percutaneous deployment of the DLM Roadsaver® stent (Terumo, Tokyo, Japan) for the exclusion of the popliteal artery aneurism. The flow diverting effect was observed immediately with contrast stagnation in the asymmetrical part of the aneurism sac (grade C2 of the O'Kelly-Marotta flow diversion scale). The procedure was uneventful, with the regaining of an adequate foot perfusion and palpable pulse at the posterior tibial artery. On the 2nd postoperative day, the patient was diagnosed with a symptomatic form of COVID-19 infection and transferred to a dedicated facility. At a one-month follow-up, the patient had no symptoms of limb ischemia and CTA showed complete thrombosis of the aneurism sac, absence of endoleaks, and patency of the treated arterial segment. This case demonstrates the possibility of off-label use of the DLM Roadsaver® stent for hybrid treatment of popliteal artery aneurism complicated by distal embolization and critical limb ischemia.

1. Introduction

Popliteal artery aneurysms, defined as a focal dilatation with a diameter more than 50% of the reference vessel diameter, account for 85% of all peripheral aneurisms. Complications occur in up to 30% cases of untreated popliteal aneurysms and are associated with a high risk of limb loss. These include aneurism thrombosis and distal embolization, manifested by acute or chronic limb ischemia, compression syndrome, and rupture. The rate of amputation due to runoff vessel occlusion is up to 15% [1, 2].

All symptomatic popliteal artery aneurisms require treatment because of the high incidence of limb loss. Asymptomatic aneurisms with a diameter greater than 2 cm are considered indication for elective aneurism repair. Open repair via a medial or posterior approach represents the standard treatment for large or symptomatic popliteal artery aneurysms and consist in aneurysm exclusion with autologous or prosthetic bypass grafting. Recently, percutaneous implantation of the PTFE-covered stents is considered an alternative approach associated with low perioperative morbidity and mortality [3].

We describe a clinical case of hybrid treatment of complicated small popliteal artery aneurysm by tibial thrombectomy and off-label use of a double-layer micromesh (DLM) stent.

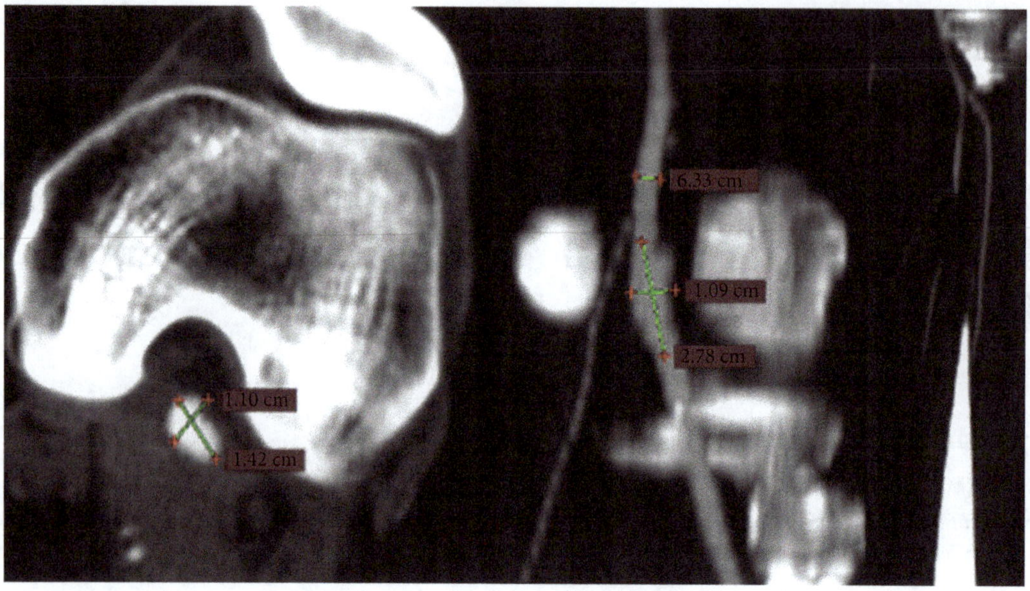

Figure 1: Computer tomography angiography demonstrating fusiform aneurysm of the left popliteal artery with a maximal diameter of 14 mm and distal occlusion of tibial and peroneal arteries.

2. Case Report

A 36-year-old male was admitted to the division of vascular surgery with clinical signs of chronic limb threatening ischemia Rutherford grade 4, with an onset of symptoms beyond 3 months. At physical examination, the left foot was hypothermic and pulseless, with a delayed capillary refill. The ankle-brachial pressure index (ABI) was 0.5. The emergency duplex ultrasound and CT angiography demonstrated an eccentric fusiform aneurysm of the left P2 popliteal artery with a maximal diameter of 14 mm, complicated by distal embolic occlusion of all three runoff vessels (Figure 1). The ipsi- and contralateral saphenous veins were considered unsuitable for bypass (<3 mm diameter), based on the results of preoperative duplex ultrasound. The decision was to perform a hybrid lower limb revascularization: open tibial thrombectomy and endovascular repair of the aneurysm. The Roadsaver® DLM carotid stent was selected for percutaneous implantation counting on its superior flexibility, easiness of deployment, and possibility of resheathing. Informed consent was obtained from the patient for off-label use of the carotid stent in the popliteal position.

During surgery, the posterior tibial artery was dissected via retromalleolar access and direct and indirect thrombectomy was performed, regaining an adequate arterial backflow. The arteriotomy was closed using an autologous venous patch. Completion angiography demonstrated a residual stenosis of the posterior tibial artery, and a balloon angioplasty was performed resulting in a satisfactory runoff (Figure 2). The intervention was continued by percutaneous implantation of an 8-40 mm Roadsaver® carotid stent in the popliteal artery via an antegrade femoral approach. The deployment was uneventful, and the immediate flow diversion effect was encountered, with the presence of the flow stagnation between the aneurism wall and the stent, corresponding to grade C2 of the O'Kelly-Marotta flow diversion scale (Figure 3). Thus, reestablishment of an adequate foot perfusion and palpable pulse on the posterior tibial artery was obtained. On the 2nd postoperative day, the patient had fever and the polymerase chain reaction test of the nasopharyngeal swab confirmed SARS-CoV-2 infection. The patient was diagnosed with a symptomatic form of COVID-19 and transferred to a dedicated facility for isolation and treatment. Taking into account the increased risk of thrombotic complications among patients infected with new coronavirus, triple antithrombotic treatment was initiated during hospitalization (clopidogrel 75 mg, dipyridamole 300 mg, and enoxaparine 60 mg). The patient was discharged on the 14th postoperative day with recommendations to continue dual antiplatelet therapy combined with 10 mg of rivaroxaban per day for one month.

At a one-month follow-up, the patient was completely asymptomatic, with palpable pulse at the posterior tibial artery, slightly delayed capillary refill (3 sec), and an ABI of 0.9. The CT angiography showed complete exclusion of the aneurism and preserved patency of the posterior tibial artery (Figure 4).

3. Discussion

The primary aim of the intervention for complicated popliteal artery aneurysm is the complete aneurysm exclusion and revascularization of the lower limb. Surgical bypass to the distal popliteal or infrapopliteal arteries using a good-quality saphenous vein is considered a preferential approach. If autologous conduit is not available, the prosthetic conduit can be used, yielding comparable primary and secondary patency [4]. During the last decades, endovascular techniques have gained popularity in popliteal artery aneurysm repair as an alternative to an open surgical approach. In the presented case, we preferred an "endovascular first" approach considering the young age of the patient and the absence of adequate saphenous conduit. In our view, open repair would exclude the possibility of endovascular reintervention if the synthetic graft would have eventually occluded.

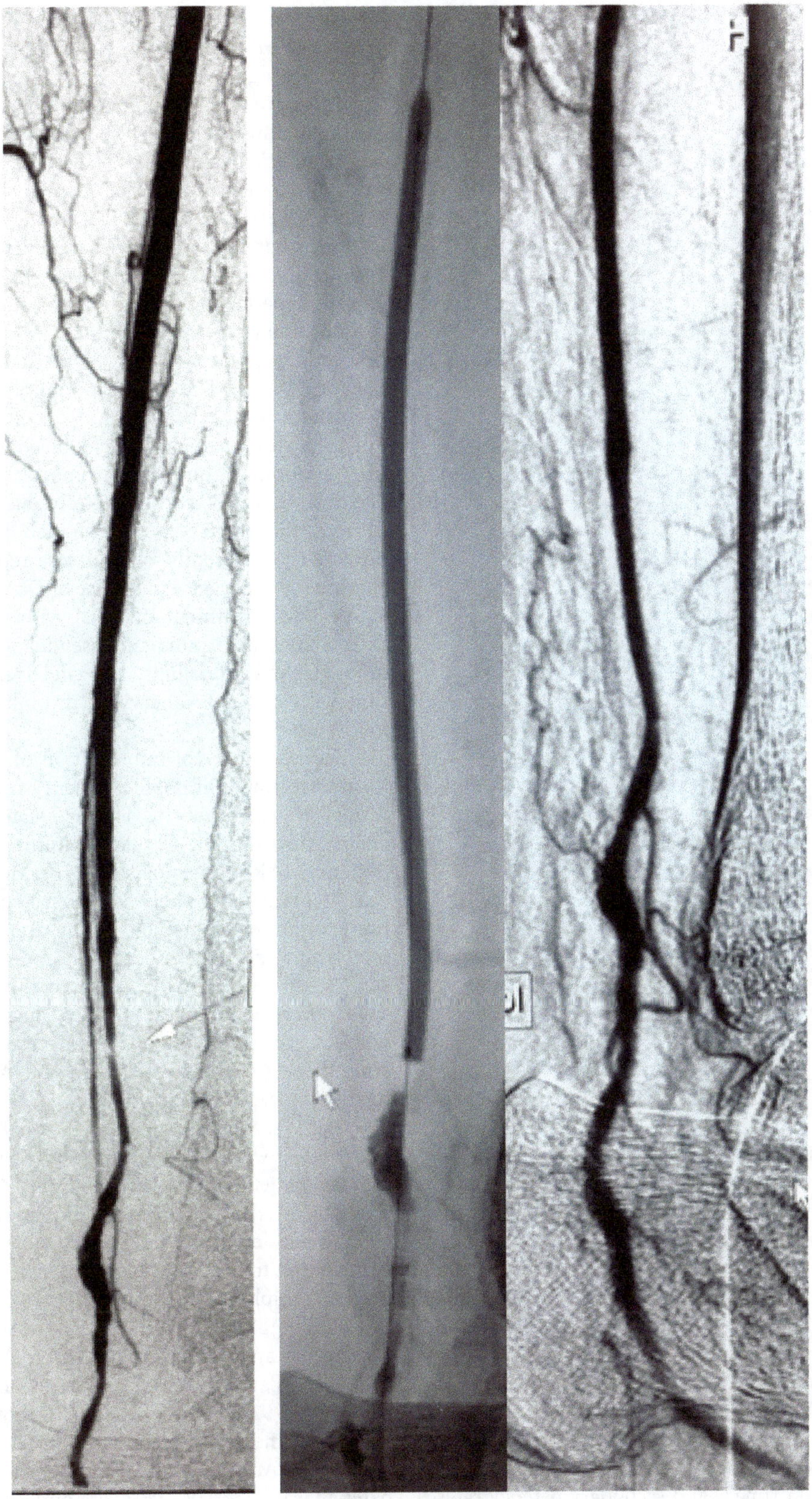

(a) (b)

FIGURE 2: Completion angiography after open thrombectomy: residual stenosis of the posterior tibial artery treated with balloon angioplasty.

Recent studies show that percutaneous implantation of covered stents is a safe and effective technique for the treatment of popliteal artery aneurysms, especially in high-risk patients. The advantages of endovascular treatment include shorter hospital stay and operative time compared to open surgery. Disadvantages include a higher 30-day graft

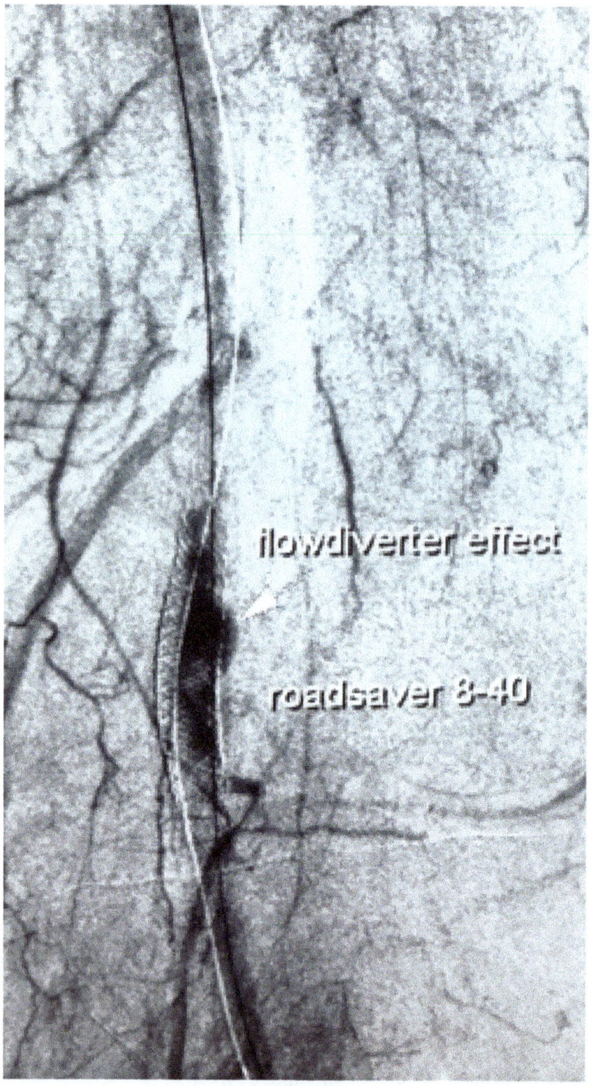

Figure 3: Flow diversion effect after stent implantation: flow stagnation between the aneurism wall and the stent, corresponding to the grade C2 of the O'Kelly-Marotta scale.

thrombosis rate (9% in the endovascular treatment group vs. 2% in the open surgery group) and a higher 30-day reintervention rate (9% in the endovascular treatment group versus 4% in the open surgical treatment group) [1, 5]. A meta-analysis of 14 studies, reporting 4880 popliteal aneurism repairs, demonstrated better primary patency for open surgery compared to endovascular treatment with no difference in secondary patency at one and three years [6].

A systematic review by Patel et al., regarding the current status of Hemobahn/Viabahn endografts for the treatment of popliteal aneurysms, reported outcomes from 514 PAAs. There was considerable heterogenicity in reporting standards among studies. Pooled primary and secondary patency rates were 69.4% (95% CI 63.3% to 76.2%) and 77.4% (95% CI 70.1% to 85.3%), respectively, at 5 years. Five studies (including only one randomized controlled trial) compared surgical to endovascular repair with no difference in primary patency on evidence synthesis (hazard ratio 1.30, 95% CI 0.79 to 12.14, $p = 0.189$) [7].

Another promising endovascular approach for popliteal artery aneurism repair is the use of uncovered stents with a flow diverting effect.

There are a small number of published studies regarding the use of flow diversion effect in the peripheral arterial circulation, especially in the popliteal arterial segment. In a review, by summarizing the data of 12 published articles, the flow diverters were used for the treatment of extracranial arterial aneurysms in 35 patients. The aneurysms were located in the hepatic ($n = 12$), splenic ($n = 6$), renal ($n = 5$), celiac ($n = 4$), superior mesenteric ($n = 3$), subclavian ($n = 2$), gastroduodenal ($n = 1$), and popliteal ($n = 1$) arteries and in the descending thoracic ($n = 1$), suprarenal ($n = 1$), and infrarenal aorta ($n = 2$). The 30-day mortality was 5.7%. Three stent occlusions occurred, and none of them have clinical consequences. Thirty patients were followed up for a mean interval of 9.2 months. Complete thrombosis of the aneurism sac occurred in 90.6%, and diameter reduction was observed in 81% of the aneurysms. No branch vessel occlusion was observed [8]. Recently, several case reports were published sharing the experience in the use of DLM stents (Roadsaver®, Casper) for treatment of renal, visceral, and supra-aortic extracranial aneurysms and pseudoaneurysms. All authors report technical feasibility and effectiveness of the intervention with complete aneurysm thrombosis at a short-term follow-up [9–12].

The experience of implantation of flow diverting stents for the treatment of popliteal aneurysms is also limited, and results are not uniform. Thakar treated 6 popliteal artery aneurysms using the Cardiatis Multilayer Aneurysm Repair System (MARS). Imaging studies performed after the procedure demonstrated aneurysm exclusion, graft patency, and preservation of branch and runoff arterial flow. There were one symptomatic stent occlusion and one leak through the stent struts into the sac with no branch outflow identified. Two other symptomatic stent occlusions were diagnosed within a 6-week follow-up period, resulting in 3 occlusions among the 6 devices deployed [13]. A similar study performed by Serracino-Inglott showed a primary patency of 50% and secondary patency in only two-thirds of the patients. However, the author states that "…one must note that the patient I managed who ended up with two blocked popliteal MARS had been diagnosed with metastatic lung carcinoma, and it is therefore possible that this may have contributed to a pro-thrombotic state, even though he was on dual antiplatelet therapy" [14].

Ucci et al. reported 23 consecutive patients with 25 popliteal artery aneurysms treated with multilayer flow modulators (Cardiatis). Complete aneurysm sac thrombosis occurred in 92.9% of the cases at 18 months. Freedom from sac enlargement was 100% (with 17 cases of aneurysm sac shrinkage). At 1, 6, 12, and 24 months, the estimated primary patency was 95.7%, 87.3%, 77%, and 70.1%, respectively. At the same intervals, primary assisted patency was 95.7%, 91.3%, 86%, and 86%, respectively, and secondary patency was 100%, 95.7%, 90.3%, and 90.3%, respectively. The collateral vessel patency was preserved in 72.4%. The authors report one case of stent fracture in an asymptomatic patient [15]. Promising results of percutaneous treatment of

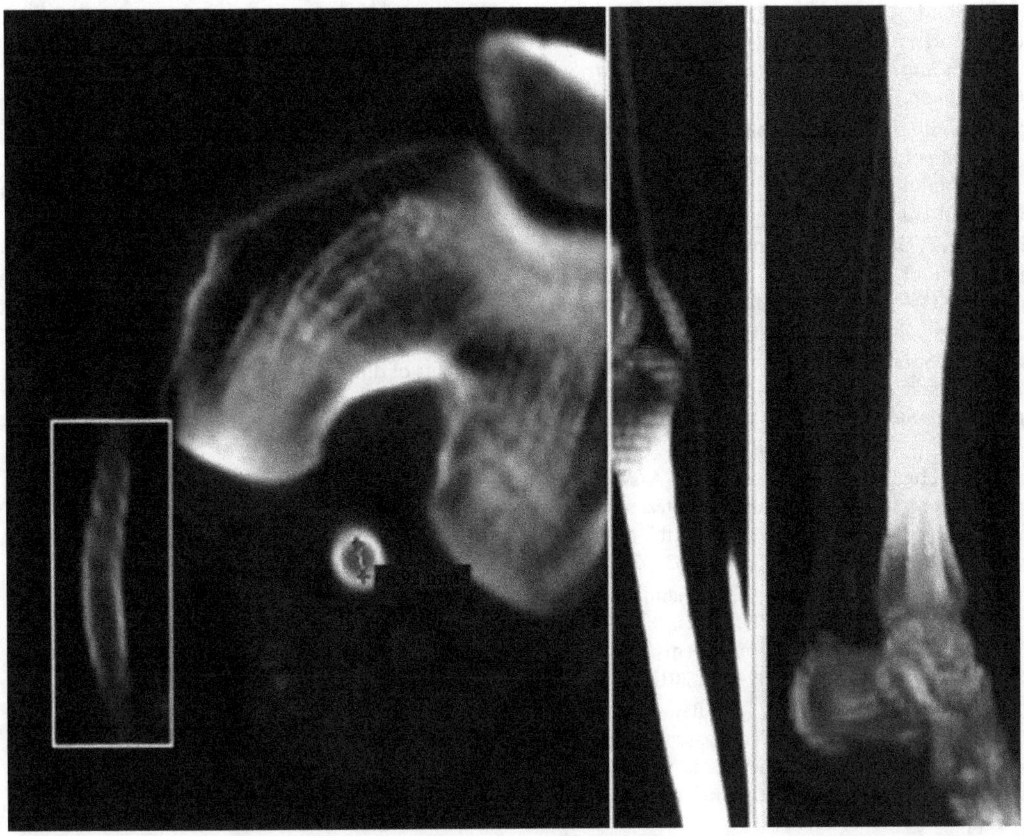

FIGURE 4: Follow-up CT angiography: complete exclusion of the aneurism and preserved patency of the posterior tibial artery.

popliteal aneurysm are also reported with the use of the nitinol interwoven-wire Supera stent (Abbott Vascular, Illinois). The authors achieved 100% technical success, freedom from sac enlargement and prevention of distal embolization. However, complete sac thrombosis at a one-year follow-up was observed only in 34% of the cases [16].

While uncovered stents seem to be effective in preventing aneurysm expansion and distal embolization, there is a risk of stent occlusion, especially in patients with prothrombotic states. The infection with new coronavirus is associated with a significant rate of arterial and venous thrombosis, and anticoagulation is recommended for all hospitalized patients [17]. However, current evidence regarding the optimal antithrombotic treatment of COVID-19 patients undergoing endovascular interventions is still lacking. Considering low bleeding risk and high cumulative risk of thrombosis (caused by stent implantation, single-vessel runoff, and SARS-CoV-2 infection) in our patient, we decided to use the triple therapy: two antiplatelet agents combined with a direct anticoagulant. The similar approach is recommended by current guidelines for patients with acute coronary syndrome and SARS-CoV-2 infection [18]. During in-hospital treatment, the enoxaparine was used as the anticoagulant of choice in order to prevent possible interactions with antiviral drugs. After discharge, it was replaced with prophylactic dose of rivaroxaban due to the possibility of oral administration. Dipyridamole was used as a component of dual antithrombotic therapy considering its potential benefits in the treatment of SARS-CoV-2 virus infection. Several publications mentioned the ability of this drug to suppress SARS-CoV-2 replication *in vitro* and improve the clinical course of the disease [19, 20].

4. Conclusion

The existing body of evidence regarding the use of flow diverting stents for the treatment of popliteal artery aneurisms is scarce, and there are not any previous reports of Roadsaver® carotid stent implantation for this purpose. The authors believe that their initial experience with off-label use of the Roadsaver® stent for the hybrid treatment of complicated popliteal artery aneurisms is promising and can serve as a background for further studies.

Consent

No written consent has been obtained from the patient as there is no patient identifiable data included in this case report.

References

[1] M. M. Kassem and L. Gonzalez, "Popliteal artery aneurysm. 2020," in *Stat Pearls [Internet]. Treasure Island (FL)*, Stat Pearls Publishing, 2020.

[2] A. Cervin, H. Ravn, and M. Björck, "Ruptured popliteal artery aneurysm," *British Journal of Surgery*, vol. 105, no. 13, pp. 1753–1758, 2018.

[3] O. Grip, K. Mani, M. Altreuther et al., "Contemporary treatment of popliteal artery aneurysms in 14 countries: a Vascunet report," *European Journal of Vascular and Endovascular Surgery*, vol. 60, no. 5, pp. 721–729, 2020.

[4] H. Chang, F. J. Veith, C. B. Rockman et al., "Comparison of outcomes for open popliteal artery aneurysm repair using vein and prosthetic conduits," *Annals of Vascular Surgery*, vol. - S0890-5096, no. 21, 2021.

[5] D. Joshi, Y. Gupta, B. Ganai, and C. Mortensen, "Endovascular versus open repair of asymptomatic popliteal artery aneurysm," *Cochrane Database of Systematic Reviews*, vol. 12, no. 12, p. CD010149, 2019.

[6] A. E. Leake, M. A. Segal, R. A. Chaer et al., "Meta-analysis of open and endovascular repair of popliteal artery aneurysms," *Journal of Vascular Surgery*, vol. 65, no. 1, pp. 246–256.e2, 2017.

[7] S. R. Patel, C. O. Hughes, K. G. Jones et al., "A systematic review and meta-analysis of endovascular popliteal aneurysm repair using the Hemobahn/Viabahn stent-graft," *Journal of Endovascular Therapy*, vol. 22, no. 3, pp. 330–337, 2015.

[8] G. S. Sfyroeras, I. Dalainas, T. G. Giannakopoulos, K. Antonopoulos, J. D. Kakisis, and C. D. Liapis, "Flow-diverting stents for the treatment of arterial aneurysms," *Journal of Vascular Surgery*, vol. 56, no. 3, pp. 839–846, 2012.

[9] K. Akkan, E. Ilgit, K. Karaman et al., "The new double-layer micromesh stent (Roadsaver®): use in endovascular treatment of supraaortic and visceral artery aneurysms and pseudoaneurysms," *CardioVascular and Interventional Radiology*, vol. 40, no. 9, pp. 1338–1343, 2017.

[10] C. Kabbasch, C. Bangard, T. Liebig, P. Majd, A. Mpotsaris, and A. Faymonville, "The Dual Layer Casper Micromesh Stent: Taking Advantage of Flow-Diverting Capabilities for the Treatment of Extracranial Aneurysms and Pseudoaneurysms," *CardioVascular and Interventional Radiology*, vol. 39, no. 3, pp. 472–476, 2016.

[11] P. van Veenendaal, J. Maingard, H. K. Kok et al., "Endovascular flow-diversion of visceral and renal artery aneurysms using dual-layer braided nitinol carotid stents," *CVIR Endovascular*, vol. 3, no. 1, p. 33, 2020.

[12] M. Massara, S. Notarstefano, G. De Caridi, R. Serra, R. Prunella, and G. Impedovo, "Endovascular treatment of a carotid pseudoaneurysm using the new double-layer micromesh stent (Roadsaver®)," *Annals of Vascular Surgery*, vol. 59, pp. 308.e15–308.e18, 2019.

[13] T. Thakar and A. Chaudhuri, "Early experience with the multilayer aneurysm repair stent in the endovascular treatment of trans/infragenicular popliteal artery aneurysms: a mixed bag," *Journal of Endovascular Therapy*, vol. 20, no. 3, pp. 381–388, 2013.

[14] F. Serracino-Inglott, "Popliteal artery aneurysms and the multilayer stent: are there problems ahead?," *Journal of Endovascular Therapy*, vol. 20, no. 3, pp. 389–392, 2013.

[15] A. Ucci, R. Curci, M. Azzarone et al., "Early and mid-term results in the endovascular treatment of popliteal aneurysms with the multilayer flow modulator," *Vascular*, vol. 26, no. 5, pp. 556–563, 2018.

[16] A. Lauricella, S. Gennai, T. Covic et al., "Outcome of endovascular repair of popliteal artery aneurysms using the Supera stent," *Journal of Vascular and Interventional Radiology*, vol. 32, no. 2, pp. 173–180, 2021.

[17] M. E. Canonico, R. Siciliano, F. Scudiero, G. D. Sanna, and G. Parodi, "The tug-of-war between coagulopathy and anticoagulant agents in patients with COVID-19," *European Heart Journal - Cardiovascular Pharmacotherapy*, vol. 6, no. 4, pp. 262–264, 2020.

[18] B. Bikdeli, M. V. Madhavan, D. Jimenez et al., "COVID-19 and Thrombotic or Thromboembolic Disease: Implications for Prevention, Antithrombotic Therapy, and Follow-Up," *Journal of the American College of Cardiology*, vol. 75, no. 23, pp. 2950–2973, 2020.

[19] X. Liu, Z. Li, S. Liu et al., "Potential therapeutic effects of dipyridamole in the severely ill patients with COVID-19," *Acta Pharmaceutica Sinica B*, vol. 10, no. 7, pp. 1205–1215, 2020.

[20] K. F. Aliter and R. A. Al-Horani, "Potential therapeutic benefits of dipyridamole in COVID-19 patients," *Current Pharmaceutical Design*, vol. 27, no. 6, pp. 866–875, 2021.

28

Isolated Persistent Left Superior Vena Cava Revealed by an Associated Asthma

I. Bachouch,[1] N. Belloumi,[1] M. Attia,[2] F. Chermiti Ben Abdallah,[1,3] S. Hantous Zannad,[2,3] and S. Fenniche[1,3]

[1]*Pulmonology Department Pavilion 4, Abderrahmen Mami Hospital, Tunisia*
[2]*Department of Radiology, Abderrahmen Mami Hospital, Tunisia*
[3]*Faculty of Medicine of Tunis, University of Tunis El Manar, Tunisia*

Correspondence should be addressed to N. Belloumi; nidhalbelloumi@gmail.com

Academic Editor: Nilda Espinola-Zavaleta

Background. Persistent left superior vena cava (PLSVC) is a rare anomaly of the thoracic venous system. *Case Report.* We present a case of a patient with isolated asymptomatic PLSVC, who was diagnosed because of dyspnea revealing an associated asthma. An 18-year-old male patient complained of paroxystic sibilant dyspnea. He did not have any anomaly in physical examination. The chest X-ray revealed cardiomegaly with a widening of lower mediastinum. The electrocardiogram does not show any anomaly. Echocardiography showed the PLSVC. The thoracic contrast computed tomography of the chest showed ecstasies of the right cardiac cavities and a double superior vena cava. The patient did not have similar family cases. Respiratory functional explorations led to the diagnosis of an associated asthma. Currently, he is followed up periodically. Asthma was improved with inhaled corticosteroid treatment. *Conclusion.* PLSVC is rare but can have important clinical implications. Associated severe cardiac malformations must be systematically sought.

1. Background

Persistent left superior vena cava (PLSVC) is an uncommon vascular anomaly. It is usually asymptomatic and had no hemodynamic implications, so it is frequently detected when cardiovascular imaging is performed for an unrelated reason [1]. It affects about 0.1 to 0.5% of the general population [1]. PLSVC can be isolated or associated with other cardiac malformations, such as atrial septal defect, endocardial cushion defect, or tetralogy of Fallot [1]. In this case report, we present a patient with isolated PLSVC with no other cardiac abnormalities, who was diagnosed because of dyspnea revealing associated asthma.

2. Case Presentation

A 18-year-old male patient presented with symptoms suggesting asthma. He was a high school student with no tobacco consumption. He did not have any exposure to bronchial irritative agents. He had a medical history of recurrent lower respiratory tract infections from birth until the age of 3 years. At the age of 13 years, paroxystic dyspnea attacks began to occur. He did not have any associated respiratory or general symptoms. Physical examination revealed normal vital signs. Respiratory, cardiac, and abdominal physical examination was normal. Complete blood count and basic metabolic panel tests were normal. The chest radiograph revealed cardiomegaly (cardiothoracic ratio = 0.6) with a widening of the lower mediastinum. The electrocardiogram does not show any anomaly. The thoracic contrast computed tomography of the chest showed ecstasies of the right cardiac cavities and a double superior vena cava (Figures 1 and 2). Echocardiography showed normal size left ventricle, dilated straight cavities without pulmonary arterial hypertension signs, no atrium septal defect, nondilated inferior vena cava, and an aspect in favor of persistent left superior vena cava. Flexible bronchoscopy showed a diffuse mucosal inflammation of the right bronchial tree without any bronchus

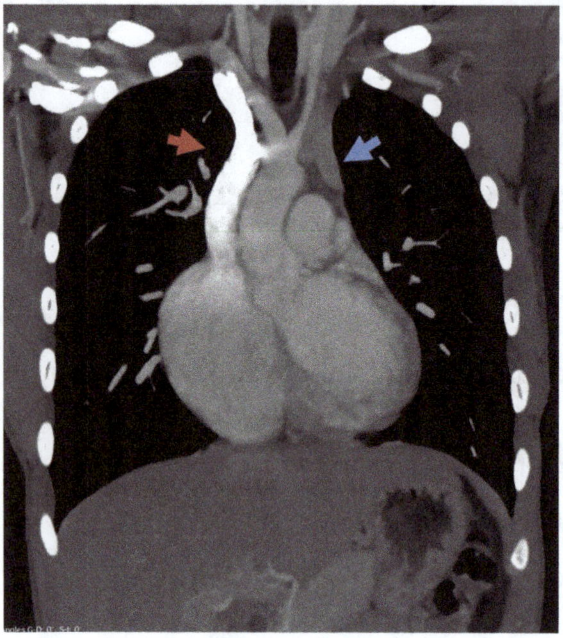

Figure 1: Coronal slide of the chest. Red arrow = right superior vena cava; blue arrow = persistent left superior vena cava.

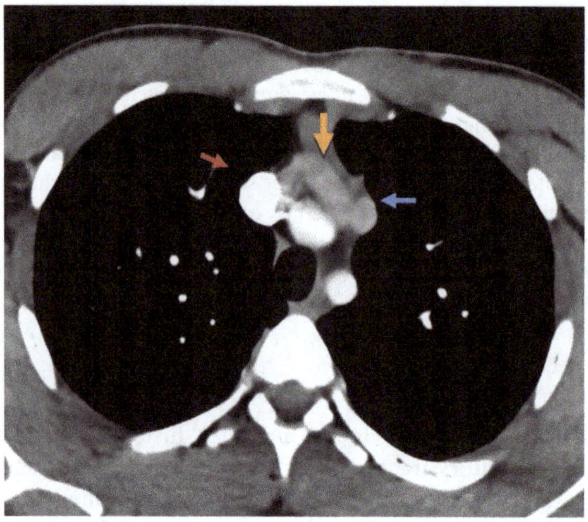

Figure 2: Sagittal slice of the chest. Red arrow = right superior vena cava; blue arrow = persistent left superior vena cava; orange arrow = left innominate vein.

obstruction. Endoscopy showed also the presence of a supernumerary bronchus in the right side of the right stump bronchus. The patient had normal spirometry. The methacholine challenge test showed mild bronchial hyperresponsiveness. The patient did not have similar family cases of congenital abnormalities. Currently, he is followed up periodically. By putting on 200 μg inhaled beclomethasone twice daily, asthma was improved.

3. Discussion

PLSVC is an uncommon vascular anomaly but is considered the most common congenital anomaly of the thoracic venous system [2]. The incidence is about 0.1 to 0.5% of the total population [2].

Four anatomic types of PLSVC were described: in the first type, there is an anastomosis between the left and right superior vena cava through the innominate venous trunk. In the second type, left and right superior vena cavae are completely separated [3]. In the third type, right superior vena cava is absent or completely atrophied. In this case, blood drainage is realized through the left superior vena cava. In the fourth type, left and right superior vena cava are separated, each one presenting its own correspondent azygos vein [3]. In our case report, imaging showed the first category of the previously described classification.

Most of PLSVC are asymptomatic and have no hemodynamic abnormalities [4]. It can be detected accidentally during imaging for unrelated symptoms or in the context of a process of intravascular invasive procedure [4]. However, in some cases, there is abnormal sinus rhythm or bradycardia present in 36% of cases [5]. This cardiac rhythm disorder can lead to indication of pacemaker implantation because of sick sinus syndrome resulting from histological abnormalities caused by an enlarged coronary sinus. This arrhythmia can be caused by histological modifications in the atrioventricular sinus. The existence of multiple electric nodes between PLSVC, coronary sinus, and right atrium can also lead to this arrhythmia [6]. Tachyarrhythmia can be caused by electric generating capacity of the PLSVC, interatrial conduction delay, or atrial arrhythmia secondary to coronary sinus dilation [6]. In our case, we did not note any hemodynamic abnormalities, and electrocardiogram does not show any anomaly.

Clinical cyanosis can be also a manifestation of PLSVC (8% of patients) due to the left to right shunt. In this case, patients always suffer from septal defect, ventricular septal defect, or other cardiovascular malformations. Echocardiography in our case does not show any atrial or ventricular septal defect or other cardiovascular malformations. Contrast echography after administration of agitated saline solution should have been undertaken to document shunts between right and left cavities.

The detection of PLSVC is important when the left subclavian vein is used for catheterization procedures like Swan-Ganz catheterization and usage in renal dialysis [2, 4], in chemotherapy, or in cardiac stimulator placement [7, 8]. These investigations can be complicated by left subclavian vein thrombosis, cardiac arrhythmia, perforation of the coronary sinus, cardiac tamponade, cardiogenic shock, or even death [4].

When using a central venous catheter, drugs can directly enter in the systemic circulation when they are applied from the left brachiocephalic vein [4]. PLSVC can also be complicated by paradoxical embolism secondary to right-to-left shunt due to draining PLSVC into the right atrium either directly or via an unroofed coronary sinus [4]. A PLSVC can also cause problems in pacemaker implantation or cardiopulmonary bypass [8].

The possibility of associated severe cardiac malformations to PLSVC leads us to indicate further cardiologic investigations such as transthoracic contrast echocardiography, transesophageal echocardiography associated with contrast saline solution, MRI, or cardiac computed tomography with contrast solution [9]. The only limitation of thoracic contrast computed tomography is radiation exposure. MRI could be a best alternative significantly superior to both transthoracic and transesophageal echocardiography [9, 10]. In our case, symptoms suggest the diagnosis of asthma. However, the aspect of widening of lower mediastinum in chest radiograph (unusual in asthma patients) led us to practice thoracic contrast computed tomography that revealed the presence of PLSVC.

4. Conclusions

PLSVC is a very rare vascular anomaly. It is usually asymptomatic, incidentally detected after cardiovascular imaging whatever was the reason. To confirm the diagnosis, magnetic resonance imaging can be a best alternative significantly superior to both transthoracic and transesophageal echocardiography. PLSVC may have important clinical implications especially during certain catheterization procedures or in the case of associated severe cardiac malformations.

References

[1] O. Uçar, L. Paşaoğlu, H. Ciçekçioğlu, M. Vural, I. Kocaoğlu, and S. Aydoğdu, "Persistent left superior vena cava with absent right superior vena cava: a case report and review of the literature," *Cardiovascular Journal of Africa*, vol. 21, no. 3, pp. 164–166, 2010.

[2] H. He, B. Li, Y. Ma et al., "Catheterization in a patient with end-stage renal disease through persistent left superior vena cava: a rare case report and literature review," *BMC Nephrology*, vol. 20, no. 1, p. 202, 2019.

[3] B. D. Sarodia and J. K. Stoller, "Persistent left superior vena cava: case report and literature review," *Respiratory Care*, vol. 45, no. 4, pp. 411–416, 2000.

[4] C. Savu, C. Petreanu, A. Melinte et al., "Persistent left superior vena cava–accidental finding," *In Vivo*, vol. 34, no. 2, pp. 935–941, 2020.

[5] U. Bartram, S. Van Praagh, J. C. Levine, M. Hines, A. S. Bensky, and R. V. Praagh, "Absent right superior vena cava in visceroatrial situs solitus," *The American Journal of Cardiology*, vol. 80, no. 2, pp. 175–183, 1997.

[6] E. Occhetta, G. Dell'Era, A. Degiovanni, and C. Sartori, "Persistence of left superior vena cava and focal right atrial tachycardia: challenges and interventional treatment," *Cor et Vasa*, vol. 57, no. 5, pp. e354–e358, 2015.

[7] J. Kang, B. Liu, and W. Sun, "Two successful insertions of peripherally inserted central catheters in a patient with persistent left superior vena cava: a case report," *Medicine*, vol. 98, no. 38, article e16988, 2019.

[8] T. Li, Q. Xu, H.-T. Liao, D. Asvestas, K. P. Letsas, and Y. Li, "Transvenous dual-chamber pacemaker implantation in patients with persistent left superior vena cava," *BMC Cardiovascular Disorders*, vol. 19, no. 1, 2019.

[9] C. Mărginean, C. O. Mărginean, I. Muntean et al., "Ultrasonographic features of the persistence of superior left vena cava and pathological cardiac associations in fetus. Case series," *Medical Ultrasonography*, vol. 18, no. 2, pp. 214–217, 2016.

[10] S. A. Horvath, N. Suraci, J. D'Mello, and O. Santana, "Persistent left superior vena cava identified by transesophageal echocardiography," *Reviews in Cardiovascular Medicine*, vol. 20, no. 2, pp. 99-100, 2019.

A Rare Case of Bilateral Posterior Tibial Artery Aneurysm Presenting as Unilateral Acute Limb Ischemia

Andrew T. Hattam and Mayur Krishnaswamy

Vascular Surgery Unit, Department of Surgery, University Hospital Geelong, Barwon Health, Geelong, Victoria, Australia

Correspondence should be addressed to Mayur Krishnaswamy; mkrish@barwonhealth.org.au

Academic Editor: Ayman El-Menyar

True aneurysms of the tibial arteries are extremely rare. Of the few previously described tibial artery aneurysms, there are scant reports of isolated true aneurysms of the posterior tibial artery (PTA). In this report, we describe the second documented case of bilateral true PTA aneurysms. Unique aspects of this case are that the aneurysmal PTA were the only patent tibial arteries bilaterally, the aneurysms were degenerative in nature, and initial patient presentation was due to aneurysm thrombosis causing acute foot ischemia. The clinical and radiological features of this case, as well as surgical decision making and management, are discussed.

1. Introduction

Aneurysms of the tibial arteries are uncommon, with true aneurysms of the tibial arteries being extremely rare. Of the few previously described tibial artery aneurysms, there are scant reports of isolated true aneurysms of the posterior tibial artery (PTA) [1]. To our knowledge, there is only one report to date of a patient with bilateral true aneurysms of the PTA [2]. Herein, we describe a case of bilateral true PTA aneurysms presenting as unilateral acute foot ischemia. Informed consent has been granted by the patient to report this case.

2. Case Report

A 75-year-old female presented acutely with a history of sudden onset paraesthesia and ischemic rest pain involving the left foot and ankle. Motor function was retained, capillary and superficial venous return were reduced, the foot was cold, and there were no palpable pedal pulses. The calf remained soft to palpate. There was no history of palpitations or arrythmia, and the patient was in sinus cardiac rhythm both clinically and on electrocardiography. Plain chest radiography and computed tomography angiography (CTA) excluded a proximal arterial source of embolism. Furthermore, there was no previous trauma, (local or systemic) infection or inflammation, collagen, connective tissue or genetic syndromes, or arteritis; nor was there a family history of aneurysmal disease. Positive cardiovascular risk factors included hypercholesterolaemia and hypertension. Baseline haematological and biochemical analyses were normal, as were the renal and liver function. The creatinine kinase was within normal limits. The right foot was well perfused with a palpable PTA pulse.

CTA demonstrated no significant stenosis in the supragenicular vessels bilaterally. On the symptomatic left side, the tibioperoneal trunk (TPT) and anterior tibial artery (ATA) were patent proximally, with the ATA and peroneal artery occluding in the distal calf. The dorsalis pedis was occluded; however, the plantar arteries reconstituted. Dominant flow to the foot was via the PTA, which occluded in the distal calf (Figure 1). These findings were considered reflective of embolic disease within the left-sided tibial arteries. The asymptomatic right leg demonstrated dominant flow to the ankle via the PTA. The ATA and peroneal arteries occluded in the midcalf.

Due to the acute nature of the patient's symptoms, emergent thromboembolectomy of the popliteal and tibial

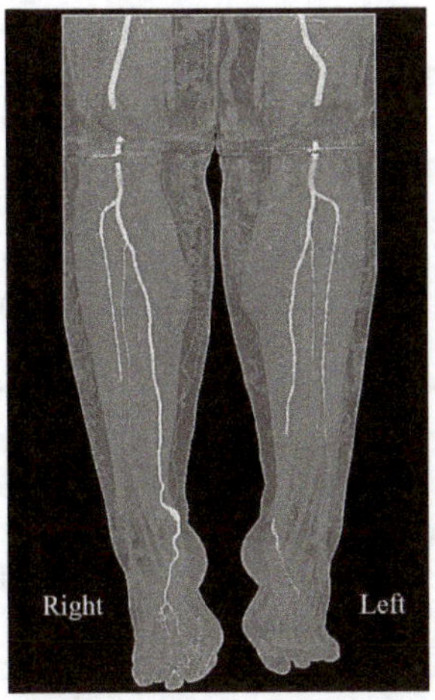

FIGURE 1: Preoperative reconstructed computed tomography angiography of the tibial arteries bilaterally, demonstrating abrupt occlusion of the left posterior tibial artery and a right-sided posterior tibial artery aneurysm. Please note that artefact from bilateral knee prostheses obstructs visualising normal flow within the popliteal arteries in this image.

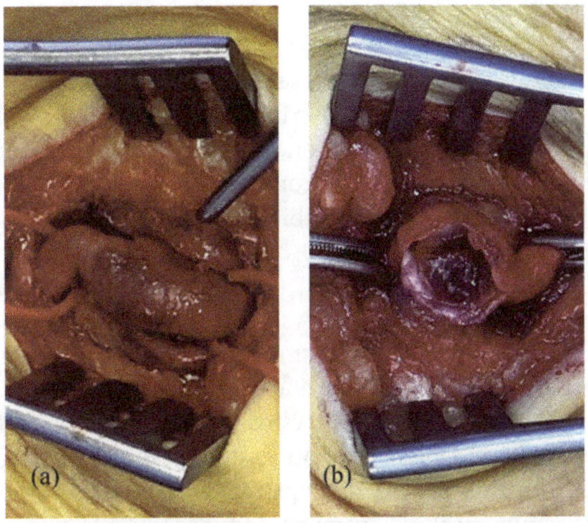

FIGURE 3: Intraoperative images demonstrating exposure of the posterior tibial artery aneurysm (a) and containing intramural thrombus (b).

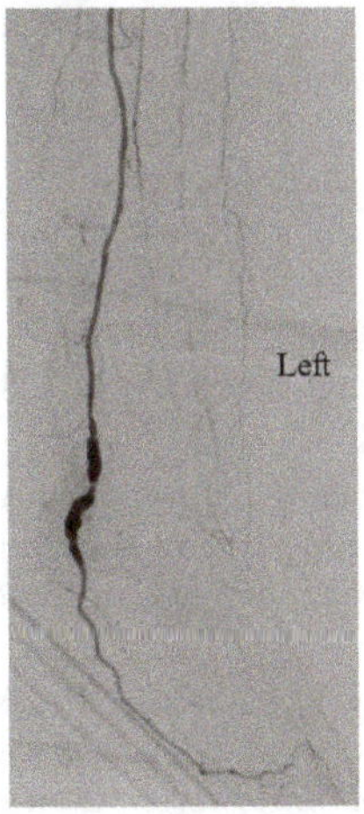

FIGURE 2: Angiography of the left posterior tibial artery aneurysm after thrombectomy.

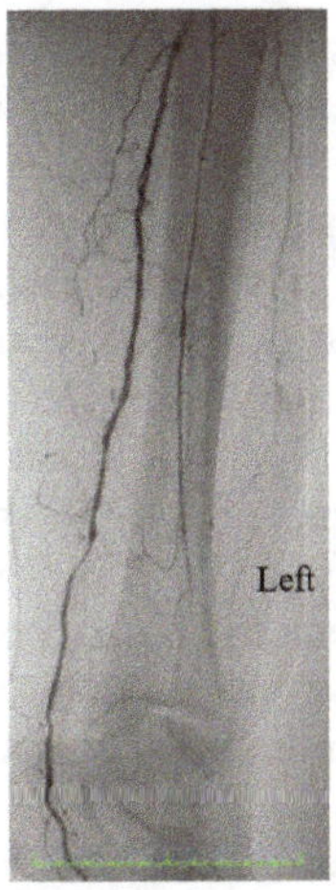

FIGURE 4: Postoperative angiography demonstrating flow to the left foot through the interposition long saphenous vein graft.

arteries was performed via a medial approach to the distal popliteal artery. Selective thromboembolectomy using Fogarty catheters for each tibial artery was unsuccessful. Urokinase was also injected into each tibial artery without effect. Subsequent exposure of the dominant PTA at the ankle demonstrated a thrombosed 10mm diameter aneurysm. A PTA thrombectomy was performed and subsequent angiography demonstrated flow to the foot via the aneurysmal PTA (Figure 2). The aneurysm was opened and demonstrated a mixture of old, organised, and fresh thrombus (Figure 3). The PTA aneurysm was excised and thrombectomy established adequate inflow and backflow to the excised PTA segment. The PTA was repaired using an interposition long saphenous vein graft (Figure 4). Postoperatively, the PTA pulse was present, the foot had brisk capillary refill, and motor and sensory function normalised. Follow-up at 16 months demonstrated the patient to have a well perfused left foot with a palpable PTA pulse.

Although the patient's contralateral foot was asymptomatic, she opted to have this repaired electively considering the aneurysmal right PTA aneurysm was the single arterial supply to the foot. Repair was performed via excision of the 8mm PTA aneurysm and a spatulated primary end-to-end PTA anastomosis. Completion angiography was satisfactory, and the right foot was well perfused with a palpable PTA pulse postoperatively. Histopathology of the right-sided PTA aneurysm demonstrated findings consistent with atherosclerotic degenerative aneurysmal disease. Specifically, there was intimal thickening, extensive lamina disruption, and broad areas of media replaced by collagenous fibrous tissue, with calcification of the media. There was no inflammation or mural necrosis seen.

3. Discussion

Most tibial aneurysms present as posttraumatic false aneurysms [1, 3, 4]. Other described aetiological mechanisms include autoimmune, infection, collagen and/or connective tissue disorders, genetic syndromes, and arteritis [5].

The number of isolated tibial aneurysms in the English literature is estimated at <50 cases, with <15 cases of isolated PTA aneurysms [1, 3]. Two previous reports have described bilateral PTA aneurysms. However, Tressider et al. [6] described mycotic aneurysms of the TPT, which involved the proximal PTA and peroneal arteries. Katz et al. [2] described bilateral PTA aneurysms with progressive bilateral calf swelling and pain. Immunohistological examination of tissue from this patient demonstrated the aneurysms to be due to a nonspecified immune-complex disease and associated collagen disorder within the arterial walls. Histology of the case described here demonstrated simple degenerative aneurysm disease. Assuming the pathological processes was mirrored in the contralateral aneurysm, this case would be the first case of bilateral degenerative PTA aneurysms in the English literature.

Most tibial aneurysms present as asymptomatic medial ankle swellings [4]. Due to their rarity, the natural history of tibial artery aneurysm disease remains incompletely characterised. Previous reports suggest symptomatic presentations are more commonly due to aneurysm thromboembolism (as occurring in this case) rather than rupture [5]. In assessing the patient for tibial artery arterial aneurysms, ultrasound Doppler studies [1], formal angiography [3], and magnetic resonance angiography [5] have been described. However, as demonstrated on CTA (Figure 1) in this case, it is difficult to characterise small vessel, noncalcific, distal tibial artery aneurysms using such imaging modalities once acute thromboembolism has occurred. Moreover, as in this case, concomitant occlusive disease of the other tibial arteries may mimic embolic disease, making diagnosis of such rare pathology more difficult. Furthermore, the very low incidence of bilateral aneurysm disease is unlikely to be able to guide clinical suspicion of such cases.

Given the rarity of tibial artery aneurysms, a standard treatment approach has yet to be established [4]. Previous authors have described relatively long-term surveillance of tibial artery aneurysms without adverse sequelae [7, 8], while others suggest surgical repair irrespective of symptoms [4]. In the emergency setting, ligation of the aneurysmal artery has been advocated [4]. However, as at least one uncompromised tibial artery is required to adequately perfuse the foot [9], the presence of ATA and peroneal artery occlusions in this case necessitated emergent reconstruction of the aneurysmal PTA to salvage the acutely ischemic foot.

The asymptomatic right leg PTA aneurysm was subsequently managed with elective surgical repair. This was performed on the basis of (1) the established natural history of the left-sided PTA aneurysm, (2) the PTA being the sole arterial supply to the foot, and (3) the established thromboembolic risk of intramural thrombus within tibial artery aneurysms identified radiologically [10].

In conclusion, tibial artery aneurysms are extremely rare and their aetiology is widely variable. Diagnosis in the emergency setting is difficult, both clinically and radiologically, after acute thromboembolic evolution. The case described herein is the second case of bilateral isolated PTA aneurysms and the first of degenerative aetiology presenting with acute foot ischemia. Consensus on the management of tibial artery aneurysms has yet to be defined. Though ligation of the aneurysmal artery is a valid surgical option in the emergency setting, we suggest reconstruction of the aneurysmal artery in circumstances where it is the sole arterial supply to the foot. The most difficult aspect of this case was diagnosis of an extremely rare tibial artery aneurysm in the acute setting. Although rare, clinicians should be mindful of the potential for tibial aneurysms at routine clinical examination, as diagnosis and management appear to be easier and safer, in the elective setting.

References

[1] D. Singh, "A rare case of symptomatic true aneurysm of posterior tibial artery," *Indian Journal of Vascular and Endovascular Surgery*, vol. 5, no. 4, pp. 289–291, 2018.

[2] S. G. Katz, R. D. Kohl, and N. Razack, "Bilateral infrapopliteal artery aneurysms," *Annals of Vascular Surgery*, vol. 6, no. 2, pp. 168–170, 1992.

[3] T. Kanaoka and H. Matsuura, "A true aneurysm of the posterior tibial artery: a case report," *Annals of Thoracic and Cardiovascular Surgery*, vol. 10, no. 5, pp. 317-318, 2004.

[4] J. Sagar and M. Button, "Posterior tibial artery aneurysm: a case report with review of literature," *BMC Surgery*, vol. 14, no. 37, 2014.

[5] Y. Tshomba, M. Papa, E. M. Marone, A. Kahlberg, N. Rizzo, and R. Chiesa, "A true posterior tibial artery aneurysm: A case report," *Vascular and Endovascular Surgery*, vol. 40, no. 3, pp. 243–249, 2006.

[6] G. C. Tresidder and R. P. Warren, "A case of bilateral mycotic aneurysm of the posterior tibial artery treated successfully by excision," *British Journal of Surgery*, vol. 41, no. 167, pp. 333-334, 1953.

[7] P. G. Borozan, H. S. J. Walker III, and G. J. Peterson, "True tibial artery aneurysms: Case report and literature review," *Journal of Vascular Surgery*, vol. 10, no. 4, pp. 457–459, 1989.

[8] J. Yao, "Multiple arterial aneurysms: a seven-year follow-up," *Journal of Contemporary Surgery*, vol. 31, pp. 73–78, 1987.

[9] R. F. Bedford and H. Wollman, "Complications of percutaneous radial-artery cannulation: an objective prospective study in man.," *Anesthesiology*, vol. 38, no. 3, pp. 228–236, 1973.

[10] D. Mukherjee, "Posterior approach to the peroneal artery," *Journal of Vascular Surgery*, vol. 19, no. 1, pp. 174–178, 1994.

30

Endovascular Embolization of a Dissected External Carotid Artery Pseudoaneurysm in a Young Female with Neurofibromatosis Complicated by Preeclampsia

Sasha Lalla,[1] Rajeev Seecheran,[2] Valmiki Seecheran,[3] Sangeeta Persad,[3] Ronald Henry,[1] and Naveen Anand Seecheran[2]

[1]*Advanced Cardiovascular Institute, Port of Spain, Trinidad And Tobago*
[2]*University of the West Indies, St. Augustine, Trinidad And Tobago*
[3]*North Central Regional Health Authority, Mt. Hope, Trinidad And Tobago*

Correspondence should be addressed to Naveen Anand Seecheran; nseecheran@gmail.com

Academic Editor: Ayman El-Menyar

Carotid artery pseudoaneurysms are infrequently encountered in clinical practice. Major contributory etiologies include blunt trauma, infections, cystic medial necrosis, fibromuscular dysplasia, arteriosclerosis, and congenital abnormalities. The authors report an exceedingly rare case of a dissected external carotid artery pseudoaneurysm in a 26-year-old female patient with neurofibromatosis complicated by preeclampsia at 28-week period of gestation, safely and successfully treated by coil embolization.

1. Introduction

Neurofibromatosis type-1 (NF-1) is an autosomal dominant genetic disorder that results from a mutation of the neurofibromin one gene, located on chromosome 17 (17q11.2). It is a multisystemic disorder with complete penetrance and an estimated prevalence of 1 in 3500 births. The prevalence of NF-1-associated vascular lesions ranges from 0.4 to 6.4%, according to a previous clinical series [1].

The spectrum of vasculopathies includes stenoses, aneurysms, and arteriovenous malformations; involving the aortic, renal, mesenteric, carotid-vertebral, subclavian-axillary, iliofemoral, intracerebral, and coronary arteries. Renal artery involvement is the most common [1].

Due to the rarity of NF-1-associated vasculopathy, clinical characteristics and management strategies have not yet been well ascertained. The authors report an exceedingly rare case of a dissected carotid artery pseudoaneurysm in a 26-year-old female patient with neurofibromatosis complicated by preeclampsia at 28-week period of gestation, safely and successfully treated via an endovascular coil embolization technique.

2. Case Report

A 26-year-old female with a medical history of neurofibromatosis type-1 and 28-week gestational age complicated by preeclampsia was referred to the cardiovascular center for evaluation of an expanding, pulsatile, tender mass on the right neck. On admission, her vital signs reflected a hypertensive emergency with systolic blood pressures of 200s mmHg, tachycardia of 112 beats per minute, tachypnea of 20 breaths per minute with oxygen saturation of 98% on room air. On physical examination, there were several features consistent with her preexisting diagnosis of NF-1, which included multiple "*café-au-lait*" macules and neurofibromas throughout her chest and abdomen, with both axillary and inguinal freckling [2].

Routine blood investigations were normal, 12-lead electrocardiography indicated a sinus tachycardia with left ventricular hypertrophy which was also visualized on an inpatient transthoracic echocardiogram. A computerized tomography scan revealed a dissected pseudoaneurysm of the right external carotid artery (ECA). In the interim, she was treated with an intravenous nitroglycerin infusion and

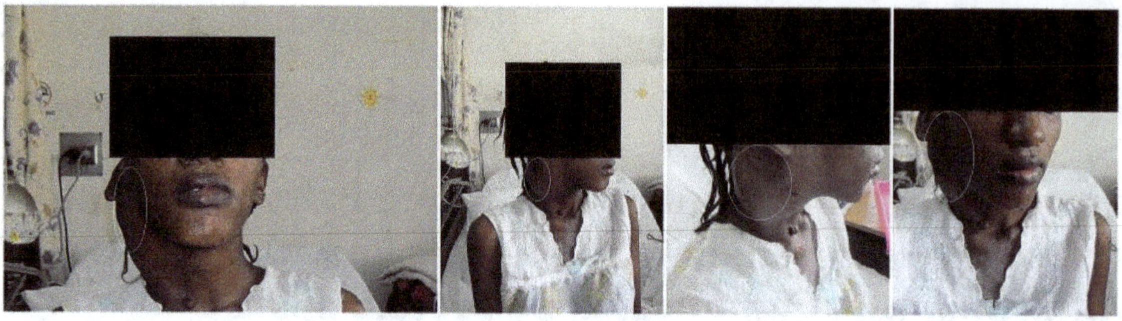

FIGURE 1: Facial depiction of the hematoma. Frontal series of the right neck hematoma (eclipsed in white), resulting from dissection of the right external carotid pseudoaneurysm.

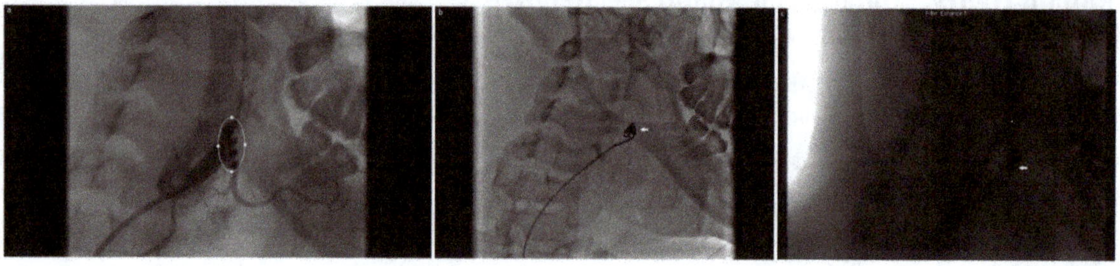

FIGURE 2: Right carotid artery cineangiography series. (a) Preintervention: the white ellipse encircles the external carotid artery dissection with contrast extravasation. (b) Intervention: The white arrow indicates successful coil embolization with 0.018" and 0.035" Tornado® embolization coils (Cook Medical® LLC, Bloomington, IN, USA). (c) Postintervention: the white arrow indicates complete occlusion of the external carotid artery distal to the superior thyroid branch; with no antegrade flow within the aneurysm.

hydralazine to achieve near-normotensive pressures over the ensuing 12 hours (see Figure 1). Subsequently, on the second day of hospitalization, selective carotid angiography demonstrated a dissected pseudoaneurysm of the right ECA measuring 2.7 cm, arising in association with the occipital branch with contrast extravasation (see Figure 2(a)). Ad-hoc successful coil embolization was achieved with 0.018" and 0.035" Tornado® embolization coils (Cook Medical LLC, Bloomington, IN, USA) (see Figure 2(b)). At the conclusion of the procedure, cineangiography revealed complete occlusion of the vessel distal to the superior thyroid branch with no further opacification of the aneurysm (see Figure 2(c)).

3. Discussion

NF-1 diagnostic criteria include the presence of two or more of the following criteria: six or more "*café-au-lait*" macules, two or more neurofibromas of any type, or one plexiform, neurofibroma; axillary or inguinal freckling; two or more Lisch nodules, optic pathway gliomas, distinctive bone lesions such as sphenoid dysplasia or thinning of the long bone cortex, with or without pseudoarthrosis, and a first degree relative diagnosed with NF-1 (see Table 1) [2].

ECA pseudoaneurysms are exceedingly rare within the general population as evidenced by the paucity of case reports, and consequently, optimal management strategies are not well established. The estimated prevalence is approximately 0.07% with a resultant mortality rate of 33% and only a handful of cases specifically involving the external carotid artery [3, 4].

Generally, these lesions accounted for only 1.4% of aneurysms in a recent review [5]. Intracranial aneurysms are also rare in cases with NF-1. Baldauf et al. identified 28 cases of intracranial aneurysms associated with neurofibromatosis predominantly located in the left internal carotid artery circulation with a female preponderance [6]. These clinical features were diametrically opposite in our patient as she displayed right external carotid artery involvement.

The pathophysiology of carotid pseudoaneurysm formation is usually attributed to penetrating or blunt trauma, usually from motor vehicle accidents. Other postulated mechanisms include direct compression of the neck, hyperextension/rotation injury and injury to the base of the skull, and anastomotic disruption following carotid vascular interventions [1]. Predisposing conditions include infection, radiotherapy, poor nutritional status, and neoplasia. Head and neck malignancies treated with radiotherapy can develop multifocal iatrogenic arteriopathy in the radiation field, leading to carotid "blow-out" [4, 7].

NF-1 is caused by a heterozygous mutation in the NF1 gene, which results in a loss of functional protein, neurofibromin, which is implicated in cell growth and differentiation. The mechanisms for the vasculopathy are complex and multifactorial, including smooth muscle dysplasia and direct vascular invasion by neurofibromatosis tissue [6]. This results in intimal proliferation of spindle cells with subsequent

TABLE 1: Clinical criteria for Neurofibromatosis Type-1 (NF-1): ≥ 2 or more of the following [2].

≥ 6 "*café-au-lait*" macules
≥ 2 neurofibromas of any type or 1 plexiform neurofibroma
axillary or inguinal freckling
optic pathway gliomas
≥ 2 Lisch nodules
distinctive bone lesions such as sphenoid dysplasia or thinning of the long bone cortex, with or without pseudoarthrosis
first-degree relative diagnosed with NF-1

degenerative changes in the small vessel, including fibrosis, loss of the smooth muscle media, and elastin fragmentation. Additionally, in larger caliber vessels, neurofibromas or ganglioneuromas invade and weaken the arterial wall leading to aneurysm formation [8, 9].

The most common clinical presentation for NF-1 associated vasculopathy is renal artery stenosis with secondary hypertension [10–12]. Hypertension is present in 1% of NF1 patients and is significantly associated with mortality and morbidity [13]. Our patient did indeed present with a hypertensive crisis; however, renal artery stenosis was not diagnosed with Doppler ultrasonography.

Patients with dissected ECA pseudoaneurysms typically present with a tender, pulsatile neck mass. There may be an associated palpable thrill, audible bruit, or focal neurological deficits. Rapid enlargement of external carotid aneurysms may even result in rupture or cranial nerve entrapment [14, 15].

Diagnostic investigations include duplex ultrasonography with a sensitivity of 92%, with the significant caveat that it may incompletely visualize the distal internal carotid arteries. Computerized tomography imaging as a stand-alone modality may not be sensitive enough and often appears normal initially whereas digital subtraction angiography provides high-fidelity enhancement of the pseudoaneurysm, which may guide management strategies. Magnetic resonance angiography accurately demonstrates carotid dissection with sensitivity and specificity of 95% and 99%, respectively, as compared to 84% and 99% for magnetic resonance imaging alone [16].

Generally, the management of carotid pseudoaneurysms is not well delineated and more so focused on the internal carotid vasculature. Strategies include observation, anticoagulation, ligation of the carotid artery with or without a bypass procedure, and arterial reconstruction. With the advent and evolution of endovascular techniques, many periprocedural surgical complications such as cerebrovascular events (5-15%) and operative mortality (2-4%) have substantially decreased [17]. Of the transcatheter armamentarium, parent vessel occlusion with coil placement is currently in *vogue* with covered stent grafts becoming a viable alternative. In this clinical scenario, there was also the added complexity of the patient being of 28-week gestational age, and fetal exposure to radiation was a significant concern during fluoroscopy. A recent study indicated that the average radiation dose was circa 4100 mGy with fluoroscopy duration of 98 minutes and expended contrast media volume of approximately 130 mL [18]. The risk-benefit analysis of the alternative "open" vascular surgery and its attendant risks were considered, and, thus, the endovascular approach was favored. A systematic review indicated an endovascular procedural success of 92.8% with in-hospital mortality, stroke, and cranial nerve injury of 4.1%, 1.8%, and 0.5%, respectively. These results suggest that this approach has achieved comparable clinical outcomes to conventional surgery in patients with extracranial carotid artery aneurysms [17].

The outcome of carotid artery pseudoaneurysms is most aptly summarized by Winslow in 1926, who stated that "but it is not so much the rarity of this lesion, when it does occur that commands our attention as its propensity to imitate peritonsillar abscess, which habit of mimicry has lent on more than one occasion to lancing, with a mortal hemorrhage. The majority of the patients should recover if an aneurysm is promptly recognized and treated, but an overwhelming proportion dies under dilatory, blundering or pernicious tactics." [19].

4. Conclusion

ECA pseudoaneurysms are exceedingly rare and should be considered when a patient presents with a tender, pulsatile neck mass. Early diagnostic imaging and invasive management should be immediately pursued with a high index of clinical suspicion as illustrated in this case, where endovascular embolization proved to be a safe and effective treatment modality.

Additional Points

Key Clinical Message. The clinician should be cognizant that a pulsatile neck mass can be a dissected aneurysm in a patient with neurofibromatosis type-1 which can be safely and successfully treated via endovascular embolization.

Consent

The patient has provided written, informed consent to have the details of her case published.

Authors' Contributions

Sasha Lalla, Rajeev Seecheran, Valmiki Seecheran, Sangeeta Persad, Ronald Henry, and Naveen Anand Seecheran all contributed equally in writing the manuscript. All authors read and approved the final manuscript.

Acknowledgments

The authors acknowledge Professor Michael Ramdass, University of the West Indies, St. Augustine.

References

[1] J. M. Friedman, J. Arbiter, J. A. Epstein et al., "Cardiovascular disease in neurofibromatosis 1: report of the NF1 cardiovascular task force," *Genetics in Medicine*, vol. 4, no. 3, pp. 105–111, 2002.

[2] G. Jentarra, S. L. Snyder, and V. Narayanan, "Genetic aspects of neurocutaneous disorders," *Seminars in Pediatric Neurology*, vol. 13, no. 1, pp. 43–47, 2006.

[3] S. Nadig, S. Barnwell, and M. K. Wax, "Pseudoaneurysm of the external carotid artery-review of literature," *Head & Neck*, vol. 31, no. 1, pp. 136–139, 2009.

[4] D. J. Minion, T. G. Lynch, B. T. Baxter, and R. Lieberman, "Pseudoaneurysm of the external carotid artery following radical neck dissection and irradiation: a case report and review of the literature," *Cardiovascular Surgery*, vol. 2, no. 5, pp. 607–611, 1994.

[5] Z. Li, G. Chang, C. Yao et al., "Endovascular stenting of extracranial carotid artery aneurysm: a systematic review," *European Journal of Vascular and Endovascular Surgery*, vol. 42, no. 4, pp. 419–426, 2011.

[6] J. Baldauf, J. Kiwit, and M. Synowitz, "Cerebral aneurysms associated with von Recklinghausen/s neurofibromatosis: Report of a case and review of the literature," *Neurology India*, vol. 53, no. 2, p. 213, 2005.

[7] J. C. Yuen and D. J. Gray, "Endovascular treatment of a pseudoaneurysm of a recipient external carotid artery following radiation and free tissue transfer," *Annals of Plastic Surgery*, vol. 44, no. 6, pp. 656–659, 2000.

[8] J. L. Falcone, M. R. Go, D. T. Baril, G. J. Oakley, M. S. Makaroun, and R. A. Chaer, "Vascular wall invasion in neurofibromatosis-induced aortic rupture," *Vascular and Endovascular Surgery*, vol. 44, no. 1, pp. 52–55, 2010.

[9] S. Saitoh and S. Matsuda, "Aneurysm of the major vessels in neurofibromatosis," *Archives of Orthopaedic and Trauma Surgery*, vol. 117, no. 1-2, pp. 110–113, 1998.

[10] E. Criado, L. Izquierdo, S. Luján, E. Puras, and M. Mar Espino, "Abdominal aortic coarctation, renovascular, hypertension, and neurofibromatosis," *Annals of Vascular Surgery*, vol. 16, no. 3, pp. 363–367, 2002.

[11] G. R. Craddock, V. R. Challa, and R. H. Dean, "Neurofibromatosis and renal artery stenosis: A case of familial incidence," *Journal of Vascular Surgery*, vol. 8, no. 4, pp. 489–494, 1988.

[12] M. Halpern and G. Currarino, "Vascular lesions causing hypertension in neurofibromatosis," *The New England Journal of Medicine*, vol. 273, no. 5, pp. 248–252, 1965.

[13] S. Kothari and I. Malav, "Renal artery stenosis due to neurofibromatosis," *Annals of Pediatric Cardiology*, vol. 2, no. 2, p. 167, 2009.

[14] C. Rhee, T. Jinn, H. Jung, M. Sung, K. H. Kim, and Y. Min, "Traumatic pseudoaneurysm of the external carotid artery with parotid mass and delayed facial nerve palsy," *Otolaryngology–Head and Neck Surgery*, vol. 121, no. 1, pp. 158–160, 2016.

[15] V. M. Pereira, S. Geiprasert, T. Krings et al., "Extracranial vertebral artery involvement in neurofibromatosis type I: Report of four cases and literature review," *Interventional Neuroradiology*, vol. 13, no. 4, pp. 315–328, 2007.

[16] C. Levy, J. P. Laissy, V. Raveau et al., "Carotid and vertebral artery dissections: Three-dimensional time-of- flight MR angiography and MR imaging versus conventional angiography," *Radiology*, vol. 190, no. 1, pp. 97–103, 1994.

[17] G. S. Oderich, T. M. Sullivan, T. C. Bower et al., "Vascular abnormalities in patients with neurofibromatosis syndrome type I: clinical spectrum, management, and results," *Journal of Vascular Surgery*, vol. 46, no. 3, pp. 475.e1–484.e1, 2007.

[18] G. P. Colby, L.-M. Lin, N. Nundkumar et al., "Radiation dose analysis of large and giant internal carotid artery aneurysm treatment with the pipeline embolization device versus traditional coiling techniques," *Journal of NeuroInterventional Surgery*, vol. 7, no. 5, pp. 380–384, 2015.

[19] H. W. Pia, C. Langmaid, and J. Zierski, *Cerebral Aneurysms: Advances in Diagnosis and Therapy*, Springer Science & Business Media, 2012.

31

Intravascular Leiomyomatosis as a Rare Cause of Nonthrombotic Pulmonary Embolism

Julie Van Maercke,[1] Anne-Sophie Van Rompuy,[2] Willy Poppe,[3] Tom Verbelen,[4] Marion Delcroix,[1] and Catharina Belge[1]

[1]*Department of Respiratory Diseases, KU Leuven-University of Leuven and University Hospitals Leuven, Leuven, Belgium*
[2]*Department of Anatomical Pathology, KU Leuven-University of Leuven and University Hospitals Leuven, Leuven, Belgium*
[3]*Department of Gynecology, KU Leuven-University of Leuven and University Hospitals Leuven, Leuven, Belgium*
[4]*Department of Cardiac Surgery, KU Leuven-University of Leuven and University Hospitals Leuven, Leuven, Belgium*

Correspondence should be addressed to Julie Van Maercke; julievmaercke@hotmail.com

Academic Editor: Ayman El-Menyar

Intravascular leiomyomatosis (IVL) is a very rare condition. It is characterized by the proliferation of benign smooth muscle cells within vascular structures without invasion of these tissues. Symptoms depend on the site of origin and the extent of invasion. Rarely, this neoplasm is located in the inferior vena cava or in the pulmonary vasculature potentially causing symptoms of dyspnea, chest pain, or syncope. We report the case of a 53-year-old woman who was referred to our hospital with extensive pulmonary embolism comprising of a subtotal occlusion of the right pulmonary artery with extension into the left pulmonary artery. Due to persistent dyspnea (New York Heart Association class II) despite anticoagulation, after a six-week period, imaging was repeated and showed stable findings. As she was not responding to adequate anticoagulant therapy, intima sarcoma of the pulmonary artery was suspected, and a pulmonary endarterectomy (PEA) was performed. A smooth, white, intravascular mass was easily and completely removed. Analysis demonstrated a lesion consisting of cells without atypia, showing expression of alpha-smooth muscle actin (alpha SMA) and desmin with partial expression of estrogen receptor (ER) and progesterone receptor (PR), leading to the diagnosis of intravascular leiomyomatosis. The patient fully recovered. Complete surgical removal of the intravascular tumor is recommended to relieve symptoms and prevent possible complications. Clinicians have to be aware that in unresolved pulmonary embolism, nonthrombotic and rare causes, like an intima sarcoma or intravascular leiomyomatosis, should be considered.

1. Introduction

Pulmonary embolism is a common and potentially life-threatening medical condition. It is usually caused by a deep vein thrombosis [1]. Other causes of intravascular obstruction are described [2] but are extremely rare. This causes substantial delay in correct diagnosis and treatment, which is often only obtained by a multidisciplinary approach. We present a case of an extensive pulmonary embolism not responding to anticoagulation therapy, which revealed to be due to intravascular leiomyomatosis.

2. Case Presentation

A 53-year-old woman was referred to the cardiology department in an affiliated center suffering from dyspnea during exercise (New York Heart Association class II) which she had experienced for a three-week period. She had recently taken a two-hour flight. She had no past medical problems and no family history of cardiovascular or lung diseases. She did not take any medication. Her physical examination was unremarkable. Echocardiography showed a normal systolic and diastolic function with a systolic pulmonary

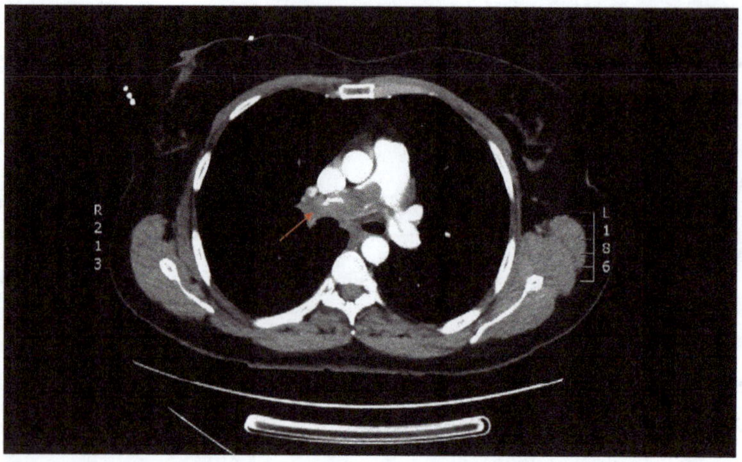

FIGURE 1: Transverse view of contrast-enhanced computed tomography images demonstrating a pulmonary embolism with subocclusion of the right pulmonary artery with extension to the left pulmonary artery and truncus pulmonalis.

artery pressure (PAPsys) of 33 mmHg. Blood count was normal besides a slightly elevated D-dimer test of 560 μg/L (0-500 μg/L). Computed tomography (CT) showed a subtotal occlusion of the right pulmonary artery and extension into the left pulmonary artery (Figure 1). Based on a diagnosis of acute pulmonary embolism, anticoagulant therapy with low molecular weight heparin (LMWH) was initiated. Although not recommended by the guidelines, screening for underlying malignancy by positron emission tomography- (PET-) CT scan was performed, which only exposed a fibromatous uterus with thrombosis of the right ovarian vein. The patient was discharged with apixaban five milligram twice daily. Due to persistent dyspnea, imaging was repeated after six weeks, showing no regression of the pulmonary embolism. As a result of this unusual outcome, she was referred to our center for treatment of chronic thromboembolic pulmonary hypertension. Based on the CT aspect with extensive proximal material in the absence of pulmonary hypertension, a nonthrombotic cause of pulmonary obstruction was suspected. Histopathological analysis of a biopsy obtained by right heart catheterization showed no microscopic or immunohistochemical evidence of an intima sarcoma. To obtain further diagnosis and treatment, a pulmonary endarterectomy (PEA) was performed. During this procedure, a smooth, white, intravascular mass was visualized (Figure 2) which was easily resected in its entirety. Macroscopic inspection of the pulmonary artery was normal. Pathological analysis of the specimen demonstrated a lesion consisting of spindle cells without atypia, showing expression of alpha SMA and desmin with partial expression of estrogen and progestogen receptors (Figure 3). Those findings led to the diagnosis of intravascular leiomyomatosis (IVL) without malignant transformation. The patient recovered completely. CT imaging of the thorax revealed no residual intravascular filling defects. Subsequently, our patient was referred to the department of gynecology. Magnetic resonance imaging (MRI) of the pelvis confirmed the presence of a fibromatous uterus without signs of malignancy. Given the postmenopausal state of the patient without strong evidence of intracaval tumor thrombosis, the gynaecologists forwent a hysterectomy. Follow-up with CT imaging of the thorax and abdomen is planned after one year.

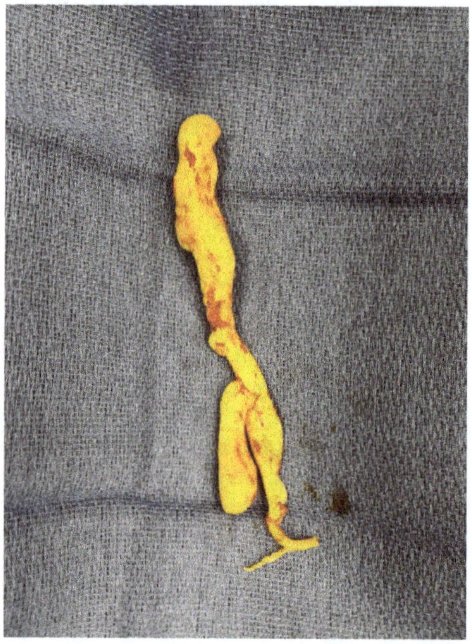

FIGURE 2: Macroscopic view of the resection specimen with a length of 15 cm and a smooth surface ("wormlike" appearance).

3. Discussion

Pulmonary embolism is a potentially life-threatening medical condition; most commonly caused by a deep vein thrombosis [1]. However, fat embolism, amniotic fluid embolism, septic embolism, tumoral embolism, and nonthrombotic pulmonary artery embolism should be considered, especially when anticoagulation treatment fails [2].

Intravascular leiomyomatosis (IVL) is a rare condition, up until now only described in case reports. It is characterized by the growth of benign smooth muscle cells within vascular structures without invading the tissue. In the majority of cases, the neoplasm originates from the uterus, with most

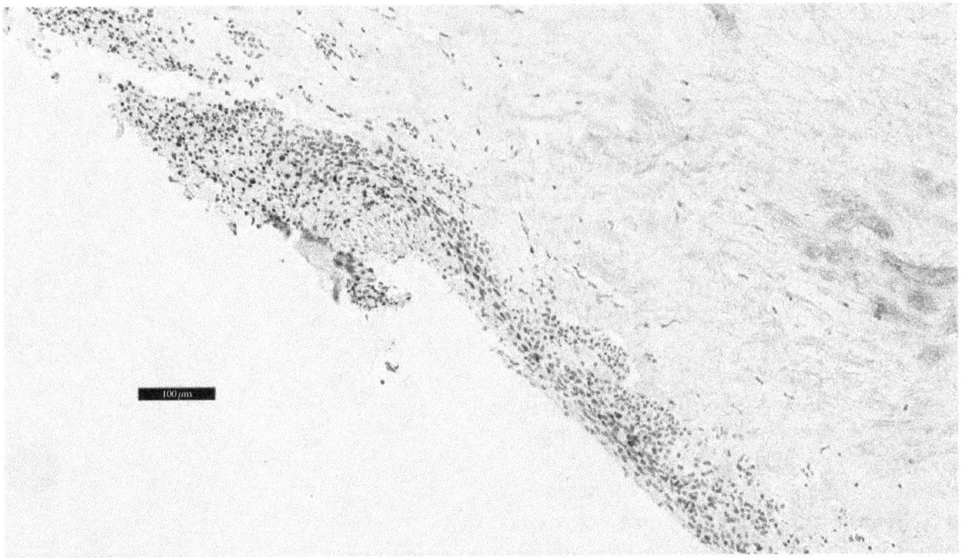

FIGURE 3: Immunohistochemical examination of the tumor (enlargement × 10) shows benign-appearing smooth muscle cells with expression of estrogen receptor (ER), marked in brown.

common extrauterine locations being the pelvic and broad ligament vessels, and more rarely, the inferior vena cava up to the pulmonary vasculature [3]. Tumors can emerge from the media of peripheral veins, by metastatic spread, or grow into the pelvic veins by direct invasion [4]. IVL with cardiac extension was first published in an autopsy report in 1907 by Durck [5].

Symptoms of IVL depend on the site of origin and the extent of intravascular invasion. In its most severe form, the tumor will migrate and further develop in the pulmonary artery which may cause symptoms of dyspnea, chest pain, and syncope.

The diagnosis of IVL as a cause of nonthrombotic pulmonary embolism is made by a multidisciplinary approach. Primarily, a comprehensive study of the past medical history must be obtained as this condition is often seen in middle-aged women with a history of hysterectomy for a fibromatous uterus [6]. Equally, anamnesis, clinical examination, and imaging by CT with contrast medium enhancement or T1-weighted magnetic resonance images (MRIs) are required [7, 8]. CT with contrast medium enhancement typically shows a hypoattenuating intravascular filling defect. In combination with a fibromatous uterus on MRI, this may suggest IVL [2], although the presence of a normal uterus on imaging does not exclude it [3]. Echocardiography is used to evaluate intracardiac extension, repercussions on the right heart function, and differential diagnosis of other intracardiac masses [9]. To differentiate from a malignant tumor, a preoperative diagnostic biopsy can be obtained [10], e.g., by right heart catheterization as was done in our case. Macroscopically, the tumor has a "wormlike" appearance. On histological and immunohistochemical examination, the tumor will show benign-appearing smooth muscle cells (desmin and alpha SMA positivity) with a weak to strong expression of estrogen receptor (ER) and progesterone receptor (PR) [3, 11].

Complete surgical removal of the intravascular tumor is recommended to relieve symptoms and prevent possible life-threatening complications depending on the location of the IVL [4]. Hysterectomy with bilateral salpingo-oophorectomy is also favored to prevent recurrence [12]. Hormonal therapy is most commonly used in patients unfit to undergo surgical treatment, in patients with incomplete resection or as neoadjuvant therapy to surgery. Tamoxifen, medroxyprogesterone, and gonadotropin-releasing hormone (GnRH) agonists in premenopausal women may be used. Results, however, are diverse ranging from minimal to meaningful response [9]. In our case, the gynecologist decided not to perform a hysterectomy since the risk of relapse was considered low due to the postmenopausal state of the patient and there was no strong evidence of important intracaval tumor thrombosis. Recurrence in patients who were treated by complete, surgical resection appears to be rare. To detect residual tumor growth or relapse, follow-up by six monthly to annual CT or MRI is advised [9, 13].

4. Conclusion

Intravascular leiomyomatosis with extension to the pulmonary arteries is a very rare condition. In case of unresolved pulmonary embolism, nonthrombotic causes, like an intima sarcoma or intravascular leiomyomatosis, should be considered.

Consent

The patient consented for publication.

References

[1] S. V. Konstantinides, G. Meyer, C. Becattini et al., "2019 ESC guidelines for the diagnosis and management of acute pulmonary embolism developed in collaboration with the European

Respiratory Society (ERS)," *European Heart Journal*, vol. 41, no. 4, pp. 543–603, 2020.

[2] Y.-H. Wu, Y.-T. Lee, C.-I. Lee, Y.-H. Tzeng, and J. Wei, "Non-thrombotic pulmonary embolism caused by intravenous leiomyomatosis," *Medicine*, vol. 98, no. 3, p. e14118, 2019.

[3] R. J. Carr, P. Hui, and N. Buza, "Intravenous leiomyomatosis revisited," *International Journal of Gynecological Pathology*, vol. 34, no. 2, pp. 169–176, 2015.

[4] S. G. Marcus, T. Krauss, R. S. Freedberg, A. T. Culliford, D. J. Weinreich, and I. Kronzon, "Pulmonary embolectomy for intravenous uterine leiomyomatosis," *American Heart Journal*, vol. 127, no. 6, pp. 1642–1645, 1994.

[5] M. J. Kocica, M. R. Vranes, D. Kostic et al., "Intravenous leiomyomatosis with extension to the heart: rare or underestimated?," *The Journal of Thoracic and Cardiovascular Surgery*, vol. 130, no. 6, pp. 1724–1726, 2005.

[6] A. Rajaii-Khorasani, M. Kahrom, M. Hashemzadeh, S. Tayebi, M. Ghazi, and A. Hamedanchi, "Pulmonary artery extension of uterine leiomyoma," *Journal of Cardiac Surgery*, vol. 27, no. 4, pp. 466–469, 2012.

[7] L. C. Bender, L. M. Mitsumori, K. A. Lloyd, and L. E. Stambaugh III, "AIRP best cases in radiologic-pathologic correlation: intravenous leiomyomatosis," *Radiographics*, vol. 31, no. 4, pp. 1053–1058, 2011.

[8] N. Fasih, A. K. Prasad Shanbhogue, D. B. Macdonald et al., "Leiomyomas beyond the uterus: unusual locations, rare manifestations," *Radiographics*, vol. 28, no. 7, pp. 1931–1948, 2008.

[9] T. D. Clay, J. Dimitriou, O. M. McNally, P. A. Russell, A. E. Newcomb, and A. M. Wilson, "Intravenous leiomyomatosis with intracardiac extension - A review of diagnosis and management with an illustrative case," *Surgical Oncology*, vol. 22, no. 3, pp. e44–e52, 2013.

[10] N. Moorjani, J. Kuo, S. Ashley, and G. Hughes, "Intravenous uterine leiomyosarcomatosis with intracardial extension," *Journal of Cardiac Surgery*, vol. 20, no. 4, pp. 382–385, 2005.

[11] G. Kir, M. Kir, A. Gurbuz, A. Karateke, and F. Aker, "Estrogen and progesterone expression of vessel walls with intravascular leiomyomatosis; discussion of histogenesis," *European Journal of Gynaecological Oncology*, vol. 25, no. 3, pp. 362–366, 2004.

[12] J. Wang, J. Yang, H. Huang et al., "Management of intravenous leiomyomatosis with intracaval and intracardiac extension," *Obstetrics and Gynecology*, vol. 120, no. 6, pp. 1400–1406, 2012.

[13] J. Du, X. Zhao, D. Guo, H. Li, and B. Sun, "Intravenous leiomyomatosis of the uterus," *Human Pathology*, vol. 42, no. 9, pp. 1240–1246, 2011.

32

Treatment of Aortic and Iliac Artery Occlusion by Catheter Thrombolysis Combined with Catheter Thrombectomy and Aortic Bifurcation Endovascular Stent Reconstruction

Xinyu Zhao, Delang Liu, Chaowen Yu, Yong Sun, and Shiyuan Chen

Department of Vascular Surgery, First Affiliated Hospital of Bengbu Medical College, Bengbu, Anhui Province, China

Correspondence should be addressed to Shiyuan Chen; 1372032523@qq.com

Academic Editor: Hiroyuki Nakajima

Aortoiliac occlusive disease (AIOD) is an occlusive disease of the infrarenal aorta and iliac arteries usually caused by stenosis or occlusion at the end of the abdominal aorta-common iliac artery. Herein, we reported a case of Trans-Atlantic Inter-Society Consensus- (TASC-) D AIOD with pale, cool, and intangible dorsalis pedis artery treated with catheter thrombolysis combined with catheter thrombectomy and aortic bifurcation endovascular stent reconstruction, which proved to be safe, effective, and minimally invasive approach. In the present paper, we discussed the physical and imaging manifestations, as well as treatments.

1. Introduction

Aortoiliac occlusive disease (AIOD) refers to the ischemic disease of lower extremities or pelvic tissue and organs caused by occlusion at the end of the abdominal aorta-bifurcation of the main iliac artery. The clinical manifestations include the disappearance of femoral artery pulsation, intermittent claudication, and impotence, which in some severe cases can cause distal limb gangrene. The most common cause of AIOD is atherosclerosis.

In the present case, due to atherosclerosis, bilateral common iliac, internal iliac, external iliac artery, and right anterior tibial artery proximal lumen occlusion were not treated in time, resulting in aortic and bilateral iliac artery thrombosis. The patient was then treated with catheter thrombolysis combined with catheter thrombectomy and aortic bifurcation endovascular stent reconstruction, which proved to be safe and effective approach.

2. Case Presentation

A 54-year-old male patient was admitted to our center on December 2, 2019. The patient presented with chills, numbness, and intermittent claudication in both lower limbs. Fontaine stage was IIa. The specialist physical examination revealed that the patient's pulsation of the left dorsalis pedis artery was weak, and the right dorsalis pedis artery was not palpable. Computed tomographic angiography (CTA) showed signs of filling defect in the proximal lumen of the common iliac, internal and external iliac arteries, and the right anterior tibial artery. They were found to have "continuity interruption" at the end of the abdominal aorta, and irregular stenosis of the local lumen of the bilateral femoral artery, deep femoral artery, popliteal artery, left anterior and posterior tibial artery, and peroneal artery was observed (Figures 1(a) and 1(c)).

During the first hospitalization, the patient refused surgical treatment and was given anticoagulation and vasodilation therapy for one week. After discharge, the patient was treated with antiplatelet aggregation and anticoagulation by oral administration of cilostazol and salgrel axetil. During the medication period, the patient developed ischemic rest pain (Fontaine stage III).

On January 8, 2020, the patient was readmitted to the hospital. Specialist physical examination revealed pale skin on both feet, the skin was also warm and cool, and the

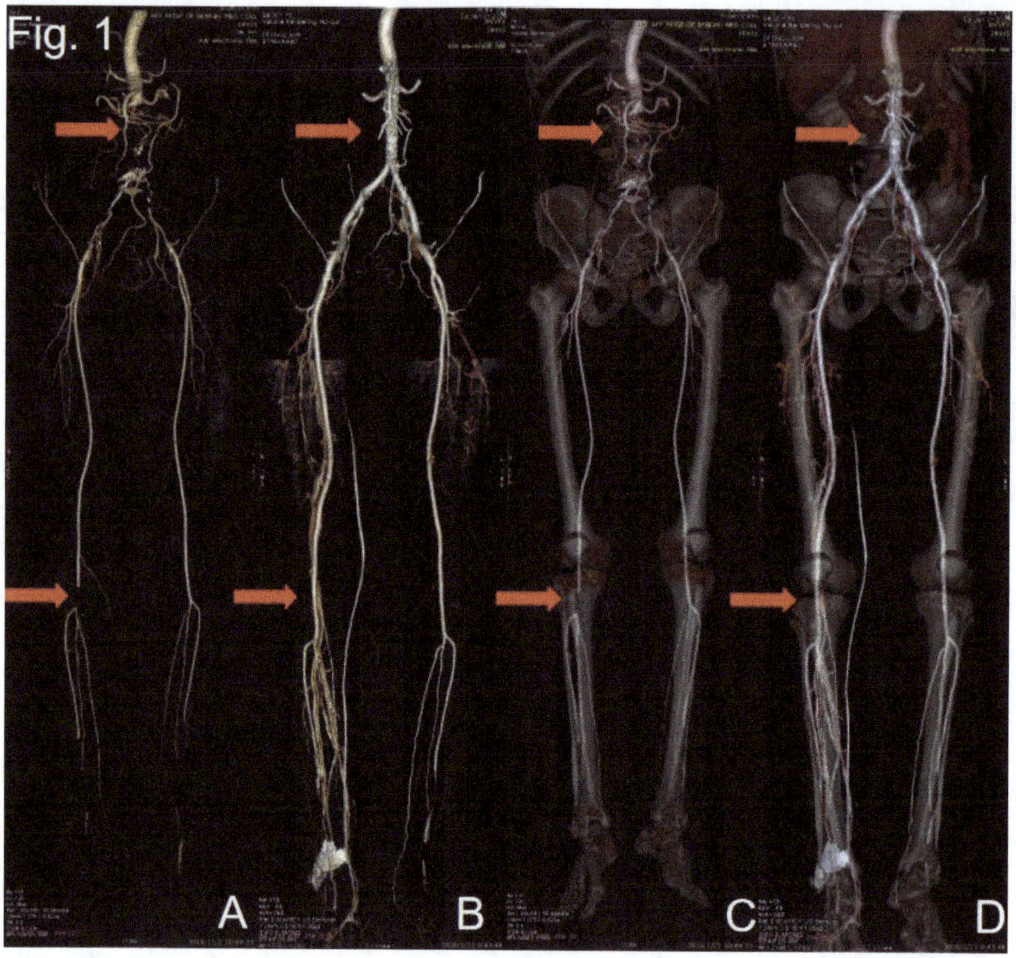

FIGURE 1: CTA before operation ((a) and (c)) after the operation ((b) and (d)). The red arrow points to the location of the lesion before and after the operation.

dorsalis pedis arteries were not palpable. Digital subtraction angiography (DSA) revealed that the right iliac artery was occluded, multiple thrombi were attached to the wall, and the abdominal aorta was occluded from the right renal artery level (Figure 2).

Through three operations that were performed at our center, we successfully opened the abdominal aorta and bilateral iliac arteries to improve the symptoms of lower limb ischemia. During the first procedure, we punctured the right femoral artery, successfully passed through the occlusive segment of the right iliac artery, and placed the end tip of the 5F 20cm UNIFUSE thrombolytic catheter into the abdominal aorta at the level of the right renal artery. Thrombolysis with 200000u urokinase was continuously given after operation. Two days later, we performed a second DSA operation. Thrombolytic catheter angiography showed that the right external iliac artery was partially developed, but the distal abdominal aorta was not seen. The possibility of blockage was considered at the tip end of the thrombolytic catheter, and the thrombolysis angiography showed that the thrombus in the proximal renal abdominal aorta was dissolved more than before. Replacement of 5F 20 cm UNIFUSE thrombolysis catheter continued thrombolysis for 24 hours (Figure 3). During the third procedure, we used thrombectomy combined with covered endovascular reconstruction of the aortic bifurcation (CERAB). The angiography of the right femoral artery showed a large filling defect below the opening of the renal artery of the abdominal aorta, the development of the right iliac artery was unobstructed, and the left iliac artery was not seen (Figure 4(a)). The 14 mm balloon was placed above the renal artery, and the balloon was filled and pulled to the end of the abdominal aorta to move the filling defect downward (Figure 4(b)). The 4F Fogarty balloon embolization tube was implanted into the end of the abdominal aorta, the arterial embolus was removed about 10 cm, and the thrombus was distally removed. The embolus of the left iliac artery was removed by the same method. The pulsation of bilateral femoral arteries was palpable after thrombectomy. The lower segment of the abdominal aorta was implanted with Medtronic ENDURANT EN LW 1616C95EE self-expanding covered stent, and the upper end was located below the opening of the right renal artery. Angiography showed that the blood flow in the stent of the abdominal aorta was unobstructed, and there was no contrast medium extravasation and filling defect. Two self-expanding covered stents (Bard Fluency 8 mm * 80 mm) were implanted in both common iliac arteries, where the proximal end of the two stents was located

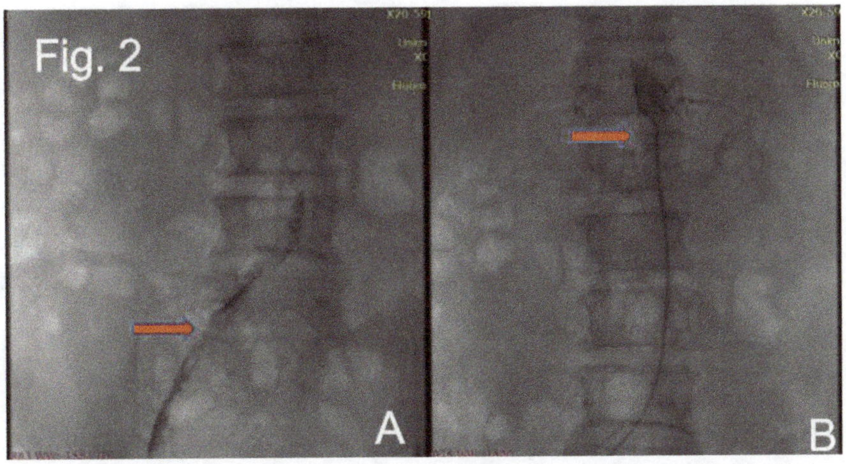

FIGURE 2: The first DSA image. Occlusion of the right iliac artery and multiple thromboses in the wall (a). Occlusion of the abdominal aorta at the level of the right renal artery (b).

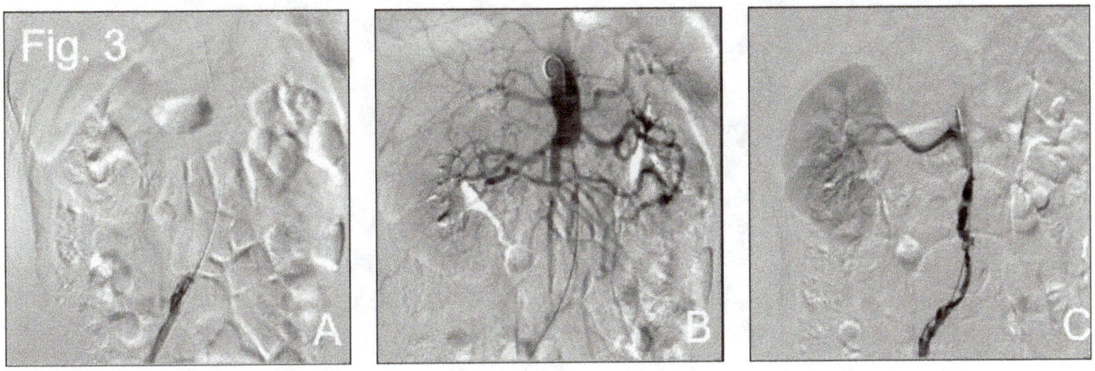

(a) (b) (c)

FIGURE 3: The second DSA image. Thrombolysis catheter blockage, partial development of right external iliac artery (a). Thrombolysis in the proximal renal abdominal aorta (b). Replacement of thrombolytic catheter angiography (c).

in the abdominal aortic stent, overlapping some 15 mm. Angiography showed that the blood flow in the abdominal aorta and bilateral iliac arteries was unobstructed, and the orifice of the bilateral iliac arteries was narrowed. The stenotic segments of bilateral iliac arteries were dilated with 8 mm balloon, and the angiographic results showed improved blood flow than before (Figures 4(c) and 4(d)). Finally, we placed 4F Fogarty thrombectomy balloon into the right popliteal artery and removed the artery 5 cm embolus. The angiography showed that the blood flow of the right popliteal artery was smooth (Figure 5).

After the operation, we examined the patient and found that the skin temperature in both feet recovered, and the bilateral dorsalis pedis arteries were palpable. Reexamination of CTA revealed that the abdominal aorta, bilateral common iliac, internal and external iliac arteries, bilateral femoral arteries, deep femoral arteries, and popliteal arteries were functioning well (Figures 1(b) and 1(d)).

After operation, the patient was orally given aspirin, 100 mg qd, Rivassaban 2.5 mg bid [1]. Also, the blood coagulation function of the patient was monitored; his prothrombin and international standard ratio were in the ideal range.

3. Discussion

Over recent years, the incidence of AIOD has been increasing year by year [2, 3]. AIOD risk factors include advanced age, smoking, obesity, diabetes, hypertension, hyperlipidemia, chronic renal insufficiency, and homocysteinemia [4]. If AIOD develops into chronic limb-threatening ischemia (CLTI), the risk of myocardial infarction, stroke, and death increases three-fold [5]. The patient reported in the present study had TASC-D type of main iliac artery occlusive disease according to TASC-II classification, and surgical treatment was recommended as the first treatment choice [4]. The total incidence of complications after AIOD surgical treatment has been reported to be about 17% to 32% [6].

AIOD treatment has gradually evolved from traditional surgical bypass surgeries to intracavitary surgery with less trauma, fewer complications, and rapid recovery [7]. We chose catheterization thrombolysis combined with catheter thrombectomy, CERAB. In this case, the signs at the first visit were mild, and the symptoms significantly aggravated after one month, suggesting that insufficient anticoagulation may lead to thrombosis of the main iliac artery. In the first

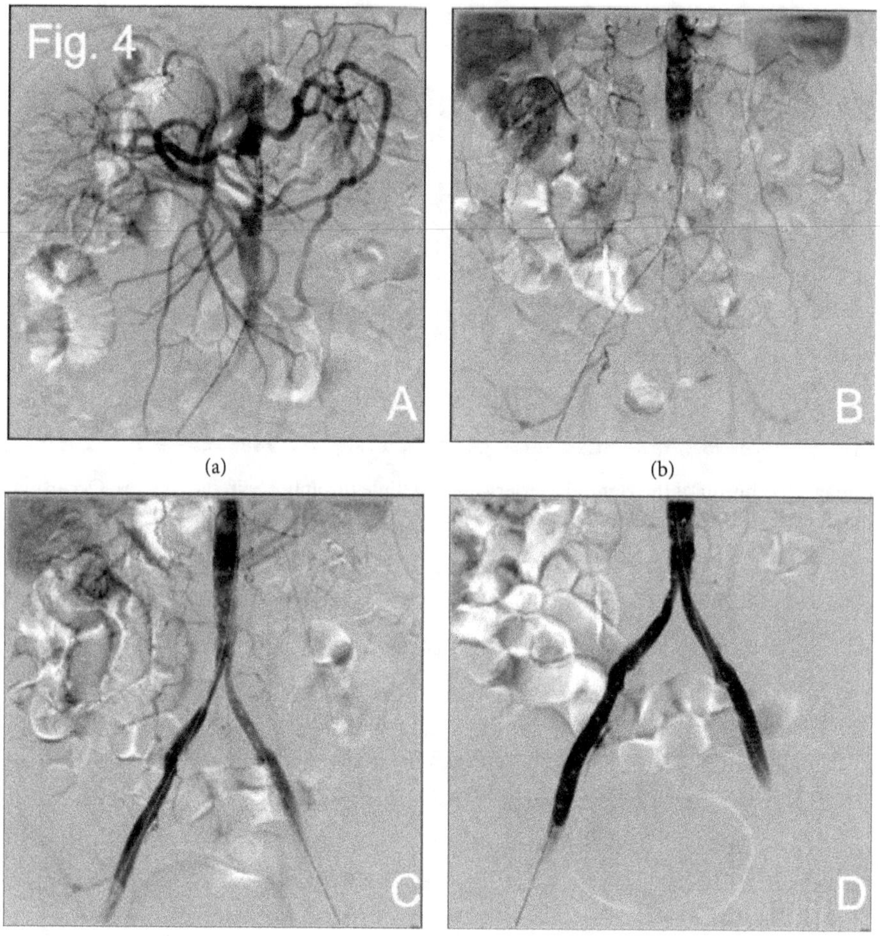

(a) (b)

(c) (d)

FIGURE 4: The third DSA image. Angiography before and after thrombectomy ((a) and (b)). Angiography before and after balloon dilatation ((c) and (d)).

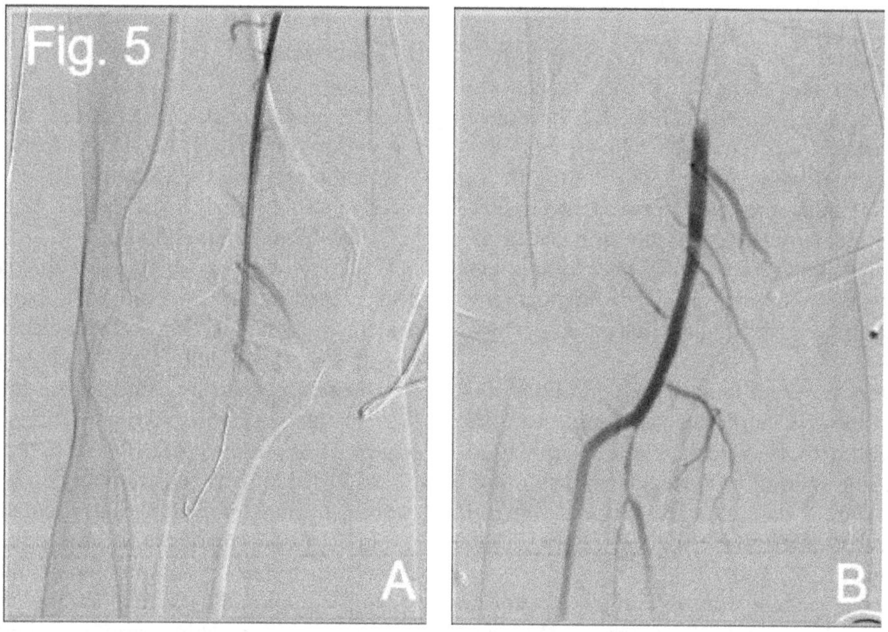

(a) (b)

FIGURE 5: Angiography of right popliteal artery before and after thrombectomy ((a) and (b)).

angiography, there was a long segment occlusion in the lumen of the right iliac artery and fresh thrombus in the wall. Blind balloon dilatation and stenting may lead to thrombus shedding, failure of opening, and similar, eventually resulting in adverse consequences. We used vertebral artery catheter combined with hard slippery guide wire to successfully pass through the occlusive segment of iliac artery and insert thrombolytic catheter. After two thrombolysis, the aortic occlusive segment adjacent to the renal artery disappeared, which in turn reduced the level of stent placement and the possibility of stent affecting the renal artery. The diameter of the abdominal aorta of the patient was large, and there was no matching thrombectomy catheter. We used a 14 mm balloon instead of a thrombectomy catheter and successfully removed the aortic-iliac artery thrombus. Considering that the patient had long aortic-bilateral iliac artery stenosis, we used CERAB [8], a technique with a high medium- and long-term patency rate in the reconstruction of complex AIOD [9, 10]. After bilateral femoral artery angiography, the path map was made to determine the opening of the bilateral internal iliac artery, after which the bilateral common iliac artery stent was implanted into the lower segment of the abdominal aorta. The use of covered stents can effectively reduce arterial perforation, rupture, acute or chronic bleeding, and avoid intimal hyperplasia and in-stent restenosis. On the other hand, it can avoid stenosis and thrombosis caused by mural thrombus shedding of occlusive disease [11, 12]. The use of covered stents can also increase the risk of covering collateral vessels or internal iliac arteries [11]. Finally, we used balloons to dilate the abdominal aorta-double iliac artery stents so as to protect the contralateral iliac artery and further avoid embolism caused by dissection, plaque displacement, and shedding.

4. Conclusion

Herein, we described a case of a patient with TASC-D aortic and iliac artery occlusion who experienced significant improvement in lower limb ischemia after three operations. We believe that catheter thrombolysis combined with catheter thrombectomy and covered endovascular reconstruction of the aortic bifurcation is a safe, effective, and minimally invasive method for the treatment of long-segment aortic iliac artery occlusion.

Consent

The patient has consented to the submission of the case.

Authors' Contributions

Xinyu Zhao and Delang Liu contributed equally to this paper.

Acknowledgments

This work was supported by grants from Bengbu Science and Technology Innovation Guidance Project (20180314).

References

[1] M. P. Bonaca, R. M. Bauersachs, S. S. Anand et al., "Rivaroxaban in peripheral artery disease after revascularization," *The New England Journal of Medicine*, vol. 382, no. 21, pp. 1994–2004, 2020.

[2] F. G. Fowkes, D. Rudan, I. Rudan et al., "Comparison of global estimates of prevalence and risk factors for peripheral artery disease in 2000 and 2010: a systematic review and analysis," *Lancet*, vol. 382, no. 9901, pp. 1329–1340, 2013.

[3] P. Song, D. Rudan, M. Wang, X. Chang, and I. Rudan, "National and subnational estimation of the prevalence of peripheral artery disease (PAD) in China: a systematic review and meta-analysis," *Journal of Global Health*, vol. 9, no. 1, article 010601, 2019.

[4] L. Norgren, W. R. Hiatt, J. A. Dormandy, M. R. Nehler, K. A. Harris, and F. G. R. Fowkes, "Inter-society consensus for the management of peripheral arterial disease (TASC II)," *Journal of Vascular Surgery*, vol. 45, no. 1, pp. S5–S67, 2007.

[5] T. W. Rooke, A. T. Hirsch, S. Misra et al., "2011 ACCF/AHA focused update of the guideline for the management of patients with peripheral artery disease (updating the 2005 guideline)," *Vascular Medicine*, vol. 16, no. 6, pp. 452–476, 2011.

[6] M. T. Menard and M. Belkin, *Aortoliac disease: direct reconstruction//Cronenwett JL, Johnston KW. Rutherford's vascular surgery*, Elsevier, Philadelphia, 8th ed edition, 2013.

[7] Y. Lun, J. Zhang, X. Wu et al., "Comparison of midterm outcomes between surgical treatment and endovascular reconstruction for chronic infrarenal aortoiliac occlusion," *Journal of Vascular and Interventional Radiology*, vol. 26, no. 2, pp. 196–204, 2015.

[8] F. A. B. Grimme, P. C. J. M. Goverde, P. J. E. M. Verbruggen, C. J. Zeebregts, and M. M. P. J. Reijnen, "First results of the covered endovascular reconstruction of the aortic bifurcation (CERAB) technique for aortoiliac occlusive disease," *Journal of Vascular Surgery*, vol. 62, no. 5, pp. 1371-1372, 2015.

[9] B. P. Mwipatayi, S. Sharma, A. Daneshmand et al., "Durability of the balloon-expandable covered versus bare-metal stents in the covered versus balloon expandable stent trial (COBEST) for the treatment of aortoiliac occlusive disease," *Journal of Vascular Surgery*, vol. 64, no. 1, pp. 83–94.e1, 2016.

[10] C. Shen, Y. Zhang, C. Qu, J. Fang, X. Liu, and L. Teng, "Outcomes of Total Aortoiliac Revascularization for TASC-II C&D Lesion with Kissing Self-Expanding Covered Stents," *Annals of Vascular Surgery*, vol. 68, pp. 434–441, 2020.

[11] B. P. Mwipatayi, S. Thomas, J. Wong et al., "A comparison of covered vs bare expandable stents for the treatment of aortoiliac occlusive disease," *Journal of Vascular Surgery*, vol. 54, no. 6, pp. 1561–1570.e1, 2011.

[12] S. S. Sabri, A. Choudhri, G. Orgera et al., "Outcomes of covered kissing stent placement compared with bare metal stent placement in the treatment of atherosclerotic occlusive disease at the aortic bifurcation," *Journal of Vascular and Interventional Radiology*, vol. 21, no. 7, pp. 995–1003, 2010.

33

Carotid Paraganglioma in Adolescence-Clinical Picture-Surgical Technique and Review of the Literature

Thomas Kotsis,[1] **Panagitsa Christoforou**,[1] **and Constantinos Nastos**[2]

[1] *Vascular Division, 2nd Department of Surgery, National & Kapodistrian University of Athens Medical School, "Aretaieion" Hospital, Athens, Greece*

[2] *2nd Department of Surgery, National & Kapodistrian University of Athens Medical School, "Aretaieion" Hospital, Athens, Greece*

Correspondence should be addressed to Thomas Kotsis; kotsisth@otenet.gr

Academic Editor: Jaw-Wen Chen

Paraganglia are clusters of cells originating from the neural crest with histological and cytochemical characteristics of neuroendocrine cells. Paragangliomas of the head and neck represent less than 0.5% of all head and neck tumors and they usually occur between the ages of 40 and 50. Paragangliomas in childhood and in adolescence are extremely rare; only 23 case reports have been reported in the recent literature. In childhood, the estimation of malignant potential is 3–10%; therefore, early diagnosis and treatment of carotid body paragangliomas are mandatory. However, due to the rarity of these lesions in young patients, they are often not included in the differential diagnosis of solid masses in the neck area, a fact that may lead to misdiagnosis or delay in treatment. We present, herein, two extremely rare cases of patients in adolescence who were diagnosed with a carotid body paraganglioma and were treated surgically in our unit. One of the patients was diagnosed and treated at the age of 15 years while the other had a long-standing tumor in the neck that was followed up by a general surgery outpatient service as a branchial cleft cyst at the age of 15 years and was eventually treated surgically 8 years later. Carotid body tumor was not considered in the initial differential diagnosis because of its rarity at this age range.

1. Introduction

Paraganglia are clusters of cells with histological and cytochemical characteristics of neuroendocrine cells originating from the neural crest [1]. Paragangliomas of the head and neck represent less than 0.5% of all head and neck tumors [2]. Sporadic paragangliomas appear more frequent in female than male, at the age of 40 to 50 years, while familial paragangliomas present earlier and more commonly in male [3]. Pediatric paragangliomas are even more rare entities and only a few cases have been reported in the recent literature [4].

We present two cases of carotid body paragangliomas (CBP) that occurred during adolescence; one of the patients had a delayed treatment, as a neck mass initially observed at childhood was considered to be a branchial cleft cyst, for which he had annual surveillance at a general surgery outpatient service.

The clinical picture, the imaging investigations, the differential diagnosis, and the surgical treatment are discussed in the current manuscript, along with a review of similar published cases.

2. Material and Methods

2.1. Search Methods. We searched the PubMed and Cochrane Library databases with no language restrictions. Studies or case reports were published between 1968 and 2018.

2.2. Selection Criteria. We performed a literature search with the keywords "Paraganglioma", "Carotid body paraganglioma", "Head and neck paraganglioma", and "Chemodectoma", without limitations to the dates or the article types. According to the database and the used terms, many studies and incidents were reported. Our research focuses on carotid body paragangliomas in adolescence, so more specific investigation with the keywords "adolescence carotid body paraganglioma" and "pediatric carotid body paraganglioma" has revealed only 23 published case reports.

2.3. Data Collection and Analysis. Two reviewers independently assessed the risk of bias. They extracted the characteristics and results of the various studies that were discussed. In case of any disagreements that had occurred during data extraction, the third reviewer was asked to decide.

2.4. Main Results. During the literature search, many investigations found to be referred to multiple incidents, including a number of pediatric people treated with CBP. In some of these series, there is no reference of the exact number of pediatric patients being treated, nor the preoperative, intraoperative, and postoperative management of these patients.

The search produced 21 papers that were reviewed (Table 1). Information about the number of cases with neck paragangliomas at pediatric age group, the year of publication, the patients age and gender, the presenting symptoms, the size of the tumor, the Shamblin type, the malignancy, the cranial nerve injury, the treatment, and the follow-up period with no complications were identified and tabulated.

3. Case Reports

We report two cases of carotid paraganglioma in young age that have been operated in our department in the last 14 years, with a diagnosis of carotid body paragangliomas diagnosed and treated during adolescence, by the same surgeon (first author).

3.1. Case 1. A 16-year-old girl, with a free past medical history, presented with a palpable mass on the left side of the neck, complaining of dysphagia and cervical pain associated with dizziness. Neurologic examination was unremarkable and diagnostic tests for Epstein–Barr infection were negative. The patient underwent a thyroid ultrasound (US), which did not reveal any significant findings from the thyroid gland. However, a 27.5mm oval shaped, well-defined, hypoechoic, solid lesion was found at the left carotid triangle. The lesion showed high vascularity. Magnetic resonance imaging (MRI) of the neck followed showing an ovoid mass measuring 26x21x30mm between the left internal and external carotid arteries. A computed tomography angiography (CTA) was also performed with similar findings, suggesting the diagnosis of a CBP (Figures 1 and 2). The patient was electively admitted in our vascular unit in order to be treated surgically. A mass 2.5 cm was removed which was classified as Shamblin II (Figure 3). The histopathology results showed "zellballen" growth pattern of paraganglioma with central round/oval chief cells containing abundant eosinophilic granular or vacuolated cytoplasm, uniform nuclei with dispersed chromatin-nests of cells. Prominent fibrovascular stroma separated characteristic nests of paraganglioma tissue and there was no evidence of malignancy (Figure 4).

The patient had no postoperative neurologic symptoms except a transient episode of left parietal hypoesthesia. This was further investigated with an MRI of the brain and carotid ultrasound, which did not reveal sinister findings.

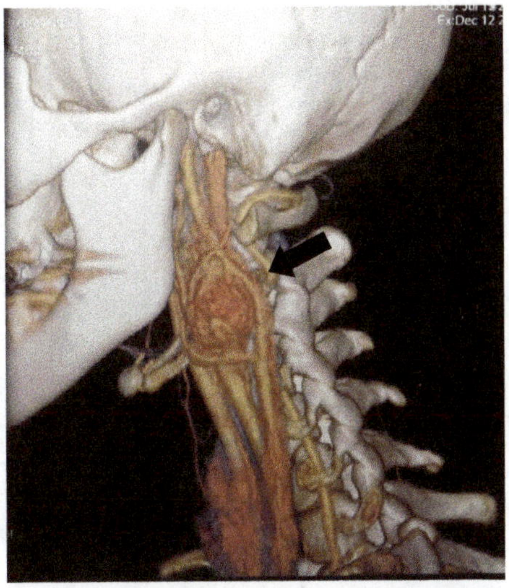

FIGURE 1: 3-dimensional (3D) cervical-computed tomography angiography (CTA), lyre sign (arrow).

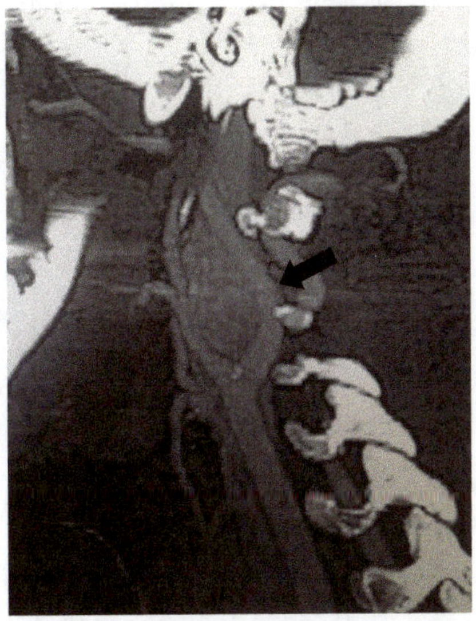

FIGURE 2: CTA-carotid body paraganglioma (CBP), lyre sign (arrow).

She had an uneventful postoperative recovery and was subsequently discharged on the 3rd postoperative day (POD).

3.2. Case 2. A 15-year-old teenage boy initially presented in a district hospital, with a swelling at the right side of his neck, without any significant clinical symptoms. Although full details of the work-up performed at the time are not available, he was diagnosed with a branchial cleft cyst and was offered surveillance with follow-up imaging. Eight years later, he visited our unit. Physical examination revealed a painless palpable well-defined mass (Figure 5) within the right carotid triangle with positive Fontaine and Kocher I signs [1]. There was no palpable lymphadenopathy. An

Table 1: Reported cases of CBPs in pediatric age group [4, 6–9, 11–26].

Year/author	Age/ Gender	Symptoms	Shamblin type	Size (mm)	Malignancy	Cranial nerve injury	Treatment	Follow-up period without complications (months)
1968/ Chambers et al [11]	12/M 14/M 9/F	NR	NR NR NR	25X25 60X60 15X20	No	No	Surgical Excision	120 120 12
1971/ Shamblin et al [12]	12/NR	NR	NR	NR	No	NR	Surgical Excision	NR
1980/ Newland et al [14]	13/F	Hypertension, Tachycardia	NR	25X80	NR	NR	Surgical Excision/ Radiotherapy, Chemotherapy	NR
1983/ Carney et al [21]	12/F	NR	NR	NR	No	No	Surgical Excision	Epithelioid myosarcoma-chondroma (24y), two nodules in left lung (30 y), well at age 31
1986/ Dickinson et al [22]	12/F	NR	NR	NR	No	XII permanent paralysis	Surgical Excision	NR
1988/ Hallett et al [6]	12/NR	Neck Mass Tumor	NR	NR	NR	Yes (not specified)	Surgical Excision	NR
1989/ Thompson et al [7]	14/F	Bilateral CBPs and Glomus Jugular Tumor	I III	20X20 Large	No	Right facial nerve paralysis No	Surgical Excision	NR
1990/ Gounot et al [16]	14/M	Right neck mass	II	35X25X15	No	No	Subadventitial Excision	12
1991/ Ophir et al [8]	12/F	Bilateral CBPS and Unilateral Jugular Tumor	III II	30X40 30X30	Family History (+)	Paralysis of IXth to XIIth cranial nerves No	Surgical Excision	96
1993/ Varudkar et al [9]	6/M	Swelling, Hypertension, Pheochromocytoma	NR	NR	No	No	Surgical Excision	NR
1999/ Hajnzic et al [25]	9/M	NR	NR	50	Metastatic Chest Paraganglioma, Pulmonary Metastasis	No	Surgical Excision Chemotherapy	Death after 4 months

Table 1: Continued.

Year/author	Age/ Gender	Symptoms	Shamblin type	Size (mm)	Malignancy	Cranial nerve injury	Treatment	Follow-up period without complications (months)
2000/ Wang et al [23]	10/NR	NR	NR	NR	No	Yes (not specified)	Surgical Excision, Preoperative Embolization	2.9
2001/ Plukker et al [24]	11/NR	NR	NR	NR	No	Yes (not specified)	Surgical Excision	NR
2003/ Takautz et al [4]	8.2/F	NR	NR	25	NR	No	Surgical Excision	118
2005/ Osborne et al [17]	16/F	Nonpulsatile Tumor	NR	NR	NR	NR	Preoperative Emboli, Subadventitial Dissection	NR
2007/ Zaupa et al [18]	15/M	Asymptomatic Mass	NR	NR	No	NR	Subadventitial Excision	NR
2007/ Sajid [26]	18/ NR	NR	NR	NR	NR	NR	Surgical Excision	NR
2008/ Georgiadis et al [13]	13/F	Painless Pulsatile Slow-Growing Mass	III	50X43X30	No	No	En Bloc Surgical Excision	9
2014/ Lopez-vasquez et al [19]	16/F	Asymptomatic Mass	NR	40X30X30	No	NR	Surgical Excision	NR
2017/Ifeoluwa et al [20]	8/F	Pulsatile Slow-Growing Mass	NR	NR	No	No	Preoperative embolization Surgical resection	Current time
2018/Hogan et al [15]	8/F	Neck mass	NR	NR	No	No	Preoperative embolization and balloon test occlusion Surgical excision	NR
2018/ our cases	16/ F	Cervical Pain, Dizziness, Dysphagia, Breathlessness and Palpable Mass	II	26x21x30	No	No	Surgical Excision	26
	15/M	Asymptomatic Mass	II	60X35	No	No	Surgical Excision	96

M: male, F: female, and NR: not reported.

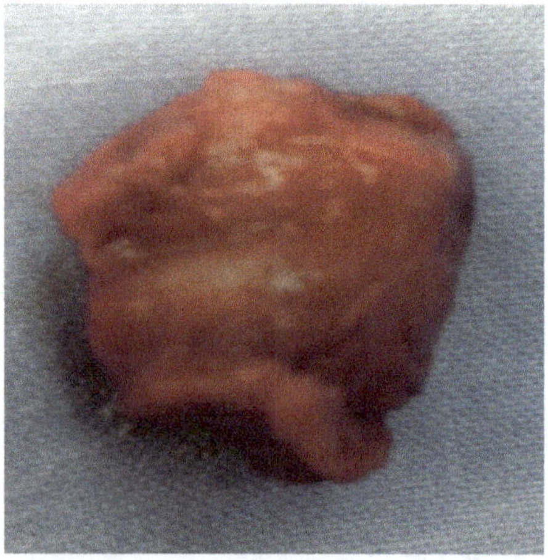

Figure 3: Paraganglioma of carotid tumor after surgical resection.

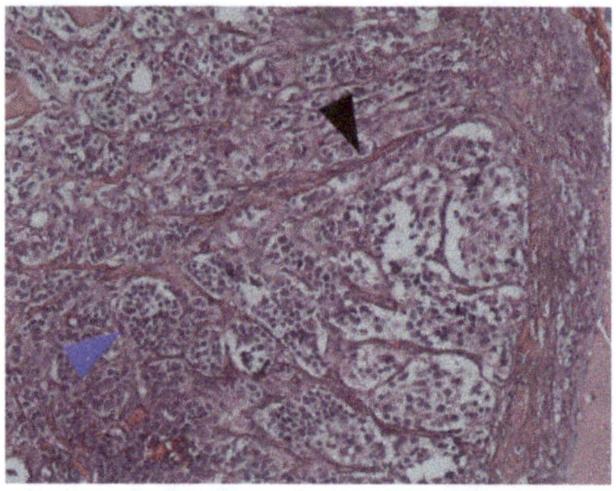

Figure 4: Histopathological appearance of CBP (16-year-old teenage girl) showing "zellballen" growth pattern of paragangliomas with central round/oval chief cells containing abundant eosinophilic granular or vacuolated cytoplasm, uniform nuclei with dispersed chromatin-nests of cells (blue arrow). Prominent fibrovascular stroma separates nests (black arrow).

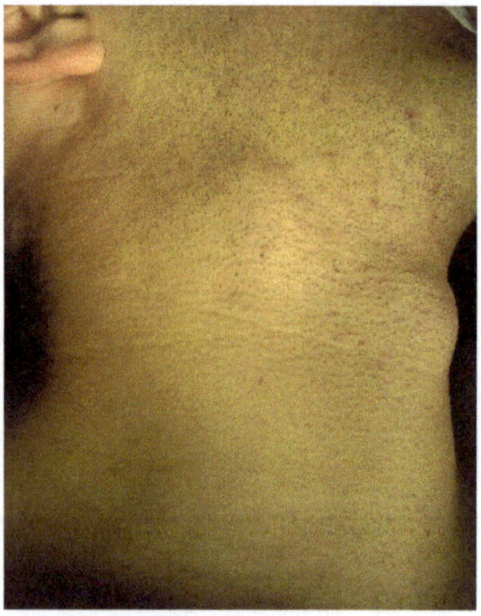

Figure 5: Painless palpable well-defined mass in the right carotid triangle.

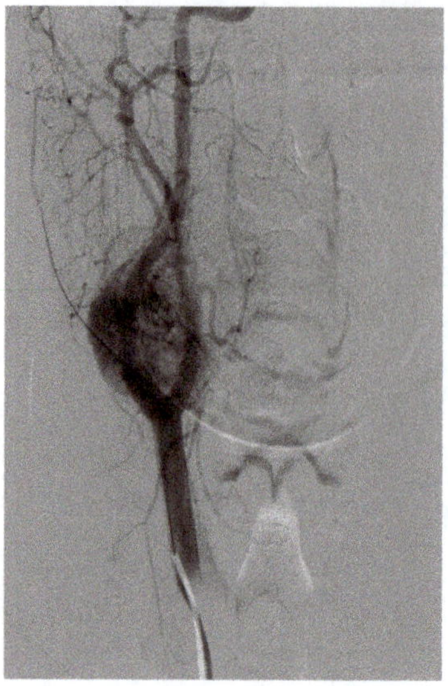

Figure 6: Digital subtraction angiography (DSA) revealed a carotid body paraganglioma in the right carotid bifurcation.

ultrasound scan was performed depicting a solid mass of mixed echogenicity in the right carotid triangle. This was suspected to be neurogenic in origin because of its location. A digital subtraction angiography (DSA) (Figure 6) followed, which revealed a 60x35mm protruding mass in the right carotid bifurcation, causing local compressive effects and posterior displacement of the vessels. The patient was admitted in our unit in order to be treated surgically. During the operation a large CBP was identified as seen in Figure 7. The tumor was classified as Shamblin II and was completely excised. Histopathology study showed a 3 cm carotid body paraganglioma with characteristic "zellballen" growth pattern and cell nests surrounded by prominent fibrovascular stroma, with no evidence of malignancy (Figure 8). The patient had an unremarkable recovery and was discharged home on the second POD.

The surgical technique adopted in both patients consisted of an oblique incision along the sternal head of the left sternocleidomastoid muscle under general anesthesia. Our strategy was to expose, dissect, and isolate the proximal common carotid artery using a vascular tape. The ansa cervicalis was also exposed early in the operation. The carotid bifurcation was exposed in a caudocranial approach. The proximal external and the proximal internal carotid arteries were isolated and controlled with vessel loops. Dissection was extended to the level of the digastor muscle in order to expose and control the distal internal carotid artery. During this process, the hypoglossal nerve was identified and preserved, by following the ansa cervicalis. The external carotid artery was cross-clamped temporarily. Finally, the tumor was removed with sharp dissection from the bifurcation with meticulous technique in order to avoid injury to the internal carotid artery and the cranial nerves. The reported plane of dissection reported as a white interface plane between the tumor and the vessels was not identified in the first patient as the tumor was severely adhering to the vessel wall and was typically

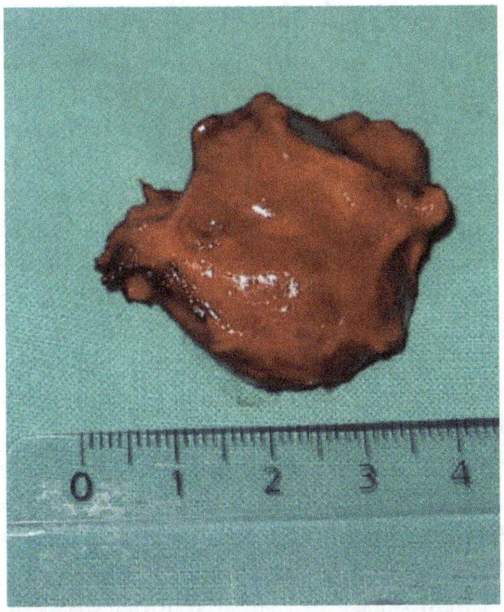

FIGURE 7: Paraganglioma of carotid tumor after surgical resection was 3 cm in diameter.

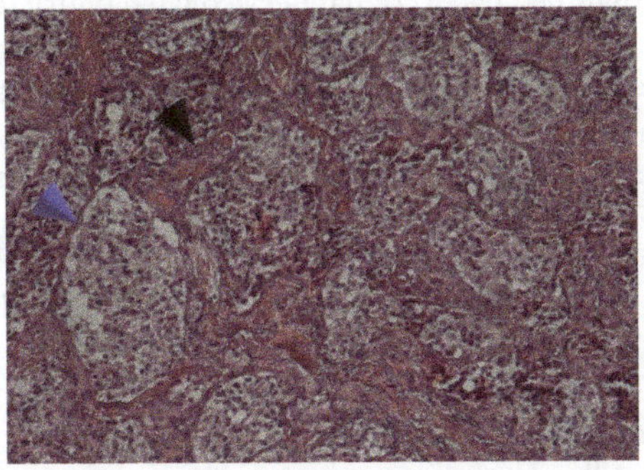

FIGURE 8: Histopathological appearance of CBP (15-year-old teenage boy) showing "zellballen" growth pattern of paragangliomas (blue arrow). Prominent fibrovascular stroma separates nests (black arrow).

found in the second patient. Following the removal of the CBP, the carotid sheath and platysma were approximated and the skin closed with a continuous subcuticular suture, after performing meticulous hemostasis (Figures 9 and 10).

Both patients had an annual postoperative follow-up with cervical ultrasound and carotid duplex ultrasonography with no evidence of local recurrence. Familial disease was excluded clinically, by screening the patient's first degree relatives with ultrasound imaging.

4. Discussion

Paragangliomas of the head and neck are quite rare tumors, and although the exact incidence is unclear they are considered to represent less than 0.5% of all head and neck tumors [2]. Paragangliomas can arise from the carotid body, the tympanic, jugular, and high vagal paraganglia. The paraganglioma of the carotid body (CBP) is the most common paraganglionic neoplasm distributed in the head and neck area. Pediatric paragangliomas are even more rare entities

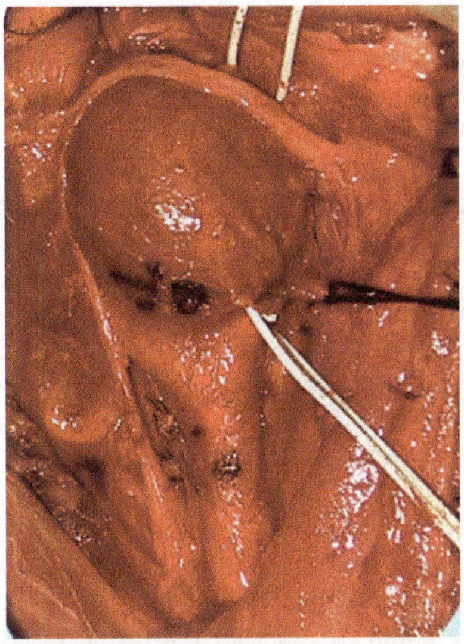

FIGURE 9: The right carotid triangle with carotid body paraganglioma.

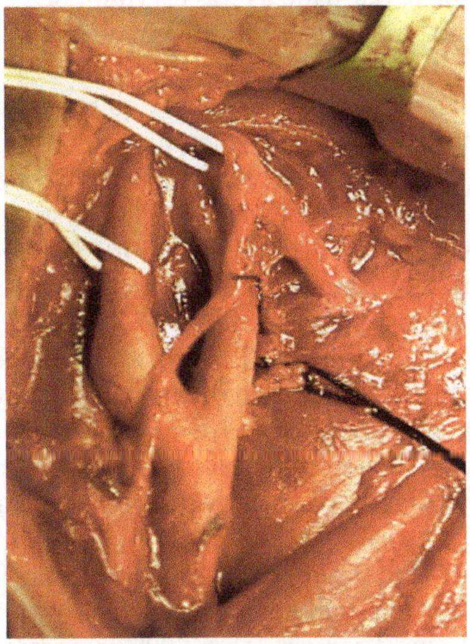

FIGURE 10: The carotid body paraganglioma of the right carotid triangle was completely excised, with preservation of the hypoglossal and vagus nerve.

and only a few cases have been reported in the recent literature (Table 1).

First recognized by Arias-Stella, CBPs occur in individuals under chronic stimulation by low environmental atmospheric partial pressure of oxygen, leading to hyperplasia of the chief cells of the carotid body [5]; Saldana et al. reported increased incidence of the tumor in Peruvian patients living in high altitudes and concluded that hypoxia was the primary stimuli leading to carotid body hyperplasia. This distinct disease may manifest with hyperplastic carotid body lesions under 1 cm and should be distinguished from typical CBP which should be treated surgically [6].

In our review of the literature we recognized 23 cervical paragangliomas involving the carotid body in children and adolescents. Mean patient age at the time of treatment was 12 years, with range 6 to 18 years (Table 1). There seemed to be a female predominance (female:male ratio, 2:1); however, some studies lack gender data and, thus, the ratio may be misleading.

Two of the patients had bilateral CBPs and at the same time presented jugular tumor [7, 8], while one patient was also diagnosed with a pheochromocytoma [9]. The overall incidence of multifocality in the sporadic form of the disease is estimated to be 5%, but this rises to 33% in familiar cases, where the disease is inherited in an autosomal-dominant pattern [10].

The incidence of familial paragangliomas is approximately 10%, and about 30% of them are caused by mutations in succinate dehydrogenase (SDH) gene [11, 12]. Presentation at young age could be associated with increased incidence of familial disease. In our review we identified one patient with familial disease and no patient with identified SDH gene mutations, although SDH mutation frequency in these patients may be underestimated, due to treatment during past decades. None of our patients was tested for SDH mutations, as this was not routinely performed in our unit during that period.

Diagnosis of these tumors can be quite challenging and most patients overlook the symptoms of the disease or are misdiagnosed with cervical lymphadenopathy, salivary gland pathology, neurofibromas, brachial cleft cysts, or lipomas [13]. Incorrect clinical diagnosis is reported in up to 30% of cases. Fine needle aspiration is not helpful as it is considered dangerous and is accompanied by a high risk of bleeding [1, 14]. Hogan et al. described a CBP in an 8-year-old female with a neck mass mistaken as reactive lymphadenopathy [15]. This is in accordance with the course of our second patient. In our review we found that most patients were either asymptomatic or had a palpable neck mass with recent increase in size [6, 13, 15–20].

The most important preoperative imaging is CTA or MRA, while digital subtraction angiography (DSA) is the mainstay of the diagnosis, with 100% reported accuracy, whereas the "lyre sign", an enhancing vascular oval mass widening the angle of the bifurcation, is essentially pathognomonic of a CBP [10]. Radionuclide perfusion scanning with 99mTc pertechnetate has also been used to diagnose CBPs, with some success, while the use of meta-iodobenzylguanidine (MIBG) scanning and xenon CT have been reported [1]. In young patients imaging modalities that incorporate radiation should be minimized if possible.

Benign tumors were found in 14 patients [7, 9, 11–13, 15, 16, 18–24], while malignancy was reported in 3 patients [8, 14, 25]. One patient had a family history of disease [8]. Biological behavior of the tumor was not reported in 5 patients [4, 6, 14, 17, 26]. One patient with malignancy died within 4 months. All patients with malignant CBPs were subjected to chemotherapy or/and radiotherapy [8, 14, 25]. Most authors agree that the only proof of malignancy is the presence of metastases. Histological appearance of a CBP is not a reliable indicator of malignancy. Many clinical, histological, and molecular characteristics have been studied in order to diagnose malignant behavior, with limited clinical utility [27]. Young age, multifocality, and family history of disease seem to be associated with malignancy [1].

Complete surgical removal of the tumor is the gold standard operation. Although this is quite straightforward in Shamblin I tumors, locally advanced tumors constitute a challenge. Radical resection is crucial due to the possibility of malignancy. According to Luna-Ortiz et al., all tumors Shamblin class II and even tumors infiltrating vessels (Shamblin class III) must be managed surgically [28]. Surgical removal of CBPs has evolved from having unacceptably high rates of mortality and morbidity, to a relatively safe operation. The incidence of cerebrovascular complications has decreased from 23% to < 5% and the perioperative mortality has decreased from 6% to 0%. Desmond et al. support that meticulous hemostasis and subadventitial dissection is the key to a successful surgical intervention [29]. However, dysfunction or permanent cranial nerve impairment remains high according to recent studies [6–8, 12, 16]. Six of the young patients identified had a cranial nerve related injury [6–8, 22–24]. One of them experienced a permanent paralysis of the hypoglossal (XII) nerve [22], and multiple nerve injuries were caused in another including paralysis of the glossopharyngeal (IX), vagal (X), spinal accessory (XI), and hypoglossal (XII) nerves [7, 8]. In three cases the number or type of cranial nerve injury was not reported [6, 23, 24].

Most patients identified by our review had CBPs that were classified as Shamblin II and III [7, 8, 13, 16]. Only one has a Shamblin I tumor [7]. Preoperative embolization (PAE) was performed in 4 patients [15, 17, 20, 23], although this modality still remains controversial with varying results. The benefits of PAE focus on the reduction of operative time and blood loss. On the other hand, it does not prevent cranial nerve injury or inpatient hospital stay. On the contrary, some authors advocate that PAE may increase local complications during surgery due to the accompanying inflammatory process, which can damage the arterial wall nearby vessels [9, 16, 23, 25]. Other authors suggest that PAE could have a potential role in Shamblin III lesions and tumors involving the carotid arteries [30]. Alternatively, a proximal covered stent can be placed in the external carotid artery preventing intracranial emboli from coils during PAE [31]. In the same session, balloon occlusion of the internal carotid artery can be performed to determine if the patient can tolerate blockage of the vessel in case of ligation, clamping, or shunting [23]. The final solution in Shamblin III CBPs is removal with excision of the entire carotid bifurcation with interposition of a vascular conduit with saphenous vein or PTFE for the ICA and ligation of the ECA [30].

5. Conclusion

Neck paraganglioma in childhood is extremely rare incidence, with only a few published cases in literature. However, CBPs must be included in the differential diagnosis of pulsatile cervical mass and imaging with US and CT or MRI needs to follow, for evaluating the nature of the mass and the relation with the adjacent vessels and the anatomic structures.

References

[1] P. B. Dimakakos and T. E. Kotsis, "Carotid body paraganglioma: Review and surgical management," *European Journal of Plastic Surgery*, vol. 24, no. 2, pp. 58–65, 2001.

[2] C. Offergeld, C. Brase, S. Yaremchuk et al., "Head and neck paragangliomas: clinical and molecular genetic classification," *Clinics*, vol. 67, Suppl. 1, pp. 19–28, 2012.

[3] S. Woolen and J. J. Gemmete, "Paragangliomas of the head and neck," *Neuroimaging Clinics of North America*, vol. 26, no. 2, pp. 259–278, 2016.

[4] T. M. Tekautz, C. B. Pratt, J. J. Jenkins, and S. L. Spunt, "Pediatric extraadrenal paraganglioma," *Journal of Pediatric Surgery*, vol. 38, no. 9, pp. 1317–1321, 2003.

[5] J. Arias-Stella and F. Bustos, "Chronic hypoxia and chemodectomas in bovines at high altitudes," *Archives of Pathology & Laboratory Medicine*, vol. 100, no. 12, pp. 636–639, 1976.

[6] J. W. Hallett Jr., J. D. Nora, L. H. Hollier, K. J. Cherry Jr., and P. C. Pairolero, "Trends in neurovascular complications of surgical management for carotid body and cervical paragangliomas: a fifty-year experience with 153 tumors," *Journal of Vascular Surgery*, vol. 7, no. 2, pp. 284–291, 1988.

[7] J. W. Thompson and S. R. Cohen, "Management of bilateral carotid body tumors and a glomus jugulare tumor in a child," *International Journal of Pediatric Otorhinolaryngology*, vol. 17, no. 1, pp. 75–87, 1989.

[8] D. Ophir, "Familial multicentric paragangliomas in a child," *The Journal of Laryngology & Otology*, vol. 105, no. 5, pp. 376–380, 1991.

[9] A. S. Varudkar, H. R. Kokandkar, G. G. Gumaste, K. S. Bhople, and N. R. Kumbhakarna, "Carotid body paraganglioma with coexistent pheochromocytoma in childhood," *Indian Journal of Cancer*, vol. 30, no. 3, pp. 109–112, 1993.

[10] V. J. Davila, J. M. Chang, W. M. Stone et al., "Current surgical management of carotid body tumors," *Journal of Vascular Surgery*, vol. 64, no. 6, pp. 1703–1710, 2016.

[11] R. G. Chambers and W. D. Mahoney, "Carotid body tumors," *The American Journal of Surgery*, vol. 116, no. 4, pp. 554–558, 1968.

[12] W. R. Shamblin, W. H. ReMine, S. G. Sheps, and E. G. Harrison Jr., "Carotid body tumor (chemodectoma). Clinicopathologic analysis of ninety cases," *The American Journal of Surgery*, vol. 122, no. 6, pp. 732–739, 1971.

[13] G. S. Georgiadis, M. K. Lazarides, A. Tsalkidis, P. Argyropoulou, and A. Giatromanolaki, "Carotid body tumor in a 13-year-old child: case report and review of the literature," *Journal of Vascular Surgery*, vol. 47, no. 4, pp. 874.e3–880.e3, 2008.

[14] M. C. Newland and B. J. Hurlbert, "Chemodectoma diagnosed by hypertension and tachycardia during anesthesia," *Anesthesia & Analgesia*, vol. 59, no. 5, pp. 388–390, 1980.

[15] A. R. Hogan, J. E. Sola, S. C. Jernigan, E. C. Peterson, and R. T. Younis, "A pediatric carotid body tumor," *Journal of Pediatric Surgery*, vol. 53, no. 7, pp. 1432–1436, 2018.

[16] E. Gounot, G. Couillault, C. Maingueneau, and J. M. Autissier, "Paraganglioma of the carotid body. Apropos of a case in a 14-year-old child," *Chirurgie Pédiatrique*, vol. 31, no. 2, pp. 125-126, 1990.

[17] R. F. Osborne, "Nonpulsatile carotid body tumor in a teenager," *Ear, Nose & Throat Journal*, vol. 84, no. 3, pp. 133-134, 2005.

[18] P. Zaupa and M. E. Höllwarth, "Carotid body paraganglioma: rare tumor in a 15-year-old adolescent boy," *Journal of Pediatric Surgery*, vol. 42, no. 4, pp. e13–e17, 2007.

[19] M. E. Lopez-Vazquez, F. J. Llamas-Macias, C. Nuno-Escobar, A. Gonzalez-Ojeda, C. Fuentes-Orozco, and M. D. Macias-Amezcua, "Carotid body paraganglioma in a teenager. Case report," *Cirugia y Cirujanos*, vol. 82, no. 3, pp. 316–322, 2014.

[20] A. Ifeoluwa, I. Lázár, É. Szövördi, and T. Karosi, "Management of carotid body tumor in pediatric patients: a case report and review of the literature," *International Journal of Pediatric Otorhinolaryngology*, vol. 93, pp. 47–52, 2017.

[21] J. Aidan Carney, "The triad of gastric epithelioid leiomyosarcoma, pulmonary chondroma, and functioning extra-adrenal paraganglioma: A five-year review," *Medicine (United States)*, vol. 62, no. 3, pp. 159–169, 1983.

[22] P. H. Dickinson, S. M. Griffin, A. J. Guy, and I. F. McNeill, "Carotid body tumour: 30 years experience," *British Journal of Surgery*, vol. 73, no. 1, pp. 14–16, 1986.

[23] S. J. Wang, M. B. Wang, T. M. Barauskas, and T. C. Calcaterra, "Surgical management of carotid body tumors," *Otolaryngology—Head and Neck Surgery*, vol. 123, no. 3, pp. 202–206, 2000.

[24] J. T. M. Plukker, E. P. Brongers, A. Vermey, A. Krikke, and J. J. A. M. Van Den Dungen, "Outcome of surgical treatment for carotid body paraganglioma," *British Journal of Surgery*, vol. 88, no. 10, pp. 1382–1386, 2001.

[25] T. F. Hajnžić, B. Krušlin, and M. Belicza, "Carotid body paraganglioma in a nine-year-old boy with extensive pulmonary metastases," *Medical and Pediatric Oncology*, vol. 32, no. 5, pp. 399-400, 1999.

[26] M. S. Sajid, G. Hamilton, and D. M. Baker, "A multicenter review of carotid body tumour management," *European Journal of Vascular and Endovascular Surgery*, vol. 34, no. 2, pp. 127–130, 2007.

[27] C. Nastos, A. Yiallourou, I. Kotsis et al., "Immunohistochemical expression patterns of S100, synaptophysin, chromogranin A and neuron specific enolase in predicting malignant behaviour in paragangliomas," *Journal of B.U.ON*, vol. 23, no. 5, pp. 1540–1545, 2018.

[28] K. Luna-Ortiz, M. Rascon-Ortiz, V. Villavicencio-Valencia, M. Granados-Garcia, and A. Herrera-Gomez, "Carotid body tumors: review of a 20-year experience," *Oral Oncology*, vol. 41, no. 1, pp. 56–61, 2005.

[29] T. H. W. Desmond and H. G. Christopher, "Current concepts in the management of carotid body tumours," *The Medical Journal of Malaysia*, vol. 65, no. 4, pp. 268–270, 2010.

[30] S. K. Kakkos, D. J. Reddy, A. D. Shepard, J. C. Lin, T. J. Nypaver, and M. R. Weaver, "Contemporary presentation and evolution of management of neck paragangliomas," *Journal of Vascular Surgery*, vol. 49, no. 6, pp. 1365.e2–1373.e2, 2009.

[31] J. M. Scanlon, J. J. Lustgarten, S. B. Karr, and J. I. Cahan, "Successful devascularization of carotid body tumors by covered stent placement in the external carotid artery," *Journal of Vascular Surgery*, vol. 48, no. 5, pp. 1322–1324, 2008.

34

Antegrade Hybrid Chimney TEVAR Endograft in a Patient with Blunt Aortic Injury: A Challenging Case with Technical Success but Unfavorable Result

Fotios Eforakopoulos,[1] Maria Giovani,[2] Petros Zampakis,[3] Christina Kalogeropoulou,[3] Fotini Fligou,[4] Nikolaos Charoulis,[1] Efstratios Koletsis,[1] and Dimitrios Dougenis[5]

[1]*Department of Cardiothoracic Surgery, University of Patras, Patras, Greece*
[2]*Department of Pediatric Surgery, Mitera Children's Hospital, Marousi, Athens, Greece*
[3]*Department of Radiology, University of Patras, Patras, Greece*
[4]*Department of Anesthesiology and Intensive Care Medicine, University of Patras, Patras, Greece*
[5]*Department of Cardiac Surgery, School of Medicine, National and Kapodistrian University of Athens, Attikon University Hospital, Athens, Greece*

Correspondence should be addressed to Fotios Eforakopoulos; feforakopoulos@hotmail.com

Academic Editor: Nilda Espinola-Zavaleta

Thoracic Endovascular Aortic Repair (TEVAR) has modified aortic medicine, particularly in patients with traumatic aortic injury (TAI). Conventional repair of TAI in the aortic arch is technically demanding as it requires cardiopulmonary bypass and deep hypothermic arrest with still a significant number of complications. Despite recent improvements in endovascular techniques, many patients have been excluded from endovascular repair due to unfavorable anatomy. To increase the feasibility of endovascular repair, adjunctive open extra-anatomical bypasses may be required to provide an adequate proximal landing zone. Several methods, for instance, chimney technique, hybrid technique, and fenestrated or branched stent-grafts, have been proposed as options to preserve the supra-aortic branches, each with its own advantages and disadvantages. We herein present a patient with complex anatomical features and blunt aortic injury, who underwent antegrade chimney stent-graft deployment through the ascending aorta, not otherwise amenable to standard retrograde delivery because of severe peripheral artery disease. The remarkable aspect, in this case, is that both stents were placed antegrade, through the ascending aorta.

1. Introduction

Traumatic aortic injury occurs in 2% of cases with blunt thoracic trauma and is considered a life-threatening condition [1]. The main cause of TAI is the movement of the mobile aortic arch against the fixed descending thoracic aorta during deceleration injury. There is a predilection for endovascular repair when anatomically possible and when institutional resources are available to support the attempt [2]. Clinical and anatomic features that support the use of TEVAR require multiple severe injuries or comorbidities with a limited life expectancy and lesions confined to the distal arch or the descending thoracic aorta. Similarly, because of severe chest or lung injuries, the patient may not tolerate one-lung ventilation, which is demanded for open surgery.

Occasionally, when supra-aortic vessels are involved, fenestrated custom-made grafts are used. These stent-grafts had to be based on the patients' individual anatomy and were thus time-consuming, limiting their application in an urgent setting. Combined hybrid techniques (both endovascular and surgical) became popular providing the possibility for arch rerouting, without cardiopulmonary bypass and hypothermic arrest. We herein present a case of a patient with a traumatic aortic transection located across the origin of the LSA who required immediate LSA revascularization because of ischemia on the left arm. The unique feature of our work is that both grafts in the descending aorta and in the LSA were placed antegrade via the ascending aorta after partial sternotomy, because of multiple atherosclerotic lesions in femoral and iliac vessels.

2. Case Report

A 79-year-old male with COPD and peripheral artery disease was transferred to our institution from a secondary hospital with the diagnosis of aortic transection, after a lone motorcyclist accident without wearing a helmet. While arriving at our emergency room, the patient was confused and complained of chest pain especially aggravated with deep breathing. Physical examinations showed stable vital signs: blood pressure (BP), 122/74 mmHg; pulse rate, 98/min; and respiratory rate, 20/min. Glasgow Coma Scale at admission was 8, so he was intubated on arrival. His injuries included subarachnoid and subdural hemorrhage, fracture of the occipital bone, mandibular fracture, rib fractures with bilateral pulmonary contusions, hemothorax in the left side, and fracture of the left femur as well. Blood loss through the chest tube at insertion was 400 ml and stabilized at 700 ml thereafter. Three-dimensional reconstruction images of contrast-enhanced computed tomographic angiography (CTA) demonstrated an intimal injury with periaortic hematoma (grade II aortic injury). It was located across the origin of the left subclavian artery (Figure 1). A multidisciplinary trauma team approach was instituted.

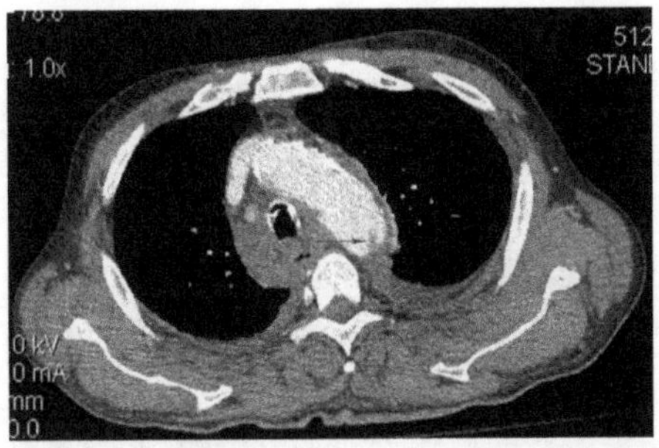

Figure 1: Preoperative CTA showed transection of the distal aortic arch.

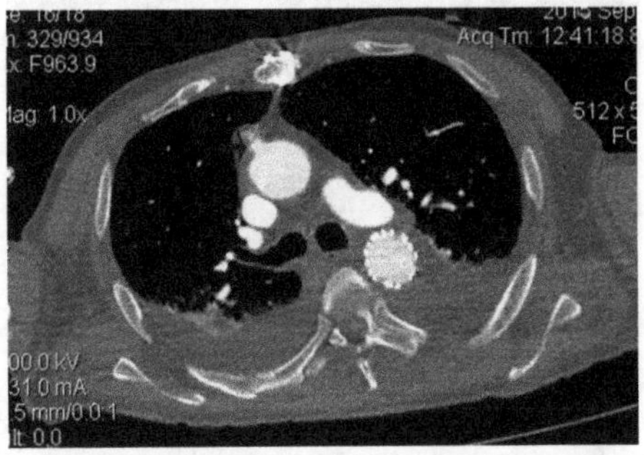

Figure 2: The first arrow indicates a graft anastomosed to the ascending aorta. The second (thin) arrow indicates endograft in the distal arch and the descending thoracic aorta.

As there is no endograft availability in our institution, orthopedists stabilized the femur, and then, we proceeded to treat the aortic injury given its severity. Fortunately, the patient was hemodynamically stable. Anti-impulse therapy was administered during the whole procedure which was held in the operating room with mobile c-arm. The patient was placed in a supine position. Aortography was performed via a catheter placed percutaneously through the brachial artery to confirm the anatomy and define the landing zones for the device. Because of multiple atherosclerotic lesions in both femoral arteries and in the left iliac artery, extraperitoneal exposure of the right iliac artery was performed. An incision was made 2 cm above and parallel to the inguinal ligament, extending from the lateral edge of the rectus sheath to a point 2 cm cephalad to the anterior superior iliac spine. After exposure of the external iliac artery, it was found that the guidewire could not be advanced in the descending thoracic aorta due to heavily calcified vessels. It was decided to proceed with partial sternotomy in order to place the stent-graft to the proper position in an antegrade fashion.

After completion of partial sternotomy, lowering the blood pressure, a partial clamp was placed on the ascending aorta and an 8 mm Goretex thin-walled, ringed graft was anastomosed in end to side fashion to the aorta (Figure 2). An access sheath was placed in the ringed graft, and a guidewire is advanced through the sheath under fluoroscopic guidance from the ascending to the descending aorta. A Conformable Gore TAG stent-graft 34 mm × 10cm was positioned by advancing it over a stiff guidewire (Lunderquist). Its position was confirmed with repeated aortography especially in LAO 30 projection. Before device deployment, the patient's blood pressure was lowered again to lessen the arterial impulse and minimize the potential for misplacement during deployment. The device was then deployed, and completion aortogram was performed to confirm patency of the endograft and successful exclusion of the transection (i.e., no endoleak). However, the LSA was covered and the elimination of arterial pulse with a decrease in oxygen saturation of the left hand was noted. The limb became pale and cold, so a placement of additional Gore Viabahn Endoprosthesis 10 mm × 10cm in the covered LSA was decided (Figure 3). The arterial pulse and oxygen saturation were immediately restored. The guidewires and introducer sheaths were removed, and the arteriotomies were repaired. Transesophageal echocardiography and angiography were used together to position and deploy the device precisely.

Subsequently, the patient was admitted to the ICU for deep sedation and ventilator management. Postoperative CTA disclosed appropriate position of stent-grafts and adequate flow to the left arm (Figure 4). On the POD 10, the patient's oxygenation worsened, and purulent sputum with fever made an appearance. We, therefore, arrived at a diagnosis of ventilator-associated pneumonia (VAP), and his PaO_2/FiO_2 ratio deteriorated, and multiple organ failure was developed. He required continuous venous-venous hemofiltration for severe acute kidney injury. Finally, the patient deceased on POD 22.

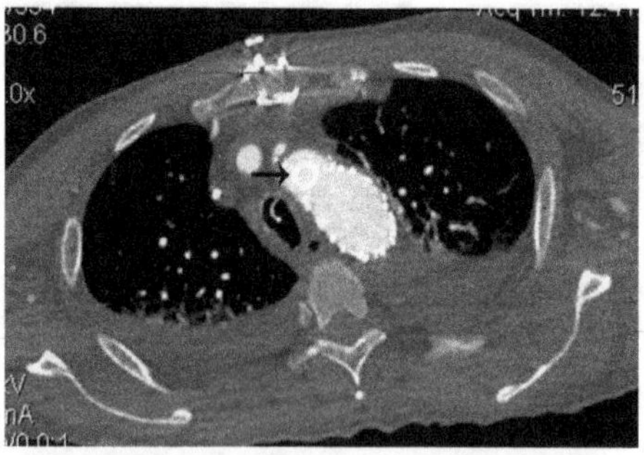

Figure 3: The proximal end of the chimney graft in the aortic arch.

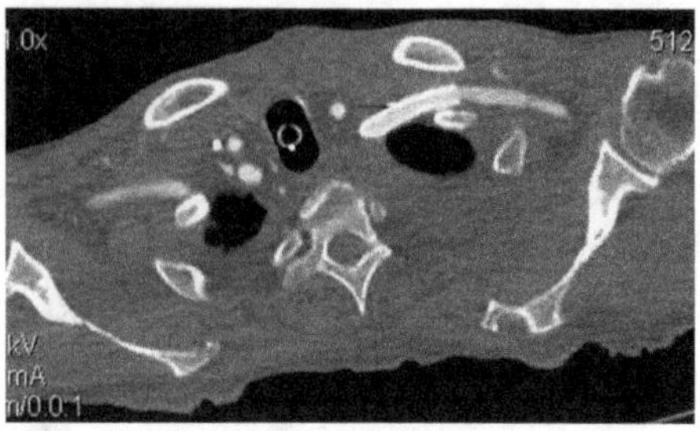

Figure 4: Postoperative CTA showed the proper position of the chimney graft inside the LSA (arrow) and the patency of the vessel.

In this patient, we did not administer antiplatelet drugs nor heparin during stent-graft deployment because of the traumatic brain injury.

3. Discussion

Patients on whom blunt aortic injury is in close proximity to the origin of the left subclavian artery (<2 cm distance) should undergo intentional coverage of this vessel. This procedure is needed in approximately 20% of cases and is usually well-tolerated [3, 4]. However, total coverage of the LSA increases the incidence of stroke (1,2%), of left upper limb ischemia (4%), and of patients requiring additional procedure (2,9%) [5]. Ischemic lesions and vertebrobasilar insufficiency are usually related to the left vertebral artery diameter < 3 mm [6]. Stroke can present in patients with dominant left vertebral artery and coronary steal syndrome in cases of patients who have a left internal mammary coronary bypass graft. When carotid-subclavian bypass for LSA revascularization is performed prior to its coverage, no instances of stroke, limb ischemia, spinal cord ischemia, endoleak, or death have occurred (hybrid procedure) [7]. Rarely, patients may evolve debilitating arm claudication symptoms later, at which time, an elective extra-anatomic procedure can be performed. Spinal drainage should be performed in cases of extensive coverage of the thoracic aorta, a history of prior open or endovascular aneurysm repair, or presence of internal iliac artery atherosclerotic lesions, with the potential risk for paraplegia [7–12].

Hybrid aortic repair is usually achieved gradually. The first stage is to bypass critical vessels supplying the brain or the left upper limb that will later be covered by the stent-graft, using an open approach. This is in general known as a "debranching" procedure. However, the open repair of the aortic arch remains the "gold standard" but the hybrid repair is an acceptable alternative. When the device is deployed in zone 2 (distal to the left common carotid origin but proximal to the subclavian artery), an extra-anatomical LCCA-LSA bypass or a transposition of the LSA into the LCCA before the positioning of the device would be enough for a safe sealing of the endograft. A substantial alternative to the hybrid approach is the use of fenestrated or chimney grafts.

Chimney graft technique permits the landing zones to be expanded to the appropriate position in the aortic arch in order to safely seal the damaged wall. Compared to the other custom-made devices, these endografts are cheaper and less complex and are proposed in urgent conditions as there is no necessity for previous device customization. Chimney endograft provides adequate blood flow to the LSA preventing both spinal cord ischemia and upper limb ischemia. This procedure can be applied in various occasions such as those with dominant vertebral artery and severe atherosclerotic right vertebral artery, those with congenital right vertebral artery dysplasia, those with left internal mammary artery (LIMA) graft, and those with left arm dialysis access [13]. Frequently, in case that the lesion is located near the LSA at the outer curvature of the arch, endoleak type Ia ensues [14]. Obviously, the radial supporting power of the aortic device is positively related to the patency of the chimney graft. The proximal landing zone of an aortic endograft must be located at the origin of the LSA; otherwise, migration of the main graft with simultaneous occlusion of LCCA or collapse of the chimney graft may be apparent [15]. Consequently, the patency of the chimney graft is affected by the distance between the proximal tip of the aortic stent-graft and the LSA origin. The perfect deployment for both devices is the proximal end of the chimney stent to be exceeded from the proximal aortic stent-graft about 1 cm.

The antegrade stent-graft placement from the ascending aorta that we present here was proved a reliable alternative in the urgent setting with difficulty in accessing the femoral and iliac vessels. An embolic complication was anticipated because of arch manipulation, but fortunately, it did not happen. Given his comorbidities and traumatic injuries, our patient was not a suitable candidate for open surgical repair and was performed endovascular repair applying an antegrade technique. To the best of our knowledge, it is the first time that antegrade implantation of chimney graft in TAI through the ascending aorta has been reported. Several groups have published small series with a transapical approach through the left ventricle to treat acute and chronic pathologies of the ascending aorta [16, 17]. The technical success is promising in selected patients [18]. However, none of them placed a chimney graft antegrade.

Other ways for the antegrade endograft placement that have been reported are the axillary approach through the right standard infraclavicular incision and direct aortic placement with elephant trunk procedure during deep circulatory arrest [19]. There are series with a small number of patients, so a study in a larger population will be required to prove the effectiveness of the antegrade technique. From the existing reports, neurologic complications appeared frequently in the antegrade hybrid approach (0%-25%) [20–23]. It is not the first time that we used antegrade positioning but it was our first attempt for antegrade placement of chimney graft. Unfortunately, the patient died 22 days after surgery because of complications that were not related to the stent-grafts. Our remaining cases will be reported in a future work.

4. Conclusion

Hybrid procedure with antegrade stent-graft deployment seems to be a promising treatment for many aortic pathologies including blunt aortic injury. A small number of reported cases and eventual neurologic complications suggest the obligation for further refinement to improve the safety of this technique.

Authors' Contributions

DD, EF, and FF provide the case. GM involved in the literature search. EF wrote the manuscript. ZP and KC performed the radiological diagnosis. DD, CN, and EF placed the stent-graft. KE revised the manuscript.

References

[1] T. C. Ungar, S. J. Wolf, J. S. Haukoos, D. S. Dyer, and E. E. Moore, "Derivation of a clinical decision rule to exclude thoracic aortic imaging in patients with blunt chest trauma after motor vehicle collisions," *The Journal of Trauma*, vol. 61, no. 5, pp. 1150–1155, 2006.

[2] N. Fox, D. Schwartz, J. H. Salazar et al., "Evaluation and management of blunt traumatic aortic injury: a practice management guideline from the Eastern Association for the Surgery of Trauma," *Journal of Trauma Nursing*, vol. 22, no. 2, pp. 99-100, 2015.

[3] S. A. Rahimi, R. C. Darling III, M. Mehta, S. P. Roddy, J. B. Taggert, and Y. Sternbach, "Endovascular repair of thoracic aortic traumatic transections is a safe method in patients with complicated injuries," *Journal of Vascular Surgery*, vol. 52, no. 4, pp. 891–896, 2010.

[4] J. C. Parodi, J. C. Palmaz, and H. D. Barone, "Transfemoral intraluminal graft implantation for abdominal aortic aneurysms," *Annals of Vascular Surgery*, vol. 5, no. 6, pp. 491–499, 1991.

[5] A. H. Sepehripour, K. Ahmed, J. A. Vecht et al., "Management of the left subclavian artery during endovascular stent grafting for traumatic aortic injury - a systematic review," *European Journal of Vascular and Endovascular Surgery*, vol. 41, no. 6, pp. 758–769, 2011.

[6] F. J. Schlösser, H. J. Verhagen, P. H. Lin, E. L. Verhoeven, J. A. van Herwaarden, and F. L. Moll, "TEVAR following prior abdominal aortic aneurysm surgery: increased risk of neurological deficit," *Journal of Vascular Surgery*, vol. 49, no. 2, pp. 308–314, 2009.

[7] R. McWilliams, "Controversies and updates in vascular surgery," *Edizioni Minerva Medica*, vol. 21, no. 2, 2014.

[8] B. W. Ullery, J. Quatromoni, B. M. Jackson et al., "Impact of intercostal artery occlusion on spinal cord ischemia following thoracic endovascular aortic repair," *Vascular and Endovascular Surgery*, vol. 45, no. 6, pp. 519–523, 2011.

[9] C. J. Keith Jr., M. A. Passman, M. J. Carignan et al., "Protocol implementation of selective postoperative lumbar spinal drainage after thoracic aortic endograft," *Journal of Vascular Surgery*, vol. 55, no. 1, pp. 1–8, 2012.

[10] P. Amabile, D. Grisoli, R. Giorgi, J. M. Bartoli, and P. Piquet, "Incidence and determinants of spinal cord ischaemia in stent-graft repair of the thoracic aorta," *European Journal of Vascular and Endovascular Surgery*, vol. 35, no. 4, pp. 455–461, 2008.

[11] J. Buth, P. L. Harris, R. Hobo et al., "Neurologic complications associated with endovascular repair of thoracic aortic pathology: incidence and risk factors. a study from the European Collaborators on Stent/Graft Techniques for Aortic Aneurysm Repair (EUROSTAR) registry," *Journal of Vascular Surgery*, vol. 46, no. 6, pp. 1103–1111.e2, 2007.

[12] A. T. Cheung, A. Pochettino, M. L. McGarvey et al., "Strategies to manage paraplegia risk after endovascular stent repair of descending thoracic aortic aneurysms," *The Annals of Thoracic Surgery*, vol. 80, no. 4, pp. 1280–1289, 2005.

[13] G. Piffaretti, G. Mariscalco, C. Lomazzi et al., "Predictive factors for endoleaks after thoracic aortic aneurysm endograft repair," *The Journal of Thoracic and Cardiovascular Surgery*, vol. 138, no. 4, pp. 880–885, 2009.

[14] B. Gehringhoff, G. Torsello, G. A. Pitoulias, M. Austermann, and K. P. Donas, "Use of chimney grafts in aortic arch pathologies involving the supra-aortic branches," *Journal of Endovascular Therapy*, vol. 18, no. 5, pp. 650–655, 2011.

[15] S. MacDonald, A. Cheung, R. Sidhu, P. Rheaume, S. M. Grenon, and J. Clement, "Endovascular aortic aneurysm repair via the left ventricular apex of a beating heart," *Journal of Vascular Surgery*, vol. 49, no. 3, pp. 759–762, 2009.

[16] H. Uthoff, L. Garcia-Covarrubias, S. Samuels, J. F. Benenati, N. L. Moreno, and B. T. Katzen, "Transapical endovascular aortic repair to treat complex aortic pathologies," *The Annals of Thoracic Surgery*, vol. 93, no. 5, pp. 1735–1737, 2012.

[17] W. Y. Szeto, W. G. Moser, N. D. Desai et al., "Transapical deployment of endovascular thoracic aortic stent graft for an ascending aortic pseudoaneurysm," *The Annals of Thoracic Surgery*, vol. 89, no. 2, pp. 616–618, 2010.

[18] E. E. Roselli, E. G. Soltesz, T. Mastracci, L. G. Svensson, and B. W. Lytle, "Antegrade delivery of stent grafts to treat complex thoracic aortic disease," *The Annals of Thoracic Surgery*, vol. 90, no. 2, pp. 539–546, 2010.

[19] W. Zhou, M. Reardon, E. K. Peden, P. H. Lin, and A. B. Lumsden, "Hybrid approach to complex thoracic aortic aneurysms in high-risk patients: surgical challenges and clinical outcomes," *Journal of Vascular Surgery*, vol. 44, no. 4, pp. 688–693, 2006.

[20] H. M. Saleh and L. Inglese, "Combined surgical and endovascular treatment of aortic arch aneurysms," *Journal of Vascular Surgery*, vol. 44, no. 3, pp. 460–466.e1, 2006.

[21] E. Weigang, J. Parker, M. Czerny et al., "Endovascular aortic arch repair after aortic arch de-branching," *The Annals of Thoracic Surgery*, vol. 87, no. 2, pp. 603–607, 2009.

[22] H. Schumacher, D. Bockler, H. Bardenheuer, J. Hansmann, and J. R. Allenberg, "Endovascular aortic arch reconstruction with supra-aortic transposition for symptomatic contained rupture and dissection: early experience in 8 high-risk patients," *Journal of Endovascular Therapy*, vol. 10, no. 6, pp. 1066–1074, 2003.

[23] G. Matalanis, M. Durairaj, and M. Brooks, "A hybrid technique of aortic arch branch transposition and antegrade stent graft deployment for complete arch repair without cardiopulmonary bypass," *European Journal of Cardio-Thoracic Surgery*, vol. 29, no. 4, pp. 611-612, 2006.

Elephantiasis and Directed Occupational Rehabilitation

Jose Maria Pereira de Godoy,[1] Henrique Jose Pereira de Godoy,[2] Ana Carolina Pereira de Godoy,[3] and Maria de Fátima Guerreiro Godoy[4]

[1] *Cardiology and Cardiovascular Surgery Department of the Medicine School in São José do Rio Preto (FAMERP), CNPq (National Council for Research and Development), Brazil*
[2] *Medicine School of Universidade Federal do Mato Grosso-Cuiabá-UFMT and Research Group in the Clínica Godoy, Sao Jose do Rio Preto, Brazil*
[3] *Pediatrics Unit Intensive Therapy of Santa Casa de São Paulo, Brazil and Research Group of Clínica Godoy, São Jose do Rio Preto, Brazil*
[4] *Medicine School in São José do Rio Preto (FAMERP) and Research Group in the Clínica Godoy, Sao Jose do Rio Preto, Brazil*

Correspondence should be addressed to Jose Maria Pereira de Godoy; godoyjmp@gmail.com

Academic Editor: Halvor Naess

The aim of the present study was to demonstrate the cure of elephantiasis over a ten-year follow-up period and novel discoveries with directed occupational rehabilitation. A 66-year-old female patient with a history of bilateral lower limb lymphedema reported the aggravation of the condition over the years, reaching stage III (elephantiasis). The physical examination confirmed elephantiasis. The circumference of the left lower limb was 106 cm. Her body weight was 106 kilograms, height was 160 cm, and the body mass index (BMI) was 41.6 kg/m^2. The patient was submitted to intensive treatment for three weeks, which led to a 21-kg reduction in weight and 66 cm reduction in leg circumference. Ten years after treatment, the patient has maintained the results with the compression stockings. Elephantiasis can be cured, although lymphedema cannot. The cure of elephantiasis depends on maintaining the treatment of lymphedema after normalization or near normalization. Directed occupational therapy stimulates the search for new activities and a life closer to normality.

1. Introduction

Lymphedema is specific type of edema in which a failure of the lymphatic system leads to the accumulation of macromolecules in the interstitial space and the retention of fluid [1]. Lymphedema can be congenital or acquired. In congenital cases, the individual is born with an altered lymphatic system that may or may not lead to lymphedema. In secondary cases, there is no problem with the lymphatic system at birth, but events occurring throughout life can cause damage to the lymphatic system, leading to failure and the formation of edema [1, 2].

This condition is divided into three clinical stages. In stage I, the patient awakens without edema, but swelling develops throughout the day. In stage II, the patient awakens with edema, which worsens throughout the day. Stage III (elephantiasis) is a more advanced stage, in which large deformities occur [1–3].

In recent years, a novel concept for the treatment of lymphedema has been developed by Godoy & Godoy aimed at the normalization or near normalization of edema in all clinical stages, including elephantiasis [3]. The researchers have developed novel manual and mechanical lymphatic drainage methods that enable the significant mobilization of macromolecules, thereby affecting the physiopathology of lymphedema [4, 5]. Another novel concept was compression stockings and braces made of grosgrain fabric, which allow a reduction in volume and the maintenance of the results [6]. Intensive, multidisciplinary treatments (eight hours per day) are other accomplishments that enable an approximately 50% reduction in volume in the first five days of treatments [3]. The multidisciplinary approach is based on directed

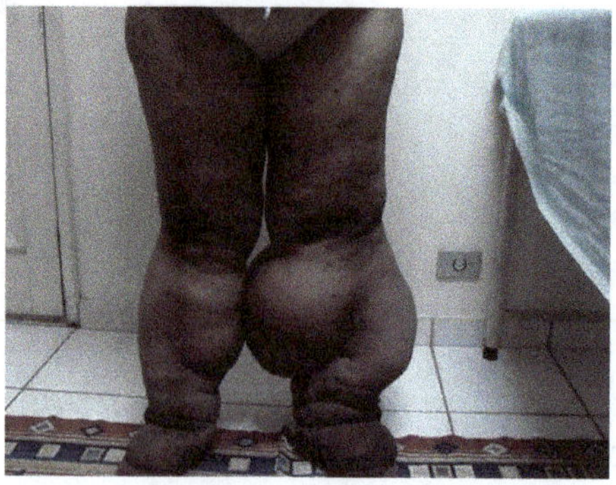

FIGURE 1: Initial condition before of treatment.

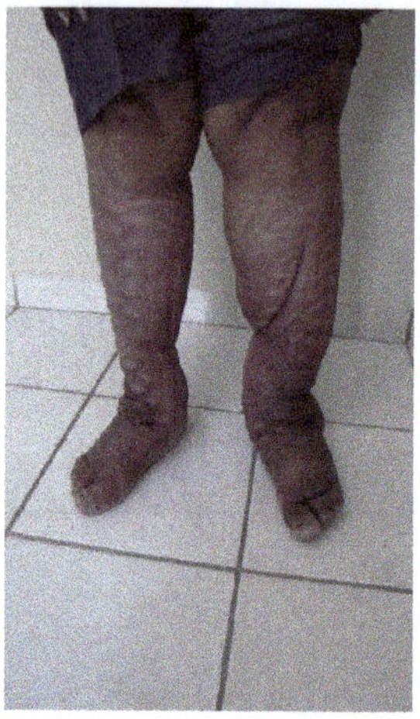

FIGURE 2: After 3 weeks of treatment.

occupational rehabilitation and the development of new skills.

The aim of the present study was to demonstrate the cure of elephantiasis over a ten-year follow-up period and novel discoveries with directed occupational rehabilitation.

2. Case Report

A 66-year-old female patient with a history of bilateral lower limb lymphedema reported the aggravation of the condition over the years, reaching stage III (elephantiasis). The patient was sent to the Godoy Clinic and reported having undergone several treatments throughout her life as well as several episodes of erysipelas. She did not marry due to the lymphedema and complained of the frequent occurrence of strangers staring at her leg, which upset her. The physical examination confirmed elephantiasis. The circumference of the left lower limb was 106 cm. Her body weight was 106 kilograms, height was 160 cm, and the body mass index (BMI) was 41.6 kg/m^2 (Figure 1).

The patient was submitted to intensive treatment for three weeks, which led to a 21 kg reduction in weight and 66 cm reduction in leg circumference (Figure 2).

Intensive treatment with the Godoy Method consisted of eight hours per day of mechanical lymphatic drainage, 15 minutes of simultaneous cervical lymphatic therapy, and hand-crafted compression stockings made from grosgrain fabric. Mechanical lymphatic therapy consisted of an electromechanical device that performs plantar flexion and extension. After three weeks of intensive therapy, the patient continued treatment at home using the compression stockings. At the follow-up evaluation, the patient was submitted to electrical bioimpedance analysis as well as circumference measurements and volumetry. The bioimpedance analysis revealed a pattern of normality, with the reduction in lymphedema. Ten years after treatment, the patient has maintained the results with the compression stockings. In occupational therapy throughout this period, the patient has been encouraged to perform activities that she has always wanted to do to improve her wellbeing. She took up belly dancing, followed by tap dancing. She reports that these activities changed her life and she is very happy for being able to realize her dream of dancing, which is an activity that she began at the age of 76 years. The study was approving Ethical Committee of Medicine School of Sao Jose do Rio Preto# 2.929.115.

3. Discussion

The present study demonstrates that elephantiasis can be cured, as the patient has been without this condition for ten years. She continues to have lymphedema, which ranges from subclinical to stages I and II, varying at different times in her life. She was orientated to improve her quality of life by performing the activities that she had always wanted to do. A certain flexibility in treatment is possible and she is able to forego the use of the stockings on some occasions, such as going to the beach and spending a week without the stockings with little edema. This flexibility enables a better quality of life. After these periods, she returns to correct treatment with the use of the compression stockings.

Another important detail was the identification of whether the patient dreamed of performing any particular activity. In this case, the choice was dance. The dance teacher was instructed by a therapist specialized in directed occupational rehabilitation for patients with lymphedema and they worked together with this purpose in mind [7]. The realization of the lifelong dream of a 76-year-old woman who had had elephantiasis was a source of joy and accomplishment. This aspect shows the extent to which occupational therapy can be useful in the rehabilitation of patients with lymphedema able to change the lives of these people and reestablish the pleasure of living, as reported by the patient in the present case. This opens an opportunity in the field of occupational therapy. There are 16 million people in the world in stage III lymphedema (elephantiasis) and millions others in the earlier stages that could benefit from this approach.

4. Conclusion

Elephantiasis can be cured, although lymphedema cannot. The cure of elephantiasis depends on maintaining the treatment of lymphedema after normalization or near normalization. Directed occupational therapy stimulates the search for new activities and a life closer to normality.

References

[1] B. B. Lee, P. L. Antignani, T. A. Baroncelli et al., "IUA-ISVI consensus for diagnosis guideline of chronic lymphedema of the limbs," *International Angiology*, vol. 34, no. 4, pp. 311–332, 2015.

[2] H. H. Keo, S. B. Gretener, and D. Staub, "Clinical and diagnostic aspects of lymphedema," *Vasa*, vol. 46, no. 4, pp. 255–261, 2017.

[3] J. M. P. de Godoy, P. A. F. Brigidio, E. Buzato, and M. F. G. de Godoy, "Intensive outpatient treatment of elephantiasis," *International Angiology*, vol. 31, no. 5, pp. 494–499, 2012.

[4] J. M. P. de Godoy, A. C. P. de Godoy, and F. G. G. Maria, "Evolution of Godoy & Godoy manual lymph drainage. Technique with linear movements," *Clinical Practice*, vol. 7, no. 4, p. 1006, 2017.

[5] K. S. de Siqueira and M. G. Karan, "Volumetric alterations utilizing the RAGodoy® device to treat lymphedema of the lower extremities," *Journal Phlebology and Lymphology*, vol. 2, pp. 16–18, 2009.

[6] J. M. P. de Godoy, A. C. P. de Godoy, and M. D. F. G. Godoy, "Godoy & Godoy compression sleeve in the treatment of arm lymphedema: New concepts for materials," *Brazilian Archives of Biology and Technology*, vol. 58, no. 6, pp. 864–868, 2015.

[7] M. F. G. Godoy, H. J. P. Godoy, and J. M. P. Godoy, "Human activity rehabilitation and occupational therapy," in *Transdisciplinary Approach to Rehabilitation of Breast Cancer Related Lymphedema*, M. F. G. Godoy, H. J. P. Godoy, and J. M. P. Godoy, Eds., pp. 169–172, Amazon, 2016.

Congenital Coronary Artery Anomalies: Three Cases and Brief Review of the Literature

Nikolaos S. Ioakeimidis,[1] Dimitrios Valasiadis,[1] Andreas Markou,[2] and Theodora Zaglavara[3]

[1]*Department of Cardiology, General Hospital of Florina "Eleni Th. Dimitriou", Egnatias 9, Florina 53100, Greece*
[2]*Department of Radiology, General Hospital of Florina "Eleni Th. Dimitriou", Egnatias 9, Florina 53100, Greece*
[3]*Department of Cardiovascular Imaging, Interbalkan Medical Centre of Thessaloniki, Asklipiou 10, Thessaloniki 57001, Greece*

Correspondence should be addressed to Nikolaos S. Ioakeimidis; ioakeimn@auth.gr

Academic Editor: Antonio Silvestro

Coronary artery anomalies (CAAs) are congenital vascular defects which can remain hidden and asymptomatic over the complete life course of an individual. They are defined as deviations from the normal coronary anatomy regarding the arterial origin, course, or both. Their incidence varies from 1.3% to 5.64% in coronary angiography cohorts, and they can be detected as incidental findings. In certain cases, CAAs can be hemodynamically significant and unfortunately can be proven lethal. Their link with sudden cardiac death, especially in otherwise healthy competitive athletes, is well established, but their prognostic significance, range of symptoms, and pathophysiology remain to be further elucidated. Here, along with a brief review of related literature, we present a series of three cases: one case of an anomalous origin of the right coronary artery (RCA) from the left coronary sinus, one case of a split RCA originating from the left coronary sinus, and one case of a dual left anterior descending (LAD) artery system.

1. Introduction and Brief Review of the Literature

Coronary artery anomalies (CAAs) are congenital defects whose hemodynamic significance, clinical presentation, and prognosis remain challenging to define. Their diagnosis is mostly incidental, and the range of symptoms they can produce is broad, varying from dyspnea to anginal complaints [1]. Numerous reports regarding their hemodynamic significance and possible lethality emerged in the 1970s, and since then, there is a growing interest to further elucidate their pathophysiology [2, 3]. Most importantly, CAAs have drawn the attention of the medical community due to the association of specific anatomical subtypes with sudden cardiac death (SCD), especially in young competitive and otherwise "healthy" athletes [4–6]. A CAA is characterized as such by taking into consideration the expected normal coronary anatomy and any possible abnormality regarding coronary artery origin, course, or both [1]. CAAs affect almost 1% of the general population, and their prevalence is found to be lower in necropsies [7]. In a cohort of 1950 patients who underwent coronary angiography, strict anatomical criteria were applied and the incidence of CAAs was found to be 5.64% [8]. Another retrospective study of 2572 multidetector computed tomography (MDCT) coronary angiograms revealed a prevalence of 2.33% [9]. The observed discrepancies between prevalence and incidence values are probably attributed to differences in the diagnostic definitions of CAAs, with some being more lenient and others stricter. Angelini et al., after careful scrutiny, provide a detailed classification of CAAs, which serves as a basis for further investigation of their clinical significance, and identify broad categories: anomalies of origination and course, anomalies of intrinsic coronary arterial anatomy, anomalies of coronary termination, and anomalous collateral vessels [7]. In their view, the characterization of anomalies as "minor" or "major," based on their clinical consequences, seems futile since large prospective studies regarding the prognostic impact of distinct CAAs are lacking. Yamanaka and Hobbs report an incidence of 1.3% in a cohort of 126,595 patients who underwent coronary angiography [10]. In their study, 87% of patients with a CAA had anomalous origin and distribution and the remaining 13% had coronary artery fistulae. The most common CAAs provided in order of decreasing incidence are split right coronary artery (RCA), ectopic RCA from the right coronary cusp, ectopic RCA from the left cusp, coronary fistulas, absent left main coronary artery (LMCA), circumflex coronary artery from the right cusp, left coronary artery (LCA) arising from the right cusp, and low origination of the RCA [7]. Regarding the link of CAAs with sudden cardiac death, it has been found that 0.6% of sudden death cases in apparently healthy young individuals could be attributed to a CAA [11]. The most common malignant anomalies reported were LCA arising from the right coronary sinus (which correlates with SCD during exertion) and RCA arising from the left coronary sinus, both following an interarterial course between the aorta and the pulmonary artery [11]. CAAs are reported as a cause of SCD in a series of young competitive athletes, being the third most common cause after definite hypertrophic cardiomyopathy (HCM) and probable HCM, accounting for 13% of deaths [12]. In the aforementioned series, the most common malignant anomaly was a left main coronary artery arising from the right coronary sinus with an interarterial course. Altered flow patterns within the anomalous vessel, which can lead to thrombus formation, reduced coronary reserve, and strangulation of the anomalous vessel by neighboring structures under specific circumstances (as in the case of an anomalous LCA with an interarterial course), have all been implicated in the pathophysiology of CAAs, trying to explain their spectrum of symptoms [7].

Here, we present a total of three cases, more specifically one case with an anomalous origin of the RCA from the left coronary sinus, one case with a split RCA originating from the left coronary sinus, and one case of a dual left anterior descending (LAD) artery system.

2. Case Presentations

2.1. Case 1: Anomalous Origin of the RCA from the Left Coronary Sinus. We present the case of a 70-year-old woman who presented at the emergency department (ED) of our non-percutaneous coronary intervention- (non-PCI-) capable hospital with a complaint of exertional dyspnea and a stabbing retrosternal pain radiating between her shoulders, both bothering her intermittently over the past three hours. The patient was overweight, and her medical history included arterial hypertension and hypothyroidism both controlled with medication. The 12-lead ECG revealed a normal sinus rhythm with ST segment depression of 1 mm at the anterior and lateral leads. High sensitivity troponin-I (hs-cTnI) was measured before admission to the coronary care unit (CCU) at 83.2 ng/L (normal value < 29 ng/L), confirming the diagnosis of non-ST elevation myocardial infarction (NSTEMI). The rest of the blood and biochemical panel was within normal limits, including a negative D-dimer assay. Chest X-ray revealed a marginally increased cardiothoracic ratio, and transthoracic echocardiography (TTE) revealed mild concentric left ventricular (LV) wall hypertrophy with a normal left ventricular ejection fraction (LVEF) and no wall motion abnormalities. Before the initiation of antiplatelets and due to the clinical description of the patient's complaint, a computed tomography (CT) angiography of the aorta was performed in order to rule out an acute aortic syndrome. No signs of aortic pathology were detected, but the CT revealed an anomalous origin of the RCA from the left coronary sinus (Figure 1). The ectopic RCA followed an interarterial course between the trunk of the pulmonary artery and the aorta. It should be noted that the CT scanner used was not technically capable of performing a CT coronary angiography (CTCA) but adequately visualized the anomaly. The patient remained hemodynamically stable during her stay, her symptoms gradually improved, and hs-cTnI was normalized. The patient was referred to a tertiary hospital for coronary angiography which confirmed the anomalous origin of the RCA (Figure 2) and did not reveal any atherosclerotic coronary lesions. A CTCA was also performed, after the classical coronary angiography, to accurately visualize the anatomy of the CAA (Figure 3). The CTCA unveiled an eccentric noncalcified plaque at the middle segment of the LAD branch of the

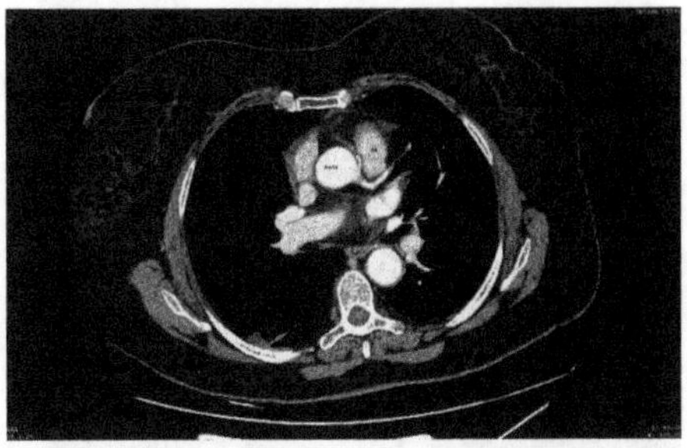

FIGURE 1: CT angiography of the aorta revealing an anomalous origin of the RCA (depicted with an "*"). The RCA exhibits an interarterial course between the aorta and the pulmonary artery (PA).

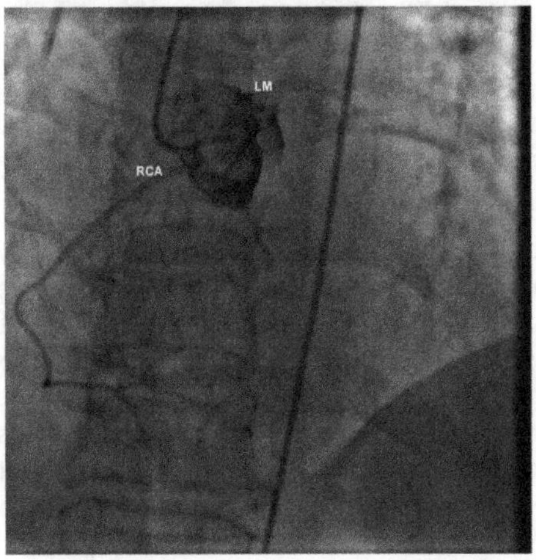

FIGURE 2: Coronary angiography confirming the anomalous aortic origin of the RCA from the left coronary sinus. LM: left main.

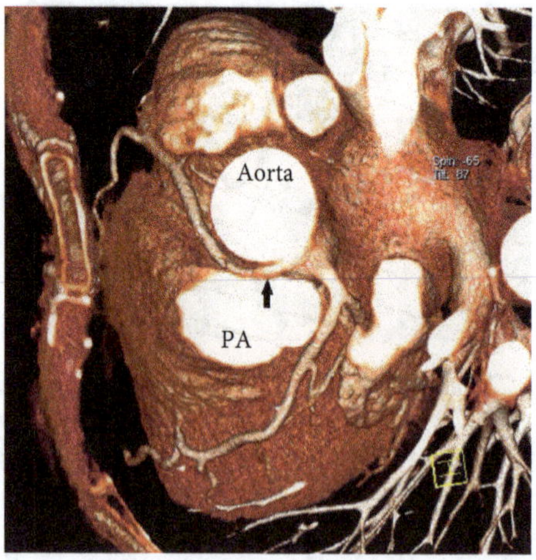

FIGURE 3: CT coronary angiography with volume-rendered 3D reconstruction of the images, revealing the interarterial course of the RCA (pointed with the arrow) between the aorta and the pulmonary artery (PA).

LCA, causing a luminal stenosis of 25-49%, which we speculate is the culprit lesion of the patient's NSTEMI, probably involving a mechanism of plaque rupture and subsequent fibrinolysis or coronary artery spasm. Finally, a dobutamine stress echocardiography study was negative for segmental wall motion abnormalities. In this case, the CAA was an incidental finding on the initial CT aortic angiography. It is probably a benign finding since the observed ischemic changes of the ECG were not compatible with the supply distribution of the RCA, and the stress echo study was unremarkable.

2.2. Case 2: Split RCA with an Anomalous Origin from the Left Coronary Sinus. We present the case of a 44-year-old man who presented at the ED of our non-PCI-capable hospital with a complaint of an intermittent burning-like sensation at the precordium during physical activity over the past two days. The patient was overweight and reported a smoking history of 30 pack-years. He was not taking any medication, and the rest of his medical history was unremarkable. The ECG revealed a normal sinus rhythm with anterior, high-lateral, and lateral repolarization disturbances (shallow inverted T waves at leads I, aVL, and V3 to V6). A measurement of hs-cTnI yielded a value of 38 ng/L (normal value < 29 ng/L), whereas the rest of the complete blood count and biochemical panel was unremarkable, apart from dyslipidemia (total cholesterol = 252 mg/dL, LDL = 155 mg/dL, and TG = 262 mg/dL). TTE revealed a reduced LVEF of 40%, increased end-diastolic LV diameter, and hypokinesis of the LV anterior, lateral, and inferolateral walls. The diagnosis of NSTEMI was confirmed; the patient was admitted to the CCU and initiated on dual antiplatelet therapy (DAPT) with aspirin and clopidogrel, low molecular weight heparin, b-blocker, ACE inhibitor, and a statin. His stay was uneventful with gradual remission of his complaint and improvement of his LV wall motion abnormalities. He was referred to a tertiary hospital for coronary angiography which revealed no atherosclerotic lesions and a split RCA with an anomalous origin from the left coronary sinus (Figures 4(a) and 4(b)). The RCA featured an initial common trunk, which then split into two distinct segments of similar caliber with one of them (RCA1 in Figures 4(a) and 4(b)) probably following a posterior course. The definition of a split RCA or a double RCA is a matter of great controversy with various anatomical descriptions, and no consensus has been reached so far [13, 14]. Unfortunately, after thorough discussion, the patient was not willing to undergo a CTCA which would visualize the anomaly in greater detail. Since coronary angiography did not reveal any atherosclerotic lesions, the patient's acute coronary syndrome (ACS) could be characterized as a myocardial infarction with nonobstructive coronary arteries (MINOCA), and based on existing evidence [15], DAPT with aspirin and clopidogrel was continued (aiming for a maximum of one year) in conjunction with an ACE inhibitor, a b-blocker, and a statin. Upon follow-up echocardiography, three months after angiography, an evident improvement of LVEF was observed (55%) along with restoration of normal wall motion.

2.3. Case 3: A Dual LAD System. We present the case of a 60-year-old man presenting at the ED of our non-PCI-capable hospital with a complaint of breathlessness at rest and on exertion over the past two days. The patient's medical history was unremarkable apart from obesity. Upon presentation, he was hemodynamically stable, and clinical examination revealed moderate wheezing and diffuse rales at lung bases bilaterally on auscultation (Killip Class II). His ECG revealed a normal sinus rhythm with a left anterior fascicular block (LAFB); shallow T wave inversion at leads I, aVL, and V6; and T wave flattening at lead V5. A measurement of cardiac troponin T (cTnT) yielded a value of 71 ng/L (normal value < 40 ng/L), and the diagnosis of a NSTEMI was highly likely. TTE revealed a reduced LVEF of 40% with no regional wall motion abnormalities. However, a difference of blood pressure values of about 20 mmHg between the two arms prompted a CT angiography of the aorta before the initiation of antiplatelet therapy. It revealed no aortic pathology but visualized a short LMCA which then split into two distinct branches of the same caliber descending toward the apex in the anterior interventricular groove, compatible with the course of the LAD artery (Figure 5). The patient was started on antiplatelets and intravenous diuretics. His stay at the CCU remained uneventful with gradual remission of symptoms and improvement of myocardial enzymes. He was referred to a tertiary center for coronary angiography which revealed an atherosclerotic lesion at the middle segment of the LCx causing a luminal stenosis of about 40% and one lesion at the second obtuse marginal branch of the LCx also causing a stenosis of 40%. Moreover, a short LMCA was confirmed (Figure 6(b), left anterior oblique caudal "spider" view), which in turn gave rise to the LCx and a common LAD trunk (which we denote as LAD-proper). The proper LAD bifurcated into two arteries, one giving rise to long septal perforators (short LAD) and one reaching the apex (long LAD), giving rise to shorter perforating arteries and diagonals (Figures 6(a) and 6(b)). The patient was discharged on DAPT (aiming for a maximum duration of one year), an ACE inhibitor, a b-blocker,

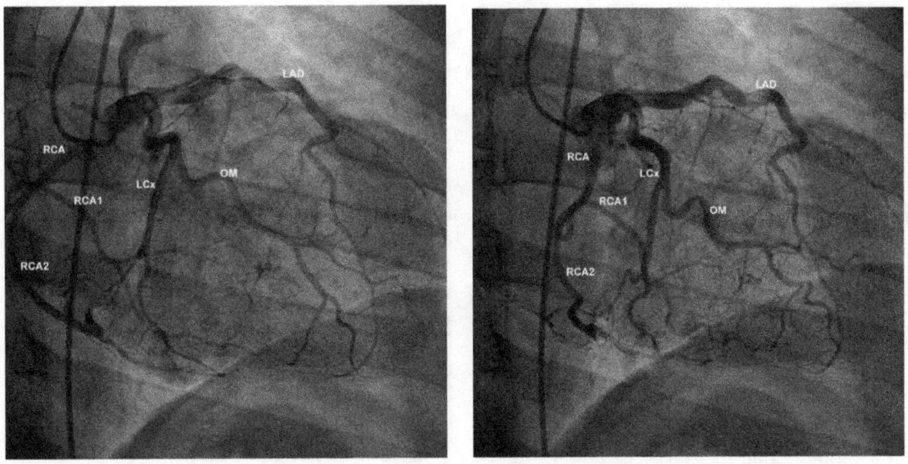

(a) (b)

FIGURE 4: (a, b) Coronary angiography (right anterior oblique projection) revealing the split RCA (marked as RCA1 and RCA2) with an anomalous origin from the left coronary sinus. The RCA and LCA were outlined simultaneously using the JL4 catheter placed at the left coronary sinus. LCx: left circumflex artery; OM: obtuse marginal artery; LAD: left anterior descending (artery).

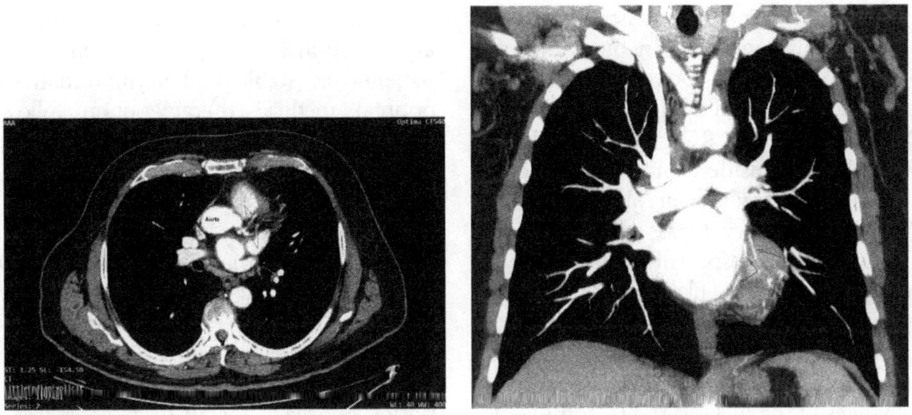

(a) (b)

FIGURE 5: CT angiography of the aorta revealing a short LMCA (a) which then splits into two distinct branches (pointed with arrows of different color) descending toward the apex in the anterior interventricular groove. The short LAD is pointed with blue arrows and the long LAD with red arrows.

a statin, and furosemide. Follow-up echocardiography was performed three months post angiography revealing a markedly improved LVEF of 52%.

Spindola-Franco et al., in 1983, classified dual LAD variants into distinct types (Types I, II, III, and IV) by studying a cohort of 2140 patients who underwent coronary angiography [16]. The prevalence of a dual LAD was 1% in their study (23 patients). Our case fits the angiographic description of a Type I dual LAD according to the abovementioned classification. Since the original classification of Spindola-Franco et al., three more dual LAD types have been described in the literature, raising the total types to seven [17, 18]. Regarding our current case, the opinion of expert interventional cardiologists who were asked to evaluate the angiographic findings was wavering between a dual LAD and a long diagonal branch, a situation that was to be expected considering the rarity of such a variant.

3. Discussion

Coronary artery anomalies remain an established cause of SCD. Presymptomatic screening protocols have been proposed especially for high-risk individuals (e.g., competitive athletes) by using novel imaging modalities like cardiac magnetic resonance [1]. The accumulation of data and the prospective study of large cohorts with CAAs, comprised of individuals detected through screening, could further elucidate the prognostic impact and pathophysiology of CAAs. The identification of highly malignant variants could prompt an early surgical intervention.

Moreover, CAAs should be taken into account in cases of an acute coronary syndrome or within the context of anginal symptoms. Considering the fact that all three patients presented to a non-PCI- and non-CTCA-capable hospital, the anomalies of Case 1 and Case 3 were discovered incidentally

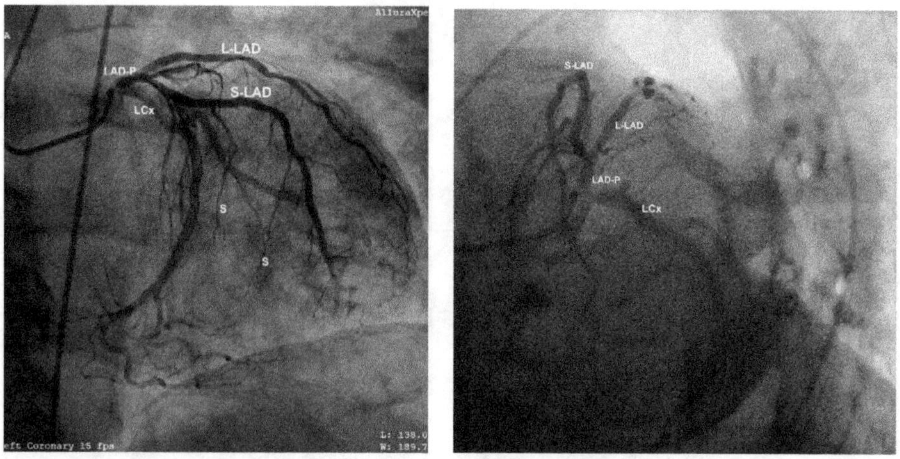

(a) (b)

FIGURE 6: (a, b) Coronary angiogram: right anterior oblique caudal projection (a) and left anterior oblique caudal "spider" projection (b). A very short LMCA, best visualized in (b), gives rise to the LCx and a common LAD trunk which we denote as LAD-P. The LAD-P bifurcates into two arteries, S-LAD, giving rise to long septal perforators, and L-LAD reaching the apex, giving rise to shorter perforating arteries and diagonals. LAD-P: left anterior descending proper; L-LAD: long LAD; S-LAD: short LAD; LCx: left circumflex artery; S: septal perforating branches.

on CT, which was prompted by emergent clinical suspicion, thus not delaying invasive management. In our view and according to the published literature, CAAs can be divided into hemodynamically significant and nonhemodynamically significant [19]. Duplication of the RCA or LAD, like in Cases 2 and 3, respectively, are considered nonhemodynamically significant anomalies, but they may perplexing surgical interventions such as coronary artery bypass grafting or percutaneous coronary interventions especially if both vessels are diseased. An interarterial course, like in Case 1 of our series, is considered significant since it can produce a wide range of symptoms under specific load circumstances. Case 1 could be classified as a MINOCA, and although the observed ischemic changes of the ECG were not compatible with the supply distribution of the ectopic RCA, we sought to investigate the "behavior" of the anomaly under increased load. This is one of the reasons we performed a stress-echo study which proved to be normal. Regarding Case 1 of our series, one could argue that a cardiac magnetic resonance (CMR) study was the imaging modality of choice to evaluate any eventual myocardial inflammation or fibrosis and simultaneously visualize the coronary anomaly. The reason it was not performed was purely financial from the patient's perspective. For the same case, an intravascular imaging modality, like optical coherence tomography (OCT) or intravascular ultrasound (IVUS), could have been used in conjunction with intracoronary functional testing in order to elucidate the behavior of the mid-LAD stenosis (detected on CTCA and graded as 25-49%) and also confirm the diagnosis of MINOCA with greater confidence. However, considering the ALARA (as low as reasonably achievable) principle of radioprotection, the patient had already undergone a CT aortography at the time of initial presentation (using a non-CTCA-capable scanner), then a coronary angiography which revealed no stenosis (therefore, no intracoronary imaging or functional tests were performed), and finally a CTCA. Subsequently, a second coronary angiography with OCT or IVUS and intracoronary functional testing was deemed excessive since the patient was stable and asymptomatic and was receiving optimal medical therapy upon follow-up examination. Regarding Case 2 (no angiographic stenosis) and Case 3 (moderate coronary atherosclerotic lesions), a thorough assessment with multimodality imaging (CMR, IVUS or OCT, and coronary functional testing) could safely confirm or exclude the diagnosis of MINOCA, according to published scientific statements [20]. However, multimodality imaging is not readily available at every tertiary site in the Greek region, which was the case for these patients. It should also be noted that the choice of a femoral catheterization approach for all three cases was based on operator experience and procedural confidence.

Data Availability

Source data used to support the findings of this study, more specifically imaging studies and laboratory investigation results, are restricted by Greek (Law 4624/2019) and European [(EU) 2016/679] regulation in order to protect patient health data as well as their privacy and anonymity. Data are available upon precisely reasoned application to the Scientific Council of the General Hospital of Florina "Eleni Th. Dimitriou," which is a public hospital of the Greek National Health System and can be contacted at postal address Egnatias 9, Florina, 53100, Greece, for researchers who meet the criteria to access confidential data.

Consent

All patients have provided written informed consent regarding the publication of their properly anonymized data in the current article.

Acknowledgments

We would like to thank cardiologist Dr. Pantelis Kligatsis, cardiologist Dr. Lykourgos Nanis, interventional cardiologist Dr. Georgios Mamadas, and interventional cardiologist Dr. Stefanos Papastefanou for their invaluable assistance regarding data collection and for their fruitful comments on the current case series.

References

[1] P. Angelini, "Novel imaging of coronary artery anomalies to assess their prevalence, the causes of clinical symptoms, and the risk of sudden cardiac death," *Circulation. Cardiovascular Imaging*, vol. 7, no. 4, pp. 747–754, 2014.

[2] M. D. Cheitlin, C. M. De Castro, and H. A. McAllister, "Sudden death as a complication of anomalous left coronary origin from the anterior sinus of Valsalva," *Circulation*, vol. 50, no. 4, pp. 780–787, 1974.

[3] A. J. Taylor, K. M. Rogan, and R. Virmani, "Sudden cardiac death associated with isolated congenital coronary artery anomalies," *Journal of the American College of Cardiology*, vol. 20, no. 3, pp. 640–647, 1992.

[4] C. Basso, C. Frescura, D. Corrado et al., "Congenital heart disease and sudden death in the young," *Human Pathology*, vol. 26, no. 10, pp. 1065–1072, 1995.

[5] C. Basso, B. J. Maron, D. Corrado, and G. Thiene, "Clinical profile of congenital coronary artery anomalies with origin from the wrong aortic sinus leading to sudden death in young competitive athletes," *Journal of the American College of Cardiology*, vol. 35, no. 6, pp. 1493–1501, 2000.

[6] R. E. Eckart, S. L. Scoville, C. L. Campbell et al., "Sudden death in young adults: a 25-year review of autopsies in military recruits," *Annals of Internal Medicine*, vol. 141, no. 11, pp. 829–834, 2004.

[7] P. Angelini, J. A. Velasco, and S. Flamm, "Coronary anomalies: incidence, pathophysiology, and clinical relevance," *Circulation*, vol. 105, no. 20, pp. 2449–2454, 2002.

[8] P. Angelini, "Coronary artery anomalies," *Circulation*, vol. 115, no. 10, pp. 1296–1305, 2007.

[9] C. Graidis, D. Dimitriadis, V. Karasavvidis et al., "Prevalence and characteristics of coronary artery anomalies in an adult population undergoing multidetector-row computed tomography for the evaluation of coronary artery disease," *BMC Cardiovascular Disorders*, vol. 15, no. 1, p. 112, 2015.

[10] O. Yamanaka and R. E. Hobbs, "Coronary artery anomalies in 126,595 patients undergoing coronary arteriography," *Catheterization and Cardiovascular Diagnosis*, vol. 21, no. 1, pp. 28–40, 1990.

[11] G. Finocchiaro, E. R. Behr, G. Tanzarella et al., "Anomalous coronary artery origin and sudden cardiac death: clinical and pathological insights from a national pathology registry," *JACC: Clinical Electrophysiology*, vol. 5, no. 4, pp. 516–522, 2019.

[12] B. J. Maron, J. Shirani, L. C. Poliac, R. Mathenge, W. C. Roberts, and F. O. Mueller, "Sudden death in young competitive athletes. Clinical, demographic, and pathological profiles," *Journal of the American Medical Association*, vol. 276, no. 3, pp. 199–204, 1996.

[13] Y.-F. Chen, T.-M. Chien, C.-W. Chen, C.-C. Lin, and C.-S. Lee, "Double right coronary artery or split right coronary artery?," *International Journal of Cardiology*, vol. 154, no. 3, pp. 243–245, 2012.

[14] S. Deora, S. Shah, and T. Patel, "Double or split right coronary artery: still a diagnostic dilemma for this rare coronary anomaly," *International Journal of Cardiology*, vol. 171, no. 3, pp. 457–459, 2014.

[15] B. Lindahl, T. Baron, D. Erlinge et al., "Medical therapy for secondary prevention and long-term outcome in patients with myocardial infarction with nonobstructive coronary artery disease," *Circulation*, vol. 135, no. 16, pp. 1481–1489, 2017.

[16] H. Spindola-Franco, R. Grose, and N. Solomon, "Dual left anterior descending coronary artery: angiographic description of important variants and surgical implications," *American Heart Journal*, vol. 105, no. 3, pp. 445–455, 1983.

[17] U. Bozlar, M. Ş. Uğurel, S. Sarı, V. Akgün, F. Örs, and M. Taşar, "Prevalence of dual left anterior descending artery variations in CT angiography," *Diagnostic and Interventional Radiology*, vol. 21, no. 1, pp. 34–41, 2015.

[18] S. Dhanse, H. Kareem, M. Sudhakar Rao, and T. Devasia, "Dual LAD system – a case report and lessons learnt from past nomenclature system," *IHJ Cardiovascular Case Reports (CVCR)*, vol. 2, pp. S4–S7, 2018.

[19] J. E. Shriki, J. S. Shinbane, M. A. Rashid et al., "Identifying, characterizing, and classifying congenital anomalies of the coronary arteries," *Radiographics*, vol. 32, no. 2, pp. 453–468, 2012.

[20] J. E. Tamis-Holland, H. Jneid, H. R. Reynolds et al., "Contemporary diagnosis and management of patients with myocardial infarction in the absence of obstructive coronary artery disease: a scientific statement from the American Heart Association," *Circulation*, vol. 139, no. 18, pp. e891–e908, 2019.

Hybrid Percutaneous Brachiofemoral Shunt and Open Abdominal Aortic Aneurysm Repair in a Kidney Transplant Recipient

Javad Salimi,[1] **Sayed Alimohammad Sadat**,[2] **Mohammad Javad Yavari Barhaghtalab**,[2] **and Hormat Rahimzadeh**[3]

[1]*Trauma and Surgery Research Center, Sina Hospital, Tehran University of Medical Science, Tehran, Iran*
[2]*Department of General Surgery, Shahid Beheshti Hospital, Yasuj University of Medical Science, Yasuj, Iran*
[3]*Department of Internal Medicine, Sina Hospital, Tehran University of Medical Sciences, Tehran, Iran*

Correspondence should be addressed to Sayed Alimohammad Sadat; alimohammad.sadat.yums@gmail.com

Academic Editor: Muzaffer Sindel

Abdominal aortic aneurysm (AAA) repair in kidney transplant recipients may cause ischemia in the transplanted kidney. As a result, various techniques have been described for protection of the renal allograft during AAA repair including temporary shunt, extracorporeal bypass, cold renal perfusion, endovascular aortic aneurysm repair (EVAR), and operation without renal allograft protection. We successfully treated a 56-year-old man, a case of kidney transplantation with AAA, using a temporary hybrid percutaneous brachiofemoral shunt using vascular prosthesis with a long 7-French (Fr) catheter sheath introducer (CSI) in the aortic arch via the right brachial artery and 8 Fr CSI in the right femoral artery that were connected together with a 7 Fr guiding catheter, before aortic cross-clamping and repair of AAA using a Dacron tube graft. The patient recovered well from the surgery without any complication and was discharged on the 6th postoperative day. To our knowledge, this is the first report of using a temporary hybrid percutaneous brachiofemoral shunt for renal allograft protection in AAA repair surgery in a patient with kidney transplantation, and we think that this temporary shunt is an easy, safe, and rapid method for renal allograft protection from ischemia.

1. Background

An arterial aneurysm is defined as a focal dilation of a blood vessel with respect to the original artery. AAA may be detected incidentally or at the time of rupture. The likelihood that an aneurysm will rupture is influenced by the aneurysm size expansion rate, continued smoking, and persistent hypertension. Treatment is recommended when it reaches 5 cm to 5.5 cm, is demonstrated as rapidly enlarging >0.5 cm over 6 months, or becomes symptomatic. Open surgical repair via a transabdominal or retroperitoneal approach has been the gold standard [1, 2].

With increasing graft survival after kidney transplantation and high rates of cardiovascular risk factors in renal transplant recipients, vascular surgeons will increasingly be faced with repairing AAAs in this patient group. It is important to avoid ischemic and reperfusion injury to the transplanted kidney. In high-risk patients, collateral perfusion reduces the risk of ischemic complications when prolonged infrarenal aortic cross-clamping is probable in open aortic and iliac aneurysm repair surgery [3–6].

Various techniques reported in literatures for decreasing the ischemic effect of aortic clamping during AAA repair are summarized in Table 1.

In this study, we report an open AAA repair surgery in a kidney transplant patient who was successfully operated with a temporary hybrid percutaneous brachiofemoral shunt using vascular prosthesis.

2. Case Presentation

A 56-year-old man with end-stage renal disease (ESRD) secondary to membranous glomerulonephritis had undergone a right-sided orthotopic renal transplantation 4 months earlier after 1.5 years of hemodialysis. His renal function was pretty good after transplantation, and he

Table 1: Techniques used for protection of the transplanted kidney during AAA repair.

Femoral V-A bypass [4]
Pump-oxygenation bypass technique [5]
Axillofemoral shunt [5, 6, 8]
Atriofemoral bypass [7]
Endovascular aneurysm repair (EVAR) [5, 7]
Topical cooling [5, 7]
Aortofemoral shunt [8]
Femorofemoral bypass with extracorporeal circulation [6–8]
Operation without renal allograft protection [9]
Femoropoliteal bypass [9]
Permanent and temporary axillofemoral bypass [7–9]
Saphenous vein branchiorenal shunt [10]
Aortoiliac shunt [7, 10]
Cold perfusion of the graft [7–9, 11]
General hypothermia [8, 9, 11]

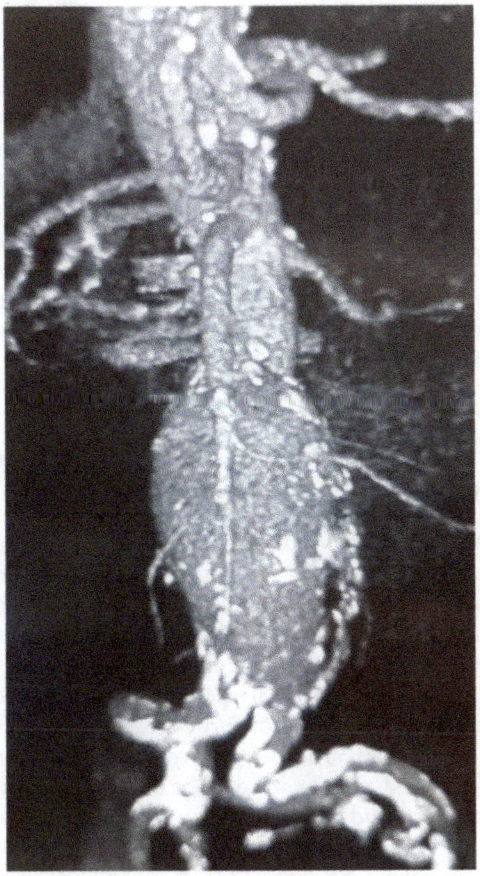

Figure 1: Abdominopelvic CT scan without contrast before AAA repair operation.

had been discharged with serum creatinine 1.6 mg/dl and had been stable over these 4 months. Renal functional scan (Tc-99m DTPA (diethylene-triamine-pentaacetate)) was normal. Past medical history was positive for hyper-

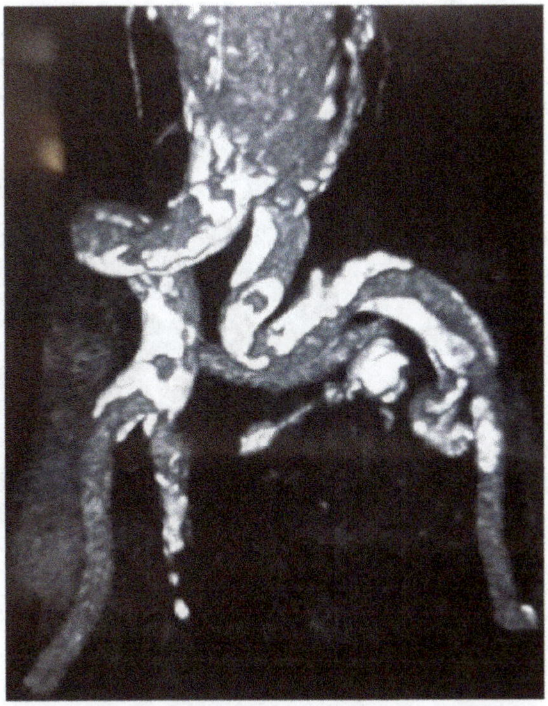

Figure 2: Abdominopelvic CT scan without contrast before AAA repair operation.

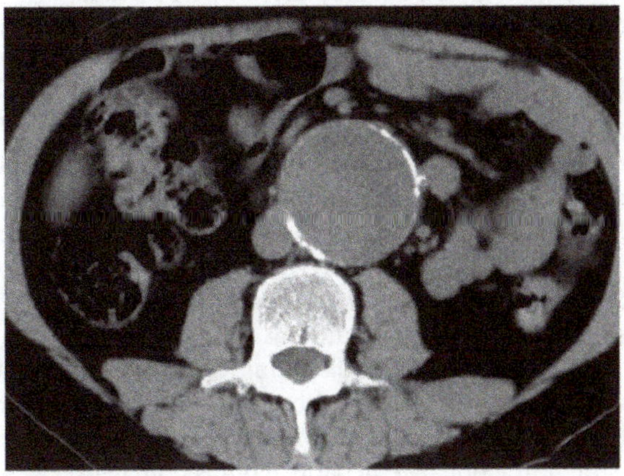

Figure 3: Abdominopelvic CT scan without contrast before AAA repair operation.

tension, hyperlipidemia, and coronary artery disease (three-vessel disease). The patient had an AAA with an anterioposterior diameter of 4.2 cm and symptom-free, so vascular surgery consultation was not done before renal transplantation. He was receiving tacrolimus, mycophenolic acid, and prednisolone after the transplantation. The patient developed with abdominal pain and raising serum creatinine (2.6 mg/dl), and abdominopelvic sonography revealed normal transplanted kidney with a large infrarenal abdominal aortic aneurysm (anterioposterior diameter of 55 mm) which did not involve the iliac arteries, and

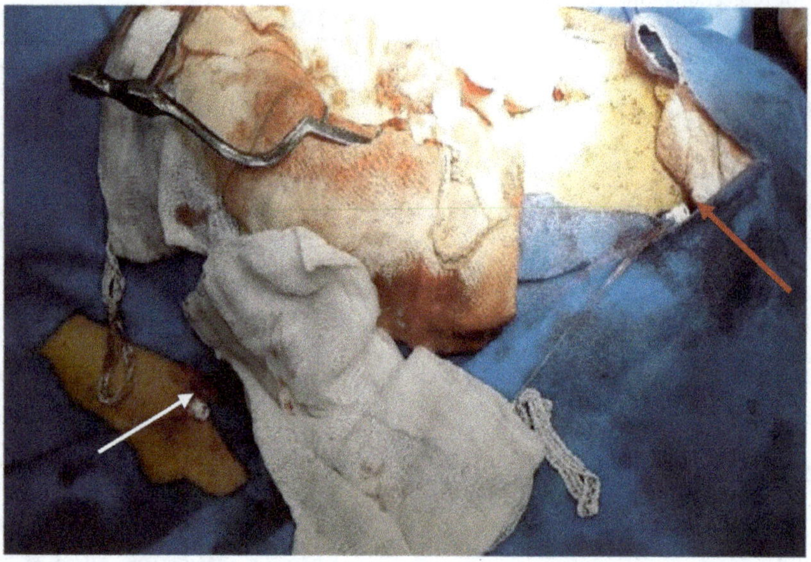

FIGURE 4: Intraoperative photography of the brachial sheath (white arrow) and femoral sheath (red arrow) used for brachiofemoral shunt during the operation.

then, computed tomography (CT) scan without contrast confirmed the diagnosis (Figures 1–3).

After appropriate hydration and medical therapy and lowering creatinine to 1.7 mg/dl, the patient was scheduled for an operation. As both iliac arteries were tortuous and calcified, they were unsuitable for the EVAR. For renal allograft protection, at first, a short 5 Fr CSI (Cordis AVANTI®+ Sheath Introducer, USA) was inserted in the right brachial artery, and then, a 65 cm 7 Fr percutaneous CSI (Epsylar-Optimed, Germany) was placed in the aortic arch under fluoroscopy on the guide of a stiff wire (Amplatz wire, Cordis, USA) via the brachial access, and an 11 cm 8 Fr CSI (Cordis AVANTI®+ Sheath Introducer, USA) was inserted in the right external iliac via the common femoral artery through a percutaneous procedure and was fixed (Figure 4).

After laparotomy and dissecting of the aorta up to the renal artery and down to both the common iliac arteries and intravenous injection of 5000 international units (IU) of unfractionated heparin, connection between both sheaths was established with a 7 Fr guiding catheter (its end was cut) and connection was covered with sterile towels and protected from compression and kinking. After confirmation of the good function of the shunt, aortic cross-clamping was done and the aneurysm was repaired with knitted Dacron prostheses 20 × 10 mm (Jotec GmbH, Hechingen, Germany) in about 35 minutes. To maintain the flow to both the lower extremity and the transplanted kidney (proximally), the common iliac artery was clamped as the end of the sheath was in the external iliac artery. Hydration was done before and during the operation, and two units of packed red blood cells were transfused. Adequate urine output of 30 cc per hour was maintained during the operation. At the end of the operation, brachial and femoral sheaths were removed, and no closure device was used.

The patient was transferred to the surgical intensive care unit (ICU) and was extubated after 4 hours. The patient developed atrial fibrillation that was controlled with intravenous amiodarone at the first day postoperation. The patient was transferred to the post-ICU vascular surgery ward at the 3rd day postoperation. There were no any other complications in the postoperative period, and the patient was discharged in stable vital sign and good condition with creatinine 1.6 mg/dl at the 6th day postoperation. The patient had no complaint during the 18-month clinical follow-up, and the last serum creatinine was 1.7 mg/dl.

3. Discussion and Conclusion

The AAA in a kidney-transplanted patient requires surgical management and is truly a life-threatening condition and has a more complicated repair. The transplanted kidney has a solitary arterial supply and lacks collateral circulation, so it is more susceptible to ischemic injury, so aortic cross-clamping may put the renal allograft at risk for ischemic damage [11]. If the period of aortic cross-clamping in open surgery is less than 50 min, slight protection may be needed and a clamp and go method could be done [6]. To minimize this risk, as was said before, there is a variety of techniques to protect the transplanted kidney in major open aortoiliac surgeries, especially AAA repair [3–11].

A different renal protecting mechanism could be the endovascular repair. The benefit is that the allograft ischemia is limited to a short time that the graft is ballooned into place, but the disadvantages are the emboli to the kidney from dislodged atherosclerotic debris during the procedure as well as the risk of contrast-induced nephropathy [7, 11].

This report is the first report of percutaneous brachiofemoral shunt for ischemic protection of the transplanted kidney in AAA repair. We think that despite the fact that this shunt can support collateral perfusion to the transplanted kidney during operation. This protective shunt is easy and safe and decreases total time of operation that is important in high-risk patients such as our patient with three-vessel coronary disease and high serum creatinine. It is obvious that this procedure needs to be developed and uses a larger shunt.

In summary, when we are not sure about the time of operation and aortic clamping and if the patient is at the high risk for operation, it is better to use protective measures to decrease ischemic effect on the transplanted kidney. This percutaneous temporary shunt is an easy and rapid way for the ischemic protection of the transplanted kidney during AAA repair or other major aortoiliac procedures.

Consent

Written informed consent was obtained from the patient for publication of this case report and any accompanying images. A copy of the written consent is available for review by the Editor-in-Chief of this journal.

Authors' Contributions

JS evaluated the patient clinically and operated the patient (main surgeon) and revised the manuscript. SAMS evaluated the patient clinically and helped to operate the patient (cosurgeon) and prepared the first version of the manuscript. MJYB helped in the revision of the manuscript. HR evaluated the patient clinically. All authors read and approved the final manuscript.

Acknowledgments

We all express our gratitude to the patient who kindly gave consent for this case to be presented in this paper.

References

[1] S. Aggarwal, A. Qamar, V. Sharma, and A. Sharma, "Abdominal aortic aneurysm: a comprehensive review," *Experimental and Clinical Cardiology*, vol. 16, no. 1, pp. 11–15, 2011.

[2] P. M. Shaw, J. Loree, and R. C. Gibbons, "Abdominal aortic aneurysm," in *StatPearls [Internet]*, StatPearls Publishing, Treasure Island (FL), 2020.

[3] E. Dregelid, "Temporary extracorporeal brachio-femoral vascular prosthesis shunt for ischemia prevention in an operation for abdominal aortic and iliac aneurysms in a patient with Marfan^|^apos;s syndrome," *Annals of Thoracic and Cardiovascular Surgery*, vol. 20, Supplement, pp. 801–804, 2014.

[4] T. Maeda, N. Watanabe, and S. Muraki, "Abdominal aortic aneurysm repair in a renal transplant recipient using a femoral V-A bypass," *Annals of Thoracic and Cardiovascular Surgery*, vol. 15, no. 6, pp. 415–417, 2009.

[5] C. J. Callaghan, I. T. Munday, N. D. Casey, S. R. Large, and M. E. Gaunt, "Abdominal aortic aneurysm repair in a renal transplant recipient: a modified pump-oxygenation bypass technique to reduce hypotension and myocardial ischaemia," *EJVES Extra*, vol. 10, no. 5, pp. 120-121, 2005.

[6] U. Sadat, E. L. Huguet, and K. Varty, "Abdominal aortic aneurysm surgery in renal, cardiac and hepatic transplant recipients," *European Journal of Vascular and Endovascular Surgery*, vol. 40, no. 4, pp. 443–449, 2010.

[7] J. H. Joh, D. H. Nam, and H. C. Park, "Endovascular abdominal aortic aneurysm repair in patients with renal transplant," *Journal of the Korean Surgical Society*, vol. 84, no. 3, pp. 189–193, 2013.

[8] M. Lepäntalo, F. Biancari, J. Edgren, B. Eklund, and K. Salmela, "Treatment options in the management of abdominal aortic aneurysm in patients with renal transplant," *European Journal of Vascular and Endovascular Surgery*, vol. 18, no. 2, pp. 176–178, 1999.

[9] J. P. Harris and J. May, "Successful aortic surgery after renal transplantation without protection of the transplanted kidney," *Journal of Vascular Surgery*, vol. 5, no. 3, pp. 457–461, 1987.

[10] R. Khan and M. Simms, "Renal protection strategies when aortic aneurysm repair necessitates renal artery re-implantation: review and a new technique," *The Internet Journal of Surgery*, vol. 7, no. 2, 2005.

[11] H. K. Kim, J. P. Ryuk, H. H. Choi, S. H. Kwon, and S. Huh, "Abdominal aortic aneurysm repair in patient with a renal allograft: a case report," *Journal of Korean Medical Science*, vol. 24, no. 1, pp. 166–169, 2009.

38

Angioembolization of Scrotal Arteriovenous Malformations: A Case Report and Literature Review

Ammar Mohammad,[1] Wael Sahyouni,[1] Taisser Almeree,[2] and Bayan Alsaid[3,4]

[1]*Department of Vascular Surgery, Al-Assad University Hospital, Damascus, Syria*
[2]*Department of Radiology, Al-Assad University Hospital, Damascus, Syria*
[3]*Department of General Surgery, Al-Assad University Hospital, Damascus, Syria*
[4]*Laboratory of Anatomy, Faculty of Medicine, University of Damascus, Damascus, Syria*

Correspondence should be addressed to Bayan Alsaid; drbayan@gmail.com

Academic Editor: Muzaffer Sindel

Arteriovenous malformations (AVMs) of the scrotum are rare lesions, usually diagnosed incidentally during the evaluation of scrotal masses or infertility. It could be presented with acute bleeding or acute pain. We are presenting a case of painless bilateral infiltrated scrotal mass (more advanced in the left side) developed dramatically over a year, no other symptoms existed. The diagnosis was made using duplex ultrasound (DUS), computed tomography arteriography (CTA), and digital subtraction angiography (DSA). Three sessions of angioembolization were performed and followed by surgical resection of the left side of the scrotum.

1. Introduction

Scrotal swelling is a very common condition in medical practice. Differential diagnosis includes benign lesions that affect any component of the scrotum (testicles, soft tissues, and vascular plexus), malignancy, metastases, and infection.

Benign vascular lesions are common in adult males. Varicoceles are the most common lesion, and the rarest is arteriovenous malformations (AVMs). These lesions may present in a broad spectrum of symptoms such as swelling, bleeding, acute pain, sensation of heaviness, and mass-like structure.

AVMs are rare congenital abnormal underdeveloped vascular lesions that grow with the child. They present with a mass-like structure with audible or tangible bruit. The duplex ultrasound study shows high systolic flow, low resistive index, and arterialization of venous waveforms. Magnetic resonance imaging (MRI) helps to define the extent of the AVM and the adjacent tissues. Angiograph shows a rapid transit shunting of contrast agent from feeding arteries to enlarged veins through an underdeveloped vascular plexus [1].

The most common locations of arteriovenous malformations (AVMs) are intracranial, followed by extracranial head and neck, extremity, and truncal and visceral sites. However, congenital scrotal AVM is a rare condition [2].

We are reporting a case of huge scrotal AMV managed by angioembolization. We also reviewed data from other similar reported cases in the medical literature.

2. Case Presentation

A 19-year-old male patient presented to our center in September 2017 with progressive diffused swelling in the scrotum. The swelling developed dramatically over the previous year with flashing skin and local warmth. There was no pain, urological symptoms, or bleeding. No medical or trauma histories were reported.

Physical examination revealed an asymmetric diffused scrotal swelling (more progressed in the left side) (Figure 1), local warmth, and scrotal skin flashing. By palpation, there was no pulse or thrill. Only the right testicle was palpable.

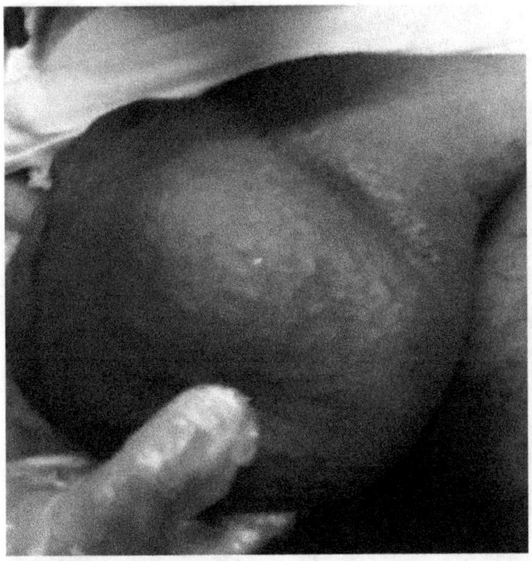

Figure 1: Left scrotal swelling.

Duplex ultrasound (DUS) showed prominent vessels exhibiting both venous and arterial components (Figure 2), with unusual high flow velocities, and dilated veins up to 1 cm in width. The skin thickness was 2 mm at its max.

Computed tomography arteriography showed a large AVM in the scrotum occupying almost all the scrotal sac indenting the testicles that look slightly small, the left testicle was encircled by the malformation. The veins seen were also dilated reaching diameters of 1 cm denoting varicoceles.

The AVM has its arterial supply from the internal iliac arteries and at least one of its veins drained in the left common femoral vein.

Digital subtraction angiography (DSA) demonstrated large AVM in the scrotum being centered mainly on the left side with multiple feeding vessels originating from the anterior division of internal iliac and common femoral arteries bilaterally more apparent from the left sides.

The feeding vessels in the left side were the internal pudendal artery, the superficial external pudendal artery arising from the common femoral artery, and the deep external pudendal artery arising from the deep femoral artery.

In the right side, the internal pudendal artery and a small branch of superficial pudendal artery were noticed.

The conventional scrotal vascular territory is divided into two parts: anterior one-third and posterior two-thirds. The anterior one-third is supplied by the superficial and deep external pudendal arteries, branching from the femoral artery. The posterior two-thirds is supplied by the internal pudendal artery, branching from the internal iliac artery [3] (Figure 3). The deep external pudendal could be a branch of the deep femoral artery.

Multiple sessions of angioembolization were performed using coils and particles followed by a total resection of the left mass. The patient was informed with all the predictive complications of the procedure.

The first session of embolization was performed in 28/9/2017 in which the left internal pudendal artery and some branches of the superficial external pudendal artery were embolized (Figure 4).

In the second session, one week later, the rest of left superficial external pudendal artery branches were embolized (Figures 5(a)–5(c)). A third session of embolization was needed after two weeks to complete the embolization of the left deep external pudendal artery (Figures 5(d)–5(f)).

Surgical resection was performed in the following day to resect the whole left side of the scrotum, the left testicle was fixed to the right side (Figure 6).

The histopathological study of resected lesions showed vascular vessels with variation in diameters, some hyaline degeneration in the vessels wall and abnormality in arteriovenous structure.

The follow-up during the next 12 months was favorable with good healing of the scrotal incision and no recurrence of lesion (Figure 7).

3. Literature Review

There are many types of vascular lesions that affect the scrotum or the testicle, Sule et al. [4] divided these into four main types:

(1) Varicoceles: common lesions that affect the spermatic cord. They consist of dilated veins with no bruit

(2) Hemangiomas: rare lesions that affect the scrotum, consist of dilated veins and capillaries with no bruit detected

(3) Lymphangiomas: rare lesions that affect the scrotum, consist of lymphatic ducts with no flow or bruit detected

(4) Arteriovenous malformations: very rare lesions that affect the scrotum, consist of abnormal microfistulas (nidus) between arteries and veins with no capillary bed, high flow, and bruit

Scrotal arteriovenous malformations are very rare. Therefore, there have been no clear recommendations on their treatment.

Until this case, there have been 17 published case reports about scrotal AVMs with variation in clinical presentation and medical management which we summarize in Table 1.

4. Discussion

Scrotal AVMs are uncommon lesions in medical practice with many types of treatment approaches. There is no medical study to support one approach over another due to the scarcity of this condition. Although embolization of feeding vessels helps in reducing the risk of massive bleeding during surgical resection in most cases, it also raises the risk of radiation complications including malignancy, sperm DNA mutations, and permanent damage to the testicular tissue.

The most common presentation was swelling or infiltrating mass [3–17], followed by pain [4, 5, 11, 13, 16, 17], and bleeding or ulceration [3–5, 8, 11, 14]. Infertility was the primary presentation in few cases [7, 10].

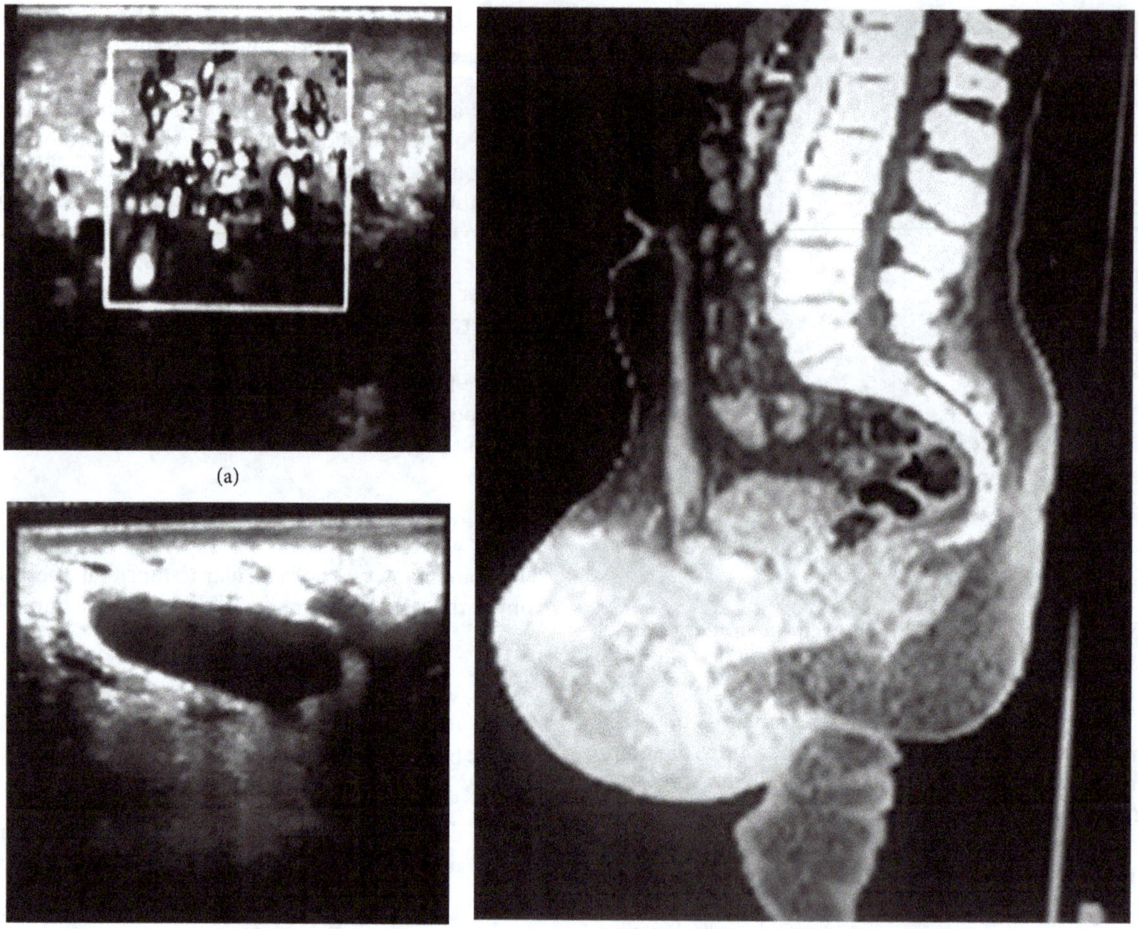

(a) (b) (c)

FIGURE 2: (a, b) Doppler ultrasound showed dilated vessels with both venous and arterial components; (c) computed tomography arteriography.

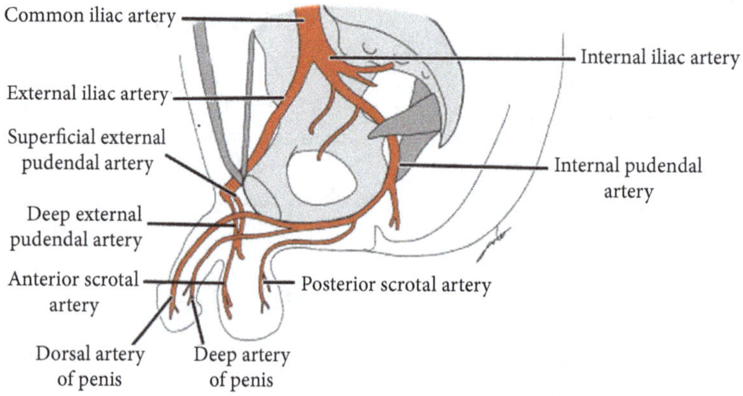

FIGURE 3: Normal blood supply of scrotum.

The main diagnostic method was DUS [3–7, 10–14, 16, 17], as we noticed before, followed by DSA [3–5, 7, 10, 12, 14, 16], especially in patients whom treated with endovascular embolization. MRI was used in some cases to confirm the diagnosis [13]. CTA is a helpful method to diagnose the lesion but not effective for establishing the management [15]; therefore, DSA is still the golden standard.

Laboratory tests were limited to the patient's condition. Although sperm analysis was commonly abnormal, it was not a routine test, especially in cases of acute pain or bleeding or with patients who refused to do the test (as in our case).

Percutaneous sclerotherapy into the nidus has been described in low-flow vascular malformation treatment. To

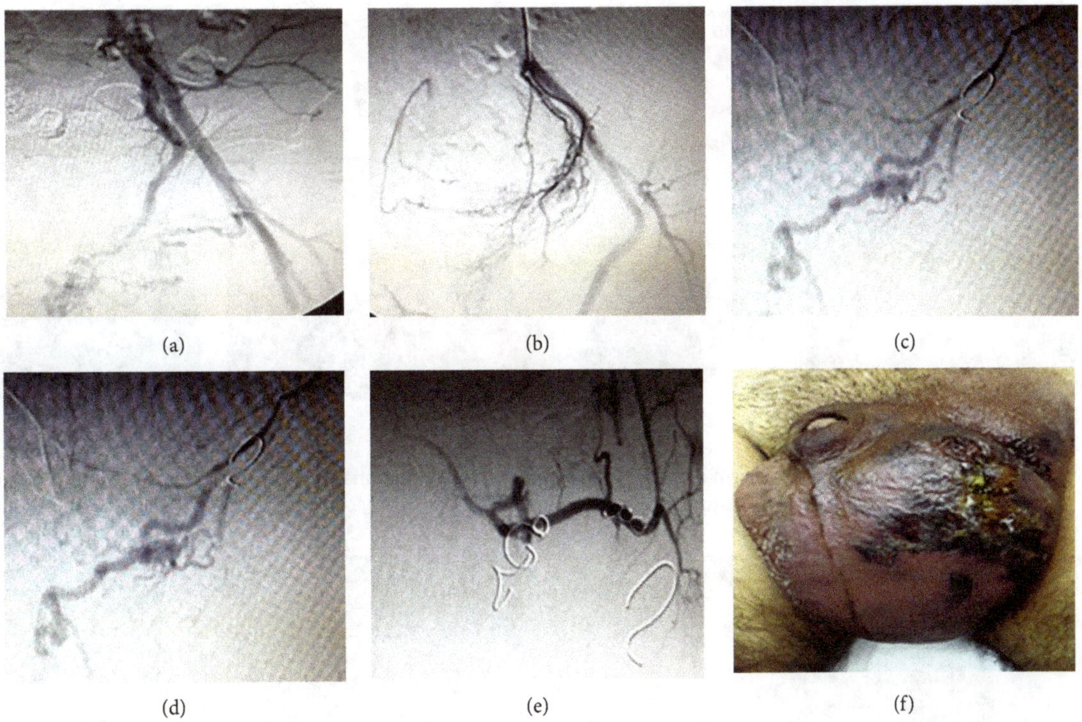

FIGURE 4: Embolization of multiple vessels: (a, b) internal pudendal artery and (c, d, e) superficial external pudendal artery. (f) View of scrotum after 24 hours.

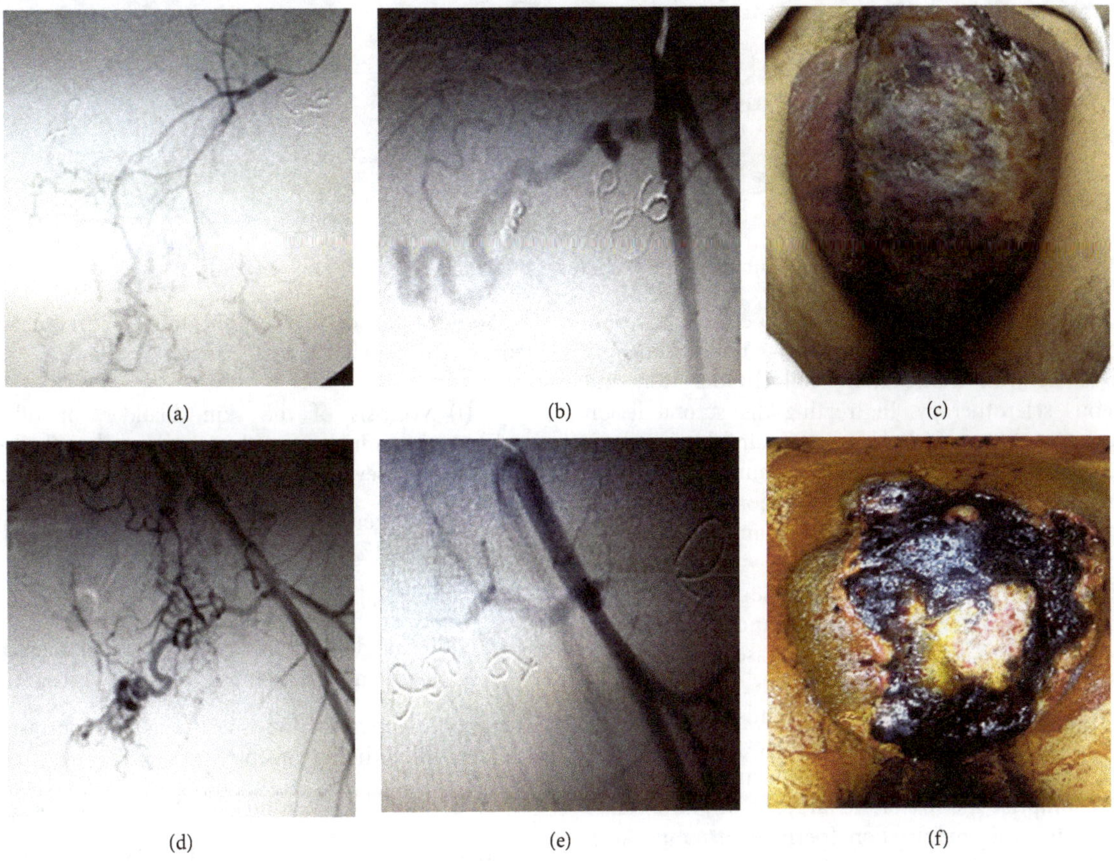

FIGURE 5: (a, b) Second session of angioembolization of the rest of superficial external pudendal artery branches; (c) affected area after 24 hours; (d) anterioposterior view of left deep external pudendal artery during the third session. (e) Final view showing no more visible feeding branches to the arteriovenous malformation. (f) Final clinically infarcted area before surgery.

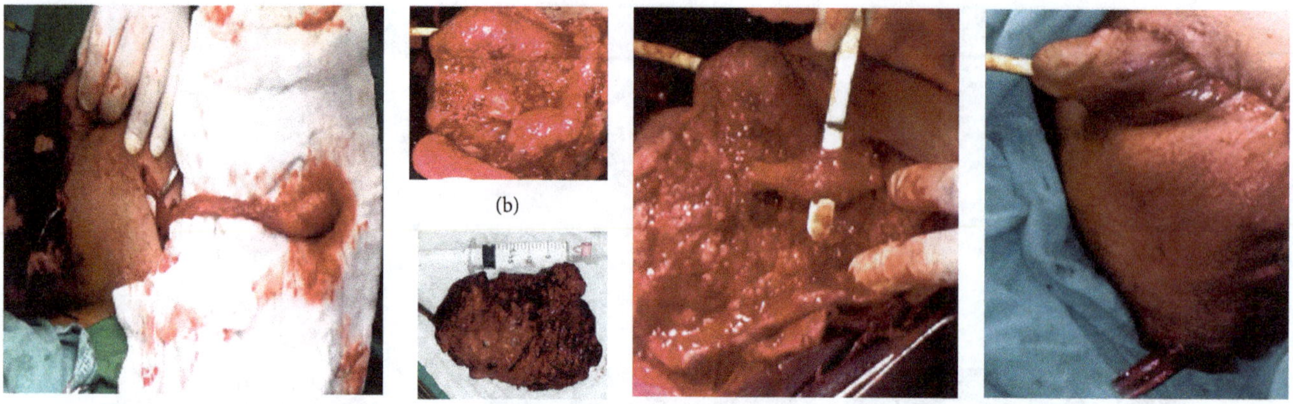

(a) (b) (c) (d) (e)

FIGURE 6: Surgical steps: (a) isolation of left spermatic cord with the testicle from inguinal incision, (b, c) resection of the lesion, and (d) insertion of the left testicle in the right side of scrotum. (e) View after surgery.

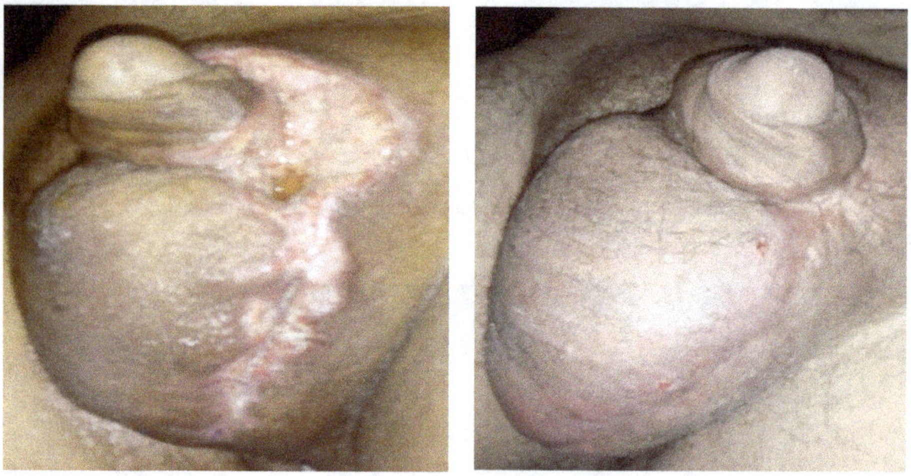

(a) (b)

FIGURE 7: After 3 months (a). After 12 months (b).

our best knowledge, the case written by So et al. is the only case report that described an endovascular method to treat a scrotal AVM with transcatheter coil embolization and percutaneous sclerotherapy. In treating the scrotal lesion with direct puncture, which is a very painful procedure, general anesthesia is required to reduce pain and minimize patient movement. In addition, compression during injection helps in localizing the sclerotherapy and reducing the embolic risk [3].

Embolization materials were variable (coils, gelatin sponge, polyvinyl alcohol sponge, butyl cyanoacrylate mixed with lipodol, particles, and onyx); in our case, we used coils and particles.

Choosing the embolization agent depends on the indication and the experience at hand. Each agent has its specific advantages and disadvantages. Factors influencing the choice of material comprise the size of the target vessel, flow velocity, and duration of embolization (permanent/temporary), see Table 2 [19].

Skin necrosis was described in some cases with angioembolization treatment. Later, surgical approach was needed to remove the necrotic tissue (as in our case).

Some of the possible complications for embolization procedure [20] in pelvic area are as follows:

(i) Necrosis of the skin, bladder, or other intra-abdominal organs has also been described especially with sever unspecified embolization

(ii) Impotence: bilateral internal pudendal artery embolization

(iii) Arterial perforation

(iv) Hemoglobinuria may develop as a consequence of the hemolysis that follows any sclerosant injection

(v) Allergic reaction due the use of contrast agent or sclerotherapy agents

(vi) Acute kidney injury due the contrast agent

(vii) Local complications in the insertion artery (hematoma, pseudoaneurysm)

(viii) Delayed malignancy due to the exposure to high dosage of radiation

Table 1: Published cases till 1/1/2019.

Author (year)	Age (years)	Presentation	Thrill/ bruit	Sperm analysis	Investigation	Management	Follow-up
Bezirdjian et al. (1989) [5]	24	Painless enlarging right scrotal mass	+	Not done	US. Arteriogram	Angioembolization (polyvinyl alcohol sponge (Ivalon)). Surgical debridement	Not mentioned
Hamid et al. (1992) [6]	55	Right scrotal swelling, pain with ulceration and bleeding	+	Azoospermia	Low s.testosterone, DUS, DSA	Angioembolization then surgery	Not commented
Sule et al. (1993) [4]	17	Intermittently bleeding pulsatile left scrotal mass	+	—	DSA	Angioembolization (gelatin sponge and coils) failed. Complete surgical resection was done	No recurrence at 2 years of follow-up
Konus et al. (1999) [7]	8	Progressively enlarging, intermittently bleeding, painful pulsatile scrotal mass	+	Not done	DUS, DSA	Angioembolization (polyvinyl alcohol sponge). Surgical excision	1 year later. No residual disease on follow-up Doppler
Kang et al. (2004) [8]	20	Acute scrotal swelling detected 4 days after a trauma	—	Not done	DUS	Surgical excision. Biopsy showed AVM	Not mentioned
Gonzalez et al. (2002) [9]	31	Left scrotal swelling with virtual azoospermia.	Not mentioned	Azoospermia	DUS, DSA	Bilateral varicocelectomy. Super selective angioembolization followed by surgical excision	3 months of follow-up, sperm analyses improved
Bandi et al. (2004) [10]	67	Recurrent scrotal AVM-bleeding nonhealing ulcer 12 years after preoperative embolization and hemiscrotectomy	Not mentioned	Not done	Not done at second presentation	Surgical excision.	Not mentioned
Choi et al. (2005) [11]		The article was inaccessible					
Monoski et al. (2006) [12]	31	Primary infertility and left scrotal fullness	—	Severe oligospermia	DSA hypertrophied internal pudendal and branch of superficial femoral a.	Bilateral varicocelectomy. Angioembolization. Surgical excision	Sperm count improved. 3 years later, successful spontaneous pregnancy
Yilmaz et al. (2009) [13]	51	Pain and throbbing sensation in right hemiscrotum	Pulsatile vessels +	Not done	Scrotal ultrasound. Confirmed at DUS	Not mentioned	Not mentioned
Jaganathan et al. (2011) [14]	2 32	2 cases both presented with scrotal swelling and bleeding	Not mentioned	Not done	DUS, DSA Emergency DUS, DSA	Selective angioembolization (poly vinyl alcohol). Parents refused surgery. Angioembolization (n-butyl cyanoacrylate mixed with lipodol)	13 months of follow-up, asymptomatic. 18 months of follow-up, no recurrence
Zachariah et al. (2012) [15]	30	Progressive swelling. One episode of acute pain before 4 mo.	—	Not done	DUS, MRI	Angioembolization was rejected. Surgical excision.	Not mentioned

Table 1: Continued.

Author (year)	Age (years)	Presentation	Thrill/ bruit	Sperm analysis	Investigation	Management	Follow-up
Key R. et al. (2013) [16]	41	Massive bleeding after a hip fracture due to trauma. With large right retro peritoneal hematoma	—	—	DUS, DSA	Several sessions of angioembolization (micro coils/emposphere's/gel foam particles/onyx	18 weeks later, no symptoms
Sato et al. (2013) [17]	38	Recurrent scrotal mass	—	—	CTA, biopsy (micro-AV fistula—AVM)	Surgical excision	10 months later, no recurrence
So WL et al. (2014) [3]	26	Scrotal pain and swelling	—	Not mentioned	DUS (AVM). DSA	Coil embolization. Subcutaneous sclerosant (sodium tetradecyl sulfate 3% with ethiodised oil (2 : 1 ratio)	3 months of review, no recurrence
Muslim et al. (2014) [18]	16	Right scrotal swelling associated with mild pain	Not mentioned	Not mentioned	DUS	Refused embolization. Surgical excision with dissecting the spermatic cord through an inguinal incision to protect it	One-year follow-up, no recurrence
Our case	19	Left scrotum swelling	+	Not performed	DUS, MCT, DSA	Three sessions of embolization, resection of scrotal lesion	One-year follow-up, no recurrence

Table 2: Types of embolization agents.

	Embolization agents
Organic	Autologous clots, fibrin
Coils	Standard coils, detachable coils, active coils
Plugs, balloons	Detachable balloon, vascular plug
Liquids, sclerosants	Alcohol, polymerizing substances (histoacryl), detergents (e.g., fibrovein, ethoxysclerol), antibiotics (e.g., doxocycline, bleomycin), precipitating substances (onyx®)
Particles	Gelfoam, polyvinyl alcohol particles, spherical particles (e.g., spherical PVA, acryl polymere)

(ix) DNA mutations of sperm cells/ovarian cells or infertility due to radiation

Conservative approach with periodic assessment was an option in some cases especially in young asymptomatic patients.

5. Conclusion

The scarcity of scrotal AVMs and the variety of medical approaches present a challenge in both diagnostic and treatment approaches.

We should think of AVMs in patients with rapidly developed lesions despite other symptoms such as pain or bleeding, without neglecting other deferential diagnoses, mainly tumors and infections.

Doppler US is very helpful for diagnosis of these lesion but is not sufficient for planning the management. Patients should be fully informed about the complications of each treatment plan in order to give an informed consent.

The management should consider the individuality of each case.

6. Limitations

We could not do a sperm count (because the patient refused). There was no intervention in the right side of the scrotum due to the hesitation of the patient.

Consent

The patient gave written informed consent to the publication of his case details and clinical photographs.

Acknowledgments

The authors thank Dr. Loay Alia, Dr. Fadi Kasoha, and Dr. Montazar Bazal from of Al-Assad University Hospital for their contribution in the surgical intervention. Also, they would like to thank Dr. Omar Tillo for linguistic revision.

References

[1] K. Hubert, J. S. Elder, and G. T. MacLennan, "Benign vascular lesions of the scrotum," *The Journal of Urology*, vol. 176, no. 5, p. 2245, 2006.

[2] J. J. Marler and J. B. Mulliken, "Current management of hemangiomas and vascular malformations," *Clinics in Plastic Surgery*, vol. 32, no. 1, pp. 99–116, ix, 2005.

[3] W. L. A. So, J. Chaganti, R. Waugh, and R. J. Ferguson, "Management of scrotal arteriovenous malformation with

transcatheter embolisation coils and percutaneous sclerotherapy under angiographic guidance," *Journal of Medical Imaging and Radiation Oncology*, vol. 59, no. 4, pp. 468–470, 2015.

[4] J. D. Sule, M. J. Lemmers, and J. M. Barry, "Scrotal arteriovenous malformation: case report and literature review," *The Journal of Urology*, vol. 150, no. 6, pp. 1917–1919, 1993.

[5] D. R. Bezirdjian, P. D. Reznikov, and J. Tisnado, "Transcatheter embolization of an arteriovenous malformation of the scrotum," *Cardiovascular and Interventional Radiology*, vol. 12, no. 5, pp. 267–269, 1989.

[6] S. Hamid, J. Aquilina, W. Davidson, and C. Dhabuwala, "Arteriovenous malformation of scrotum: a case report," *The Journal of Urology*, vol. 147, no. 1, pp. 160–162, 1992.

[7] Ö. Konus, E. Ilgit, C. Yücel, E. Özbek, and B. Önal, "Scrotal arteriovenous malformation and its preoperative embolization," *European Radiology*, vol. 9, no. 3, pp. 425–427, 1999.

[8] T. W. Kang, Y.-D. Choi, Y. Y. Jeong et al., "Intrascrotal extratesticular arteriovenous malformation," *Urology*, vol. 64, no. 3, p. 590, 2004.

[9] R. R. Gonzalez, A. J. Thomas Jr., and M. Goldstein, "Arteriovenous malformation of the scrotum causing severe oligospermia," *Fertility and Sterility*, vol. 78, article S210, 2002.

[10] G. Bandi, F. J. Bianco, and C. Dhabuwala, "Recurrent scrotal arteriovenous malformation," *Journal of Urology*, vol. 171, no. 4, p. 1628, 2004.

[11] S. H. Choi, J. H. Lee, D. J. Kim, and S. R. Cho, "Scrotal arteriovenous malformation," *Korean Journal of Urology*, vol. 46, no. 8, pp. 873–875, 2005.

[12] M. A. Monoski, R. R. Gonzalez, A. J. Thomas, and M. Goldstein, "Arteriovenous malformation of scrotum causing virtual azoospermia," *Urology*, vol. 68, no. 1, pp. 203.e5–203.e6, 2006.

[13] C. Yilmaz, M. Arslan, and M. Arslan, "Intrascrotal arteriovenous malformation simulating varicocele," *American Journal of Roentgenology*, vol. 192, no. 6, article W351, 2009.

[14] S. Jaganathan, S. Gamanagatti, A. Mukund, and A. Dhar, "Bleeding scrotal vascular lesions: interventional management with transcatheter embolization," *CardioVascular and Interventional Radiology*, vol. 34, no. S2, pp. 113–116, 2011.

[15] J. R. Zachariah, A. K. Gupta, and S. Lamba, "Arteriovenous malformation of the scrotum: is preoperative angioembolization a necessity?," *Indian Journal of Urology*, vol. 28, no. 3, pp. 329–334, 2012.

[16] R. Key and T. Bishop, "Successful use of onyx® for transcatheter arterial embolization of a scrotal arteriovenous malformation refractory to traditional embolic agents," *Radiology Case Reports*, vol. 8, no. 3, p. 846, 2013.

[17] N. Sato, T. Kuroki, Y. Tosa, T. Kusano, and S. Yoshimoto, "A scrotal arteriovenous malformation: a case report," *Modern Plastic Surgery*, vol. 4, no. 1, pp. 16–19, 2014.

[18] S. Muslim, N. Roy, and I. Alam, "Scrotal arteriovenous malformation excision–an inguinal approach," *Journal of Clinical Urology*, vol. 10, no. 3, pp. 227–229, 2017.

[19] M. Smits, "Embolization materials and tecnique 2017," January 2020, https://angiofellow.com/author/mrtnsmits/last.

[20] J. I. Bilbao, A. Martínez-Cuesta, F. Urtasun, and O. Cosín, "Complications of embolization," *Seminars in Interventional Radiology*, vol. 23, no. 2, pp. 126–142, 2006.

39

A Complicated Entity: Acute Celiac Artery Dissection with Resultant Pancreatitis, Duodenitis and Cholecystitis

Graham T. Endler, Karleigh R. Curfman, Jason H. Hwang, and John L. Gray

Duke LifePoint Conemaugh Memorial Medical Center, Johnstown PA 15905, USA

Correspondence should be addressed to Graham T. Endler; gendler@conemaugh.org

Academic Editor: Nilda Espinola-Zavaleta

Arterial dissection is a well-recognized pathology often seen in Vascular Surgery offices and Emergency Departments alike; however, visceral arterial dissection is an extremely rare, small subset of this entity. With that, an isolated celiac artery dissection as presented within this report is an exceptionally unique pathology that has scarcely been reported, and due to this, management guidelines are undefined. Given the viscera supplied by the celiac artery, many intra-abdominal structures are at risk for ischemia when damage to the celiac artery occurs, potentially witnessed by this report. Due to the exclusivity of this pathology, we are compelled to report the case of a 71-year-old male who presented with complaints of abdominal pain and was found to have an acute celiac artery dissection, which likely resulted in severe ischemic duodenitis, as well as possibly acute pancreatitis, and questionable influence on cholecystitis.

1. Introduction

The purpose of this paper is to report a unique entity and its management that occurred at our facility: acute spontaneous celiac artery dissection with resultant duodenitis, in addition to potentially acute pancreatitis and possibly cholecystitis. True splanchnic artery dissections are a less common clinical entity than aortic, carotid, and other visceral artery dissections; however, they still remain an important vascular pathology that requires appropriate and timely treatment. With continual advancements in imaging technology and endovascular techniques, recognition of these dissections has increased along with the subsequent evolution in their treatment. Celiac artery dissections in the absence of aortic artery dissections are a truly unique pathology, scantly reported in the literature. The recognition of symptoms can be masked, leading to a delay in diagnosis; the clinical picture is often complicated as well due to a lack of recommended treatment guidelines as a result of the infrequency of this entity.

Herein, we present the history of one case involving a 71-year-old male with a previously undiagnosed celiac artery dissection, whose clinical picture was complicated by the development of acute pancreatitis, duodenitis, and cholecystitis. Due to the severe ischemic duodenitis the patient developed, we feel that his celiac artery dissection was significant enough to be the cause of this pathology. In addition, while acknowledging the possibility of a passed choledocholith, given the absence of choledocholithiasis on Endoscopic Retrograde Cholangiopancreatography, we postulate that his acute pancreatitis as well as acute cholecystitis was possibly also sequelae of his celiac artery dissection. Therefore, we provide a review of his hospital course and treatment approach in conjunction with the current literature in regard to diagnosis and management.

2. Clinical Course

The patient presented is a 71-year-old male with history significant for Guillain-Barre syndrome and resolved paralysis after plasmapheresis treatments, type 2 diabetes mellitus, and hypertension, who presented with a 4-day history of nausea and intermittent, stabbing epigastric and right upper quadrant (RUQ) pain. He had previously presented to a different facility with similar complaints, for which he was diagnosed with cholelithiasis by ultrasound (US). He denied

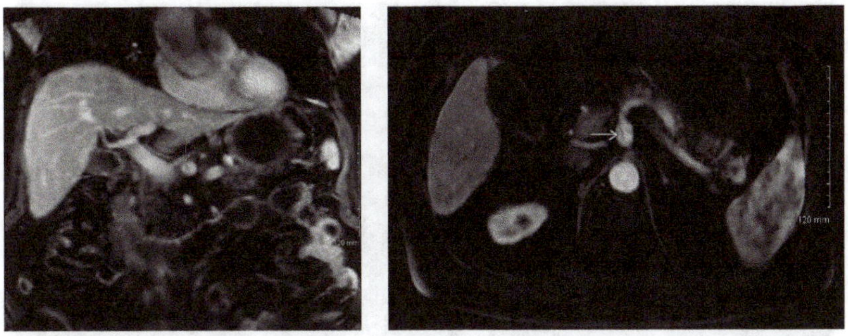

(a) (b)

FIGURE 1: (a, b) Magnetic Resonance Cholangiopancreatography (MRCP) imaging demonstrating signs of pancreatitis and a 1.4 cm celiac artery aneurysm with dissection flap. Given concerns for the possibility of gallstone pancreatitis, the patient underwent MRCP imaging which was the first study to make the diagnosis of a 1.4 cm celiac artery aneurysm and was suggestive of a dissection flap (white arrows). The MRCP was also useful in confirming the diagnosis of acute pancreatitis due to visualized peripancreatic inflammation.

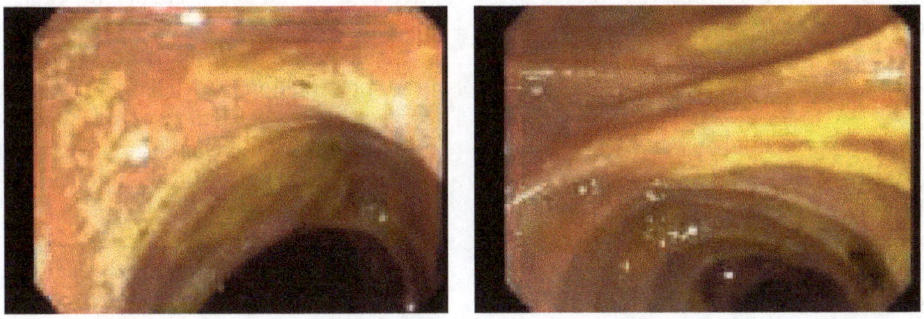

(a) (b)

FIGURE 2: (a, b) Endoscopic Retrograde Cholangiopancreatography (ERCP) showing signs of reported severe duodenitis, likely due to ischemia. After the concern for possible gallstone pancreatitis, the patient underwent an ERCP. With the ERCP, a biliary sphincterotomy and balloon sweep were performed which visualized biliary sludge, but no signs of choledocholithiasis. The ERCP was also suggestive of severe duodenitis, for which ischemic pathology was questioned and, given the patient's known celiac artery dissection, was likely sequelae of the dissection.

fevers, chills, acholic stools, and bilirubinuria and was continuing to tolerate intake despite his nausea. He had no prior similar events, no inciting causes, and no worsening or alleviating factors, he denied use of tobacco or alcohol, and his family history was only significant for aortic valvular repair in his father. On physical examination, he experienced RUQ/epigastric tenderness, no jaundice or abdominal distention, and only mild tachycardia (low 100 s). He displayed a leukocytosis (WBC 24.5), transaminitis with hyperbilirubinemia (AST 176, ALT 158, alkaline phosphatase 185, total bilirubin 2.9, direct bilirubin 1.8), and an elevated pancreatic enzyme (lipase > 1100). Abdominal US was significant for cholelithiasis, biliary sludge, and gallbladder wall thickening (1.1 cm), without pericholecystic fluid or ductal dilation. His common bile duct (CBD) measured 7.6 mm.

The diagnosis of gallstone pancreatitis was presumed and he underwent Magnetic Resonance Cholangiopancreatography (MRCP). The MRCP showed peripancreatic edema and stranding consistent with interstitial pancreatitis and, surprisingly, a 1.4 cm celiac artery aneurysm with filling defect suggestive of focal dissection flap (Figures 1(a) and 1(b)). Given concern for gallstone pancreatitis, he proceeded with Endoscopic Retrograde Cholangiopancreatography (ERCP), for which biliary sphincterotomy and balloon sweep revealed biliary sludge, but no stones. Severe duodenitis was seen on the ERCP, strongly felt to be due to acute ischemia, in correlation to the newly diagnosed celiac artery dissection (Figures 2(a) and 2(b)).

As a result of the celiac artery dissection, CT Angiography (CTA) was obtained. This demonstrated fusiform aneurysmal dilation of the proximal celiac artery with a focal dissection flap just proximal to the origin of the splenic artery, which extended to the origins of the common hepatic artery and left hepatic artery (Figures 3(a) and 3(b)). Subsequently, aneurysmal dilation was noted in the ascending aorta (4.6 cm) and left internal iliac artery (1.5 cm). Vascular Surgery was consulted and recommended intravenous anticoagulation and transition to continued oral anticoagulation once stable for discharge, with outpatient follow-up and imaging for monitoring of the dissection and aneurysms.

On hospital day 4, he underwent uncomplicated laparoscopic cholecystectomy as his pancreatitis improved with pain control, hydration, and bowel rest. He tolerated the

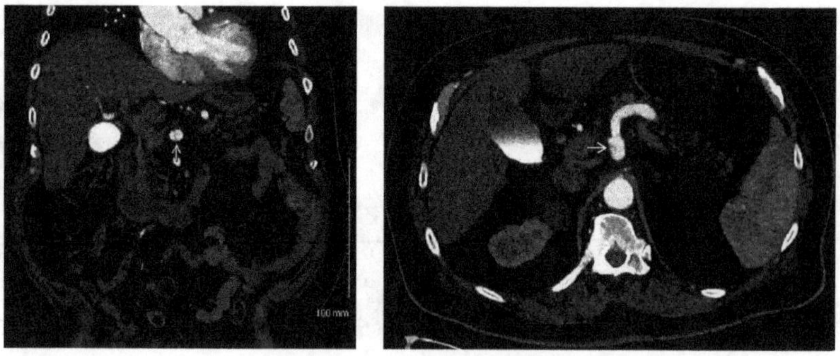

(a) (b)

Figure 3: (a, b) Computed tomography angiography (CTA) images illustrating the patient's newly diagnosed celiac artery aneurysm, confirming a dissection flap, and displaying the extent of the dissection flap. CTA imaging was obtained after suspicion was raised on MRCP for a celiac aneurysm and dissection in order to confirm and better characterize the disease. (a) demonstrates the patient's fusiform aneurysm, measuring it at 1.4 cm, as well as displays the celiac artery dissection flap. (b) evaluates the patient's confirmed celiac artery dissection, beginning just proximal to his splenic artery origin and extending to the origin of the common hepatic artery.

procedure well and the rest of his hospital course was uneventful, being discharged on day 7.

3. Discussion

Arterial dissection has been defined as the cleavage of the arterial wall by blood flow resulting in intramural hematoma between two elastic layers [1, 2]. Isolated arterial dissection, occurring in the absence of aortic dissection, has been a reported entity in the carotid and renal arteries; however, it is rarely reported in the visceral arteries [2]. As per the study produced by Vaidya and Dighe, spontaneous dissection of visceral arteries was first described by Bauersfeld in 1947; however, it reports primarily affecting the renal arteries rather than the celiac artery, as the case presented within [2]. Suspected causes of arterial dissection are numerous and include atherosclerosis, trauma, iatrogenic causes, pregnancy, fibromuscular dysplasia, infectious disease, hypertension, Marfan syndrome, and Ehlers-Danlos syndrome [2]. Spontaneous arterial dissection is more common in males, a reported 5 : 1 occurrence ratio, with an average age of 55 years old [1–3]. Approximately one-half of visceral artery dissections are asymptomatic, though presentation with abdominal pain, weight loss, hemorrhage, and more atypical symptoms like malabsorption, jaundice, or pancreatitis has been reported [4, 5]. Visceral arteries have been shown to have a decrease in dissection rates compared to the aorta and carotid arteries, with dissection of the celiac artery being very rare. As per one study, the first reported case of celiac artery dissection was in 1959, with only 13 cases reported prior to 2001 [3]. Since the advent of improved diagnostic technologies (contrast enhanced computed tomography (CT), CTA, and magnetic resonance angiography (MRA)), the number of reported cases has more than doubled, with Obon-Dent et al. reporting a total of 33 cases in their study from 2012 [3, 6]. Several risk factors described for spontaneous celiac artery dissection are represented in our case; our patient was an older male (71 years), with history of hypertension, and presenting complaint of abdominal pain. Subsequently, he was found to have a left internal iliac and aortic aneurysm, cholecystitis, duodenitis, and pancreatitis.

As described by Wollard and Ammar, pancreatitis can be a rare presentation associated with visceral artery dissection [5]. As such, few cases of reported pancreatitis due to pancreatic ischemia from celiac artery dissection have been published. At the time of production, only four prior cases of acute pancreatitis secondary to celiac artery dissection could be identified after extensive PubMed query. In two separate reports, initial imaging revealed celiac artery dissection, and in conjunction with elevated amylase and lipase, acute pancreatitis was diagnosed. These patients were treated conservatively for pancreatitis with pain control, bowel rest, and hydration as well as blood pressure control, which ultimately alleviated their symptoms without operative intervention [1, 7]. In contrast, one patient with acute pancreatitis and unremitting abdominal pain eventually required an operation. They continued to experience abdominal pain days after presenting and underwent MRA of the abdomen, which visualized a celiac artery dissection. The patient proceeded with selective angiography of the aorta and celiac artery with placement of two stents in the celiac artery, relieving her symptoms [6]. In the publication by Amabile et al., an additional patient with documented pancreatitis secondary to celiac artery dissection was identified and underwent surgical intervention, though details of further management were not described [8]. Although we are unable to prove a direct causation of the celiac artery dissection leading to acute pancreatitis in our case, given the patient's presentation and evidence of severe duodenitis, we hypothesize that pancreatitis was at least aggravated, if not caused by celiac artery dissection, with added evidence of an ERCP negative for evidence of biliary cause.

The contrast in medical and surgical treatment options for celiac artery dissection is striking. Entertainment of procedural intervention should only be employed when the patient is hemodynamically unstable, experiencing persistent symptoms of ischemia, such as abdominal pain, has failed medical therapy for blood pressure control, or if the dissection progresses [2]. Though it has been observed that surgical management should be exercised in those described circumstances, the optimal indicated procedure for celiac artery dissection has not been confirmed and procedures greatly vary in the reported studies. The study by Obon-Dent et al. employed the use of angiography and endovascular techniques to achieve remission of symptoms [6]. Two patients in the Amabile study were identified as having undergone surgical repair. One patient, similar to that of the Obon-Dent report, underwent endovascular repair with the use of covered stent in the celiac trunk, while the other required an upper aortomesenteric venous bypass for combined celiac and superior mesenteric artery dissections; both patients were symptom-free at the time of study production [6, 8]. Furthermore, Glehen et al. described several operative interventions for patients with celiac artery dissection including one patient with resection of the splenic, celiac, and left gastric arteries, another who underwent celiac artery arteriotomy, resection, side to side anastomosis of the hepatic arteries, and reimplantation onto the celiac artery ostium with a graft, and lastly a patient who underwent celiac artery arteriotomy with graft placement between the divided celiac artery and bifurcation of the splenic artery and hepatic artery [9]. Finally, to further contrast surgical management options, in the report by Fenoglio et al., their patient endured operative repair after an increase in dissection size, for which resection of the celiac artery with reconstruction and anastomosis of the gastroduodenal artery and hepatic artery was performed [10]. As described, several operative interventions for celiac artery dissection have been employed, all of which have reported a complete resolution of symptoms by the time of study publication. However, though all of these reports expressed results that were ultimately therapeutic, a concise decision on operative management as the standard of care or its suggested technique has not been agreed upon.

4. Conclusion

The case presented in this report is truly unique in pathology. As described, arterial dissection is a known diagnosis that is commonly seen in both the aorta and the carotid arteries, with a decreased presentation in the visceral arteries, especially the celiac artery. Dissection of the celiac artery has scarcely been described in literature, especially prior to the institution of evolved imaging techniques, which are now routinely employed. The pathology of celiac artery dissection in the absence of other vascular dissections is extremely rare, which speaks for the necessity of reporting the case herein. Given that the patient's celiac artery dissection resulted in the diagnosis of severe acute duodenitis and potentially acute pancreatitis and cholecystitis, we feel it is essential to report this case. The occurrence of acute pancreatitis secondary to a celiac artery dissection has only been found in the reported literature on extremely scant occasions, and though we cannot concretely confirm a causal relationship in this instance, the existence is suggested, and thus, it is vital to report details of our patient findings and management for review. It is our hope in the production of this report to provide evidence towards the pathology of celiac artery dissection regarding the presentation, symptoms, imaging, and diagnostic techniques as well as describe previously employed options of various surgical techniques and nonsurgical management for alleviation of symptoms, though a unanimous decision on management technique has yet to be established.

Consent

Written informed consent was obtained from the patient for publication of this case report, "A Complicated Entity: Acute Celiac Artery Dissection with Resultant Pancreatitis, Duodenitis, and Cholecystitis," and any accompanying images. A copy of the consent obtained is available for review by the editor of this journal

Authors' Contributions

GTE, KRC, and JHH were the contributors to conception and design, acquisition of data, and interpretation of data. KRC and GTE were responsible for manuscript writing and drafting. GTE, KRC, JHH, and JLG were responsible for revising the manuscript critically for important intellectual content. GTE, KRC, JHH, and JLG gave the final approval of the version to be published.

References

[1] N. D'Ambrosio, B. Friedman, D. Siegel, D. Katz, A. Newatia, and J. Hines, "Spontaneous isolated dissection of the celiac artery: CT findings in adults," *American Journal of Roentgenology*, vol. 188, no. 6, pp. W506–W511, 2007.

[2] S. Vaidya and M. Dighe, "Spontaneous celiac artery dissection and its management," *Journal of Radiology Case Reports*, vol. 4, no. 4, pp. 30–33, 2010.

[3] R. K. Dean, D. Gill, R. Khan, and I. Amzuta, "An uncommon dissection: adding to the evidence of celiac artery dissection," *The American Journal of Emergency Medicine*, vol. 35, no. 7, pp. 1037.e1–1037.e2, 2017.

[4] J. A. Batsis and A. S. Arora, "Celiac artery dissection: an uncommon cause of abdominal pain and weight loss," *Clinical Gastroenterology and Hepatology*, vol. 3, no. 10, p. A30, 2005.

[5] J. D. Woolard and A. D. Ammar, "Spontaneous dissection of the celiac artery: a case report," *Journal of Vascular Surgery*, vol. 45, no. 6, pp. 1256–1258, 2007.

[6] M. Obon-Dent, B. Shabaneh, K. G. Dougherty, and N. E. Strickman, "Spontaneous celiac artery dissection case report and literature review," *Texas Heart Institute Journal*, vol. 39, no. 5, pp. 703–706, 2012.

[7] J. Lund and K. Vipul, "Spontaneous celiac artery dissection leading to acute pancreatitis," *Chest*, vol. 148, no. 4, article 258A, 2015.

[8] P. Amabile, M. Ouaïssi, S. Cohen, and P. Piquet, "Conservative treatment of spontaneous and isolated dissection of mesenteric arteries," *Annals of Vascular Surgery*, vol. 23, no. 6, pp. 738–744, 2009.

[9] O. Glehen, P. Feugier, Y. Aleksic, P. Delannoy, and J. M. Chevalier, "Spontaneous dissection of the celiac artery," *Annals of Vascular Surgery*, vol. 15, no. 6, pp. 687–692, 2001.

[10] L. Fenoglio, A. Allione, E. Scalabrino et al., "Spontaneous dissection of the celiac artery: a pitfall in the diagnosis of acute abdominal pain. Presentation of two cases," *Digestive Diseases and Sciences*, vol. 49, no. 7-8, pp. 1223–1227, 2004.

Successful Endovascular Repair of a Ruptured Popliteal Artery Aneurysm: A Case Report and Literature Review

Duncan Muir[1] **and Sachin R. Kulkarni**[2]

[1]*University of Bristol Medical School, UK*
[2]*Gloucestershire Hospitals NHS Foundation Trust, Cheltenham, UK*

Correspondence should be addressed to Duncan Muir; dm14867@bristol.ac.uk

Academic Editor: Muzaffer Sindel

Introduction. It is rare for a popliteal artery aneurysm (PAA) to present with rupture. This case reports a longer-term success in the management of a large ruptured popliteal artery aneurysm with an endovascular approach, with a literature review of management of such cases. *Case Report.* An 80-year-old man presented to the accident and emergency department with pain and swelling behind the left knee and at the back of the thigh. An ultrasound scan and subsequent CT angiogram revealed a large 9.4 cm ruptured PAA. The patient had significant comorbidities deeming him unfit for a major surgical intervention of drainage of haematoma and exclusion bypass. Therefore, he underwent urgent endovascular treatment of the ruptured PAA with a covered stent graft. A follow-up duplex scan at 1 year showed a patent stent with no evidence of endoleak, and the patient remained asymptomatic. A clinical follow-up at 18- and 24-month postprocedure showed a patent stent graft and complete resolution of haematoma. *Conclusion.* Whilst open repair with exclusion bypass may still be a treatment of choice, an endovascular approach is both safe and effective in the management of a ruptured PAA in an unfit patient with an acceptable longer-term outcome.

1. Introduction

Popliteal artery aneurysms constitute the most prevalent form of peripheral arterial aneurysms, accounting for approximately 85% of all peripheral aneurysms [1]. PAAs carry a high risk of intravascular thrombosis as well as distal embolization causing critical limb ischaemia [1]. They are often asymptomatic; however, they may present with foot ischaemia, leg oedema, and pain behind the knee due to their proximity to nerves. PAA rupture is a rare but recognized presentation that requires a rapid diagnosis and treatment for limb salvage [1]. The standard treatment for such ruptures is a surgical exclusion bypass; however, a number of other management options are described in the literature [2–13]. Such options include endovascular treatment with coil embolization [10] and/or stent graft. Surgical treatment may have an additional benefit of drainage of haematoma preventing its complications as well as restoring the blood supply to the foot. However, in unfit patients, this may not be a viable option. This case report describes a successful management of ruptured PAA by an endovascular technique with a patent stent graft after 24 months in a patient unfit for major surgical intervention.

2. Case Presentation

An 80-year-old man presented with a 4-day history of swelling and pain behind the left knee with reduced mobility with very short distance intermittent claudication affecting the left calf and reduced range of knee movement. This patient in the preceding week was admitted under the care of medical specialty where a diagnosis of a spontaneous haematoma behind the thigh was made. Haematoma was thought to be a result of the patient being on oral anticoagulation (warfarin) for atrial fibrillation. The patient did not report history of trauma. He looked frail on the current admission on the vascular ward requiring support for some activities at home and had been on treatment for prostate cancer. He had previously also had coccygectomy for metastasis as well as a recent history of permanent pacemaker insertion for syncopal episodes

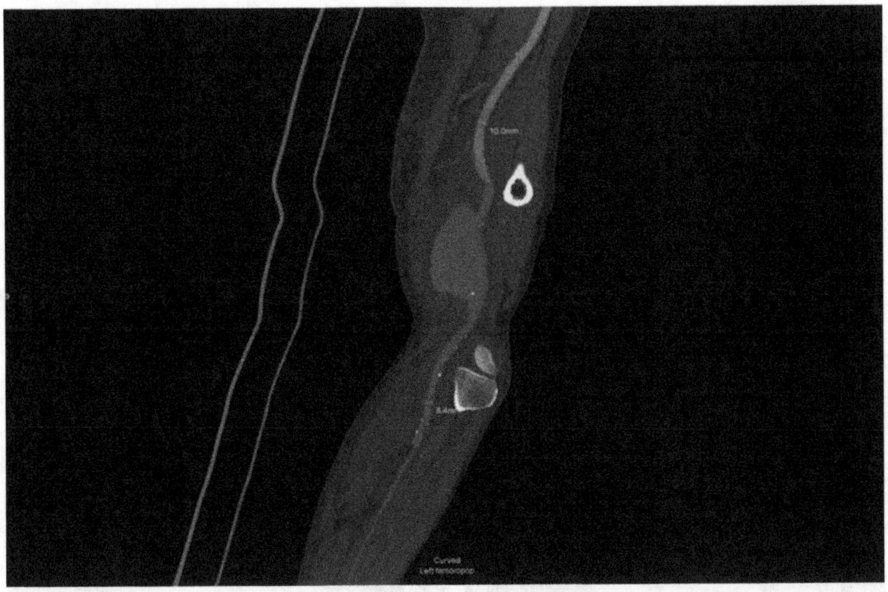

FIGURE 1: Initial CT angiogram.

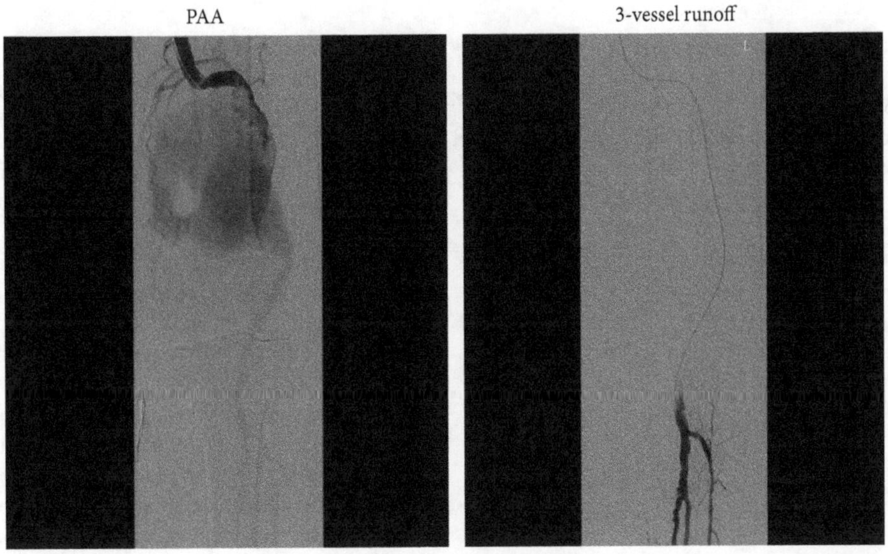

FIGURE 2: Intraoperative arteriogram.

and bradycardia. He also suffered from hypertension and was on a number of medications including warfarin. He was a lifelong nonsmoker and lived in a retirement home. There was no family history of aneurysms.

Examination revealed extensive bruising at the back of the left thigh and knee with palpable femoral and pedal pulses. The popliteal pulse was difficult to feel due to a large haematoma. The left foot was viable with fully intact sensory and motor function. There was no clinical evidence of calf compartment syndrome on the left leg. The right foot was warm with all palpable pulses in the leg.

An initial ultrasound scan revealed PAA with no evidence of popliteal or femoral vein DVT. A CT angiogram performed on the same day showed generalized arteriomegaly and the ruptured 9.4 cm PAA involving only the above-knee popliteal artery (Figure 1) and relatively disease-free 3-vessel runoff to the ankle and foot. Options to treat this patient were either a surgical exclusion bypass with evacuation of haematoma or an endovascular treatment. For a number of reasons including patient frailty, associated comorbidities, and potential feasibility of successfully treating the PAA with a stent graft due to intact 3-vessel crural runoff, decision was made to treat the aneurysm by an endovascular approach.

Under general anaesthesia, the left common femoral artery was explored with a small open incision. An initial angiogram through a 5F sheath confirmed the CT findings of ruptured PAA with 3-vessel runoff (Figure 2). The aneurysm sac was traversed using a curved catheter and a soft hydrophilic wire which was then exchanged to a stiff wire. A 5F sheath was exchanged to an 11F sheath to allow for insertion of 2 Viabahn (Gore®) covered stent grafts of 8-250 mm and 10-100 mm dimensions with a 4 cm overlap

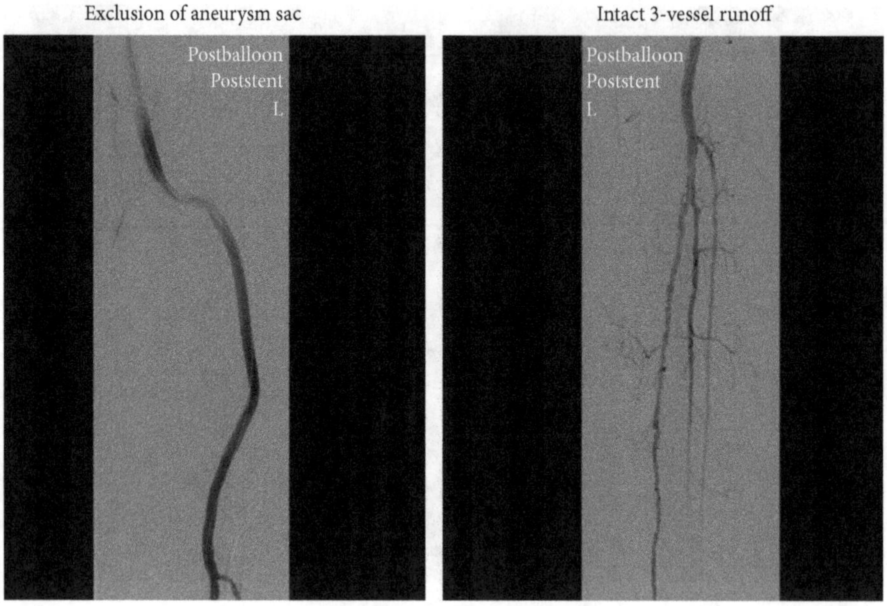

FIGURE 3: Post-stent-graft insertion.

which were postdilated with 8 and 10 mm balloons. Postcompletion angiography revealed complete exclusion of the aneurysm sac with improved filling of the runoff vessels (Figure 3). The procedure lasted for approximately 55 minutes.

The patient made a good recovery following the repair with a predischarge duplex scan demonstrating a successful exclusion of the aneurysm with good 3-vessel runoff. The patient was discharged on dual antiplatelet therapy which was continued for 6 weeks after which the patient continued on one antiplatelet and an anticoagulant treatment for AF. Subsequent 3-month surveillance duplex scans for up to a year showed a patent stent with intact distal circulation (Figure 4). Duplex surveillance was discontinued after 1 year as per local protocol; a clinical follow-up after 18 and 24 months confirmed a patent stent graft with palpable pedal pulses.

3. Discussion

This case reports successful endovascular stent graft repair for exclusion of a ruptured PAA with a patent stent graft after 24 months. It has one of the longest follow-ups with a successful outcome reported in the literature for the treatment of ruptured PAA. Rupture of a PAA is a rare clinical presentation, and literature regarding optimum management is limited, being mostly documented in the form of case reports. The patient in this case report had significant comorbidities and was frail for a surgical repair with exclusion bypass and therefore had an endovascular repair. Open cutdown of the groin rather than a percutaneous approach was performed due to nonavailability of an appropriate closure device at the time of the procedure to close the arterial puncture made for the insertion of the 11F sheath. However, in an ideal situation, the procedure would have been performed percutaneously under local anaesthesia. The patient made an uneventful recovery, and the stent graft was patent after a 24-month follow-up.

A literature review conducted at the time of submission of this case report showed 62 [2–13] reported cases of ruptured PAA. Most cases reported were males, with an age range of 55-96 and a mean age of 81. Different treatment modalities were used to treat such cases; however, the majority of the patients were treated with a standard open repair with exclusion of the aneurysm and bypass surgery. Only one case was treated with coil embolization [10], and twelve were treated by endovascular intervention [2–5, 7, 11–13]. Until recently, open surgical repair has been the approach of choice; however, endovascular repair has become increasingly popular due mostly to availability of better stent grafts with a potentially better longer-term outcome. In a similar case report, the benefit of endovascular repair in a mycotic PAA was described [3]. Extensive comorbidity and sepsis resulted in the patient being considered unfit for open repair, and therefore, an endovascular stent graft was inserted via the ipsilateral femoral artery. One week later, the patient developed an infected haematoma; however, this resolved, and the patient was eventually discharged home. Follow-up CT scans demonstrated no evidence of recurrent infection and satisfactory stent graft function. This case highlights the benefit of endovascular repair in elderly, critically ill, or septic patients.

Endovascular repair is also advocated in another case study in a patient unfit for major surgical repair [4]. In this case report, endovascular stenting was performed in a 96-year-old gentleman with a ruptured PAA. A follow-up after fifteen weeks demonstrated a patent stent graft on Doppler ultrasound and palpable pedal pulses. Literature review at the time of publication of this study concludes that whilst endovascular repair is both safe and effective, open surgical repair still remains a first-choice treatment for PAAs. Therefore, although some of the published data favor endovascular treatment, an open surgical approach is still advocated for an improved longer-term outcome for PAAs. Trinidad-Hernandez et al. [13] reviewed 25 patients

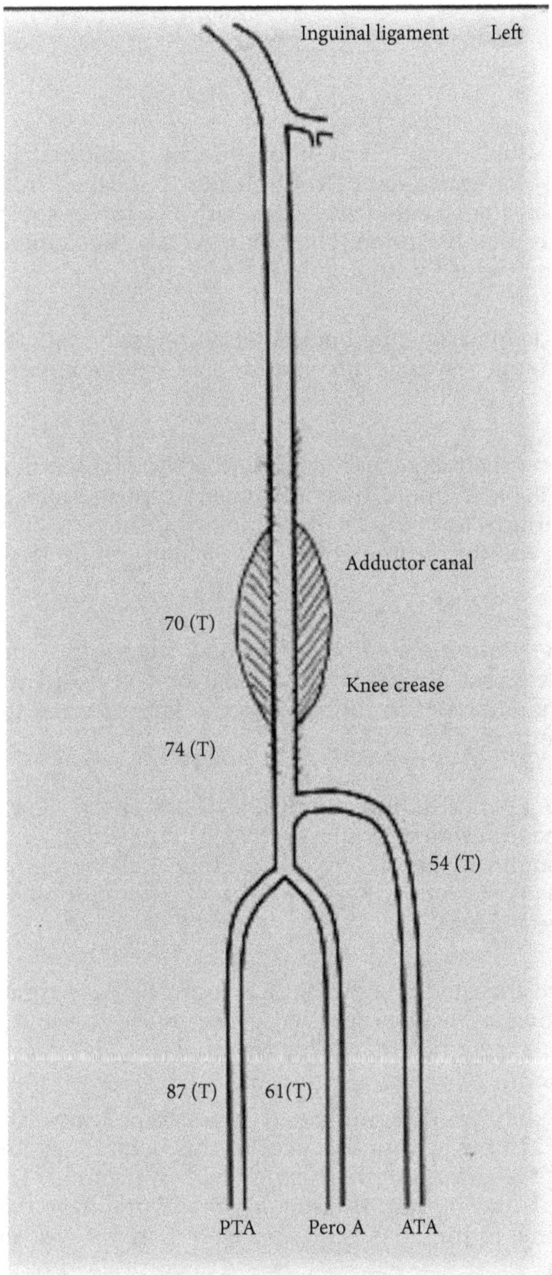

FIGURE 4: 1-year follow-up duplex scan showing the patient's stent. 3-vessel runoff with triphasic flow.

(31 limbs) treated with endovascular PAA repair of which 12 limbs were treated with emergency repair (1 ruptured and 11 thrombosed) and the rest with elective repair. Whilst endovascular repair was reportedly better for elective PAAs, major adverse events were higher in limbs that had endovascular repair as an emergency. An observational study by Coskun et al. [7] on 7 patients with ruptured PAAs supports open surgical repair to be the treatment of choice. However, these studies were not comparative studies, and therefore, a prospective randomized study for emergency presentation of PAAs may be required to better understand the treatment options.

4. Conclusion

PAA rupture is a rare, potentially limb- and life-threatening condition. On account of the small number of reported cases with relatively short-term outcome data, there is little substantiated evidence to prove which technique of repair has the best outcome. However, there is some evidence suggesting that in unfit elderly patients, an endovascular approach is both safe and effective in the treatment of ruptured PAAs.

Consent

The patient's written permission was acquired for publication of photographs.

References

[1] M. Loukas, Z. Klaassen, R. S. Tubbs, and N. Apaydin, "Popliteal artery aneurysms: a review," *Folia Morphologica*, vol. 66, no. 4, pp. 272–276, 2007.

[2] J. Akman, E. Katsogridakis, and G. A. Antoniou, "Ruptured popliteal artery aneurysms," *Vascular*, vol. 27, no. 4, pp. 430–447, 2019.

[3] M. G. Bani-Hani, L. Elnahas, G. R. Plant, A. Ward, and M. Moawad, "Endovascular management of ruptured infected popliteal artery aneurysm," *Journal of Vascular Surgery*, vol. 55, no. 2, pp. 532–534, 2012.

[4] S. L. Brown, M. Lewis, and D. R. Morrow, "Endovascular repair of ruptured popliteal artery aneurysms: a case report and review of the literature," *EJVES Short Reports*, vol. 32, pp. 24–28, 2016.

[5] A. Cervin, H. Ravn, and M. Björck, "Ruptured popliteal artery aneurysm," *The British Journal of Surgery*, vol. 105, no. 13, pp. 1753–1758, 2018.

[6] M. Cho, S. Ahn, S. L. Min, and S. K. Min, "Ruptured giant popliteal artery aneurysm," *Journal of Vascular Surgery Cases and Innovative Techniques*, vol. 3, no. 4, pp. 201-202, 2017.

[7] I. Coskun, O. S. Demirturk, H. A. Tunel, C. Andic, and O. Gulcan, "Positive clinical outcomes of the saphenous vein interposition technique for ruptured popliteal artery aneurysm," *Surgery Today*, vol. 44, no. 9, pp. 1674–1677, 2014.

[8] A. Fioranelli, E. A. Carpentieri, N. Wolosker, V. Castelli, and R. A. Caffaro, "Rupture of thrombosed popliteal aneurysm: a case report," *Annals of Vascular Surgery*, vol. 51, pp. 324.e7–324.e10, 2018.

[9] V. G. Goshko, T. P. W. Souster, and F. X. Scheuermeyer, "Man with leg pain," *Annals of Emergency Medicine*, vol. 71, no. 4, pp. 463–476, 2018.

[10] Y. Kawai, H. Morimae, and M. Matsushita, "A ruptured popliteal artery aneurysm treated with coil embolization," *Annals of Vascular Diseases*, vol. 12, no. 1, pp. 80–82, 2019.

[11] S. M. Kim and I. M. Jung, "Successful endovascular treatment of a ruptured popliteal artery aneurysm in a patient with Behcet disease," *Ann Vasc Surg*, vol. 53, pp. 274.e1–274.e5, 2018.

[12] I. P. Mikhaylov, V. N. Lavrenov, G. A. Isaev, L. S. Kokov, and E. Y. Trofimova, "Ruptures of popliteal artery aneurysms," *Khirurgiya. Zhurnal im. N.I. Pirogova*, no. 4, pp. 57–62, 2018.

[13] M. Trinidad-Hernandez, J. J. Ricotta II, P. Gloviczki et al., "Results of elective and emergency endovascular repairs of popliteal artery aneurysms," *Journal of Vascular Surgery*, vol. 57, no. 5, pp. 1299–1305, 2013, Epub 2013 Feb 1.

Permissions

All chapters in this book were first published by Hindawi Publishing Corporation; hereby published with permission under the Creative Commons Attribution License or equivalent. Every chapter published in this book has been scrutinized by our experts. Their significance has been extensively debated. The topics covered herein carry significant findings which will fuel the growth of the discipline. They may even be implemented as practical applications or may be referred to as a beginning point for another development.

The contributors of this book come from diverse backgrounds, making this book a truly international effort. This book will bring forth new frontiers with its revolutionizing research information and detailed analysis of the nascent developments around the world.

We would like to thank all the contributing authors for lending their expertise to make the book truly unique. They have played a crucial role in the development of this book. Without their invaluable contributions this book wouldn't have been possible. They have made vital efforts to compile up to date information on the varied aspects of this subject to make this book a valuable addition to the collection of many professionals and students.

This book was conceptualized with the vision of imparting up-to-date information and advanced data in this field. To ensure the same, a matchless editorial board was set up. Every individual on the board went through rigorous rounds of assessment to prove their worth. After which they invested a large part of their time researching and compiling the most relevant data for our readers.

The editorial board has been involved in producing this book since its inception. They have spent rigorous hours researching and exploring the diverse topics which have resulted in the successful publishing of this book. They have passed on their knowledge of decades through this book. To expedite this challenging task, the publisher supported the team at every step. A small team of assistant editors was also appointed to further simplify the editing procedure and attain best results for the readers.

Apart from the editorial board, the designing team has also invested a significant amount of their time in understanding the subject and creating the most relevant covers. They scrutinized every image to scout for the most suitable representation of the subject and create an appropriate cover for the book.

The publishing team has been an ardent support to the editorial, designing and production team. Their endless efforts to recruit the best for this project, has resulted in the accomplishment of this book. They are a veteran in the field of academics and their pool of knowledge is as vast as their experience in printing. Their expertise and guidance has proved useful at every step. Their uncompromising quality standards have made this book an exceptional effort. Their encouragement from time to time has been an inspiration for everyone.

The publisher and the editorial board hope that this book will prove to be a valuable piece of knowledge for researchers, students, practitioners and scholars across the globe.

List of Contributors

Antoine Berberi
Department of Oral and Maxillofacial Surgery, Faculty of Dental Medicine, Lebanese University, Lebanon

Georges Aoun and Georges Aad
Department of Oral Medicine and Maxillofacial Radiology, Faculty of Dental Medicine, Lebanese University, Lebanon

Saad Khairallah
Department of Pathology, Faculty of Medicine, Lebanese University and Director Institute National de Pathology, Lebanon

Ghassan Abi Chedid
Department of Radiology, Sacre-Coeur Hospital, Baada Lebanon and Head Department of Medical Imaging, Lebanese German University, Beirut, Lebanon

Kevin Singh Kang
Department of Cardiology, University of Pittsburgh Medical Center Hamot, Erie, PA 16550, USA

John Steven Wilson
Department of Cardiology, Meadville Medical Center, Meadville, PA, USA

Margaret R. Paulson
Division of Hospital Internal Medicine, Mayo Clinic Health Systems, Eau Claire, 2321 Stout Road, Menomonie, Wisconsin 54751, USA

Ricardo A. Torres-Guzman, Francisco R. Avila, Karla Maita, John P. Garcia, Abdullah Eldaly, Luiza Palmieri-Serrano and Antonio J. Forte
Division of Plastic Surgery, Mayo Clinic, 4500 San Pablo Road, Jacksonville, Florida 32224, USA

Jonathan C. Thompson
Division of Orthopedics, Mayo Clinic Health Systems, 1400 Bellinger Stree, Eau Claire, Wisconsin 54703, USA

Michael J. Maniaci
Division of Hospital Internal Medicine, Mayo Clinic, 4500 San Pablo Road, Jacksonville, Florida 32224, USA

Nicholas J. Murphy
Wayne State University School of Medicine, 540 E. Canfield Ave. Detroit, MI 48201, USA

Loay S. Kabbani and Alexander D. Shepard
Department of Surgery, Henry Ford Hospital, 2799 W Grand Blvd Detroit, MI 48202, USA

Farzan Siddiqui
Department of Radiation Oncology, Henry Ford Hospital, 2799 W Grand Blvd Detroit, MI 48202, USA

D. Baldwin and K. L. Chow
Department of General Surgery, University of Illinois at Chicago, Chicago, IL, USA

H. Mashbari
Department of General Surgery, University of Illinois at Chicago, Chicago, IL, USA
Department of General Surgery, Jazan University, Saudi Arabia

M. Sarhan
Department of Surgery, Division of Vascular Surgery, Advocate Christ Medical Center, Oak Lawn, IL, USA

Keisuke Nakabayashi, Shinya Hata, Nobuhito Kaneko, Akihiro Matsui, Kazuhiko Tanaka, Hiroshi Ando and Minoru Shimizu
Kasukabe Chuo General Hospital, Heart Center, Saitama, Japan

Luca Spinedi and Hans Stricker
Division of Angiology, Ospedale Regionale di Locarno, Locarno, Switzerland

Daniel Staub
Division of Angiology, University Hospital Basel, University of Basel, Basel, Switzerland

Heiko Uthoff
Gefässpraxis am See, Hirslanden Clinic St. Anna, Lucerne, Switzerland

Martine Dunnwald and Marc A. Pizzimenti
Department of Anatomy and Cell Biology, Roy J. and Lucille A. Carver College of Medicine, University of Iowa, Iowa City, Iowa, USA

Andrés-Trasahedo Estíbaliz, Labrador-Sánchez Eztizen, Flores-Robles Bryan-Josué, Pinillos-Aransay Valvanera, Laura Torrecilla Lerena and López-Martín Juan-Antonio
Rheumatology Department, San Pedro Hospital, Logroño, La Rioja, Spain

Salazar-Asencio Osman-Alberto
Neurosurgery Department, Son Espases University Hospital, Islas Baleares, Spain

A. Bianchi, S. Pozza and L. Giovannacci
Department of Visceral and Vascular Surgery, Ospedale Regionale di Lugano-CH, Switzerland

Jos. C. van den Berg
Department of Interventional Radiology, Ospedale Regionale di Lugano-CH, Switzerland

Ryo Kanamoto, Shinichi Hiromatsu, Tomoyuki Anegawa, Kanako Sakurai, Shohei Yoshida, Yusuke Shintani, Hiroyuki Otsuka, Satoru Tobinaga and Hiroyuki Tanaka
Department of Surgery, Kurume University School of Medicine, Fukuoka, Japan

Aman Berry Williams
The Townsville Hospital and Health Service, Australia

Ramanath Dukkipati
Harbor-UCLA Medical Center, Torrance, California, USA
Lundquist Research Institute, Torrance, California, USA
UCLA School of Medicine, Westwood, California, USA

Alexandre M. Benjo
Lake Side Heart and Vascular Center, Lake Havasu, Arizona, USA

Antonio Jimenez
Puerto Rico Vascular Center, Puerto Rico, USA

Ivo Lukitsch
Division of Nephrology, Ochsner Medical Center, New Orleans, Louisiana, USA

Gift C. Echefu
Baton Rouge General Medical Center, Internal Medicine Program, Baton Rouge, Louisiana, USA

Damodar R. Kumbala
Renal Associates of Baton Rouge, Baton Rouge, Louisiana, USA

Eleni Skandalou
Internal Medicine Department, General Hospital "G. Papanikolaou", Thessaloniki, Greece

Panagiotis Papadopoulos, Marianthi Kavelidou and Ioannis Skandalos
Surgical Department, General Hospital "Agios Pavlos", Thessaloniki, Greece

Stavros Kalfadis
B'Surgical Department General Hospital "G. Papanikolaou", Thessaloniki, Greece

Theodoros Tzigkalidis
Pathology Department, General Hospital "Agios Pavlos", Thessaloniki, Greece

Rayan S. El-Zein, Jeffrey Sobecki, Roy Greenberg and Robert A. Palma
Department of Internal Medicine, OhioHealth Doctors Hospital, 5100 W Broad St, Columbus, OH 43228, USA

Michael Keleher
Department of Interventional Radiology, OhioHealth Doctors Hospital, 5100 W Broad St, Columbus, OH 43228, USA

Kevin Lee
Department of Anesthesiology, The University of Toledo Medical Center, Toledo, OH, USA

Sophia Toraby
Department of Surgery, The University of Toledo Medical Center, Toledo, OH, USA

Robert Cotterman
Department of Surgery, The University of Toledo Medical Center, Toledo, OH, USA
Department of Critical Care and Trauma Surgery, ProMedica Toledo Hospital, Toledo, OH, USA

Babatunde Oriowo and John Fish
Department of Surgery, The University of Toledo Medical Center, Toledo, OH, USA
Department of Vascular Surgery, ProMedica Toledo Hospital, Toledo, OH, USA

Joe M. Das
Consultant Neurosurgeon, Department of Neurosurgery, College of Medical Sciences–Teaching Hospital, Bharatpur–10, Chitwan, Nepal

Rashmi Sapkota
Sister-in-Charge, Department of Neurosurgery, College of Medical Sciences–Teaching Hospital, Bharatpur–10, Chitwan, Nepal

Manish Mishra
Medical Officer, Department of Neurosurgery, College of Medical Sciences–Teaching Hospital, Bharatpur–10, Chitwan, Nepal

Shamir O. Cawich, Dave Harnanan and Lemuel Pran
Department of Surgery, University of the West Indies, St. Augustine Campus, Trinidad and Tobago West Indies

Brian Welch, Alex Schaal and Roberto Cantu
Flushing Hospital Medical Center, 4500 Parsons Blvd., Flushing, NY 11355, USA

Thomas F. O'Shea
Boston University School of Medicine, 72 E Concord St., Boston, MA 02118, USA

Zerrin Pulathan and Gökalp Altun
Cardiovascular Surgery Department, Karadeniz Technical University Faculty of Medicine, Trabzon, Turkey

Hassan Al-Thani, Ahmed Hussein and Ahmed Sadek
Vascular Surgery Section, Department of Surgery, Hamad General Hospital (HGH), Doha, Qatar

Ali Barah
Radiology Department, HGH, Doha, Qatar

Ayman El-Menyar
Clinical Research, Trauma and Vascular Surgery Section, HGH, Doha, Qatar
Clinical Medicine, Weill Cornell Medical College, Doha, Qatar

Slimane Idir and Jean-Pierre Becquemin
East Paris Vascular Institute (IVPE), Paul d'Égine Private Hospital (Ramsay Santé), Champigny-sur-Marne, France

Ahmed S. Zugail
East Paris Vascular Institute (IVPE), Paul d'Égine Private Hospital (Ramsay Santé), Champigny-sur-Marne, France
Department of Surgery, Faculty of Medicine in Rabigh, King Abdulaziz University, Jeddah, Saudi Arabia

Hossam I. Shaabi
Department of Vascular and Endoluminal Surgery, Nancy Regional and University Hospital Center (CHRU), Nancy, France
Department of Surgery, Faculty of Medicine, Jazan University, Jazan, Saudi Arabia

Yujiro Yokoyama
General Surgery Department, Easton Hospital, 18042, USA

Masato Nakajima
Cardiovascular Surgery Department, Yamanashi Prefectural Central Hospital, 400-8506, Japan

Enrique M. San Norberto, Liliana A. Fidalgo-Domingos, Noelia Cenizo, Álvaro Revilla and Carlos Vaquero
Department of Vascular Surgery, Valladolid University Hospital, Valladolid, Spain

James H. Taylor
Department of Cardiac Surgery, Valencia General University Hospital, Valencia, Spain

Mattia Cosenza, Luigi Panza, Anna Paola Califano, Carolina Defendini, Maria D'Andria, Roberto Romiti, Antonio Fabio Massimo Vainieri and Sergio Morelli
Department of Internal Medicine and Atherosclerosis Prevention, University of Rome, La Sapienza, Italy

Vu Hoang Vu, Nguyen Duong Khang and Le Minh Khoi
Cardiovascular Center, University Medical Center, University of Medicine and Pharmacy at Ho Chi Minh City, Vietnam

Mai Thanh Thao
Department of Radiology, University Medical Center, Ho Chi Minh City, Vietnam

Sorin Barat
Division of Vascular and Endovascular Surgery, Republican Clinical Hospital, 29 Nicolae Testemitanu Str., Chisinau, Moldova

Dumitru Casian
Department of General Surgery Nr.3, Vascular Surgery Clinic, Nicolae Testemitanu State University of Medicine and Pharmacy, 165 Stefan cel Mare si Sfant Bd., Chisinau, Moldova

I. Bachouch and N. Belloumi
Pulmonology Department Pavilion 4, Abderrahmen Mami Hospital, Tunisia

M. Attia
Department of Radiology, Abderrahmen Mami Hospital, Tunisia

F. Chermiti Ben Abdallah and S. Fenniche
Pulmonology Department Pavilion 4, Abderrahmen Mami Hospital, Tunisia
Faculty of Medicine of Tunis, University of Tunis El Manar, Tunisia

S. Hantous Zannad
Department of Radiology, Abderrahmen Mami Hospital, Tunisia
Faculty of Medicine of Tunis, University of Tunis El Manar, Tunisia

Andrew T. Hattam and Mayur Krishnaswamy
Vascular Surgery Unit, Department of Surgery, University Hospital Geelong, Barwon Health, Geelong, Victoria, Australia

Sasha Lalla and Ronald Henry
Advanced Cardiovascular Institute, Port of Spain, Trinidad And Tobago

Rajeev Seecheran and Naveen Anand Seecheran
University of the West Indies, St. Augustine, Trinidad And Tobago

Valmiki Seecheran and Sangeeta Persad
North Central Regional Health Authority, Mt. Hope, Trinidad And Tobago

Julie Van Maercke Marion Delcroix and Catharina Belge
Department of Respiratory Diseases, KU Leuven-University of Leuven and University Hospitals Leuven, Leuven, Belgium

Anne-Sophie Van Rompuy
Department of Anatomical Pathology, KU Leuven-University of Leuven and University Hospitals Leuven, Leuven, Belgium

Willy Poppe
Department of Gynecology, KU Leuven-University of Leuven and University Hospitals Leuven, Leuven, Belgium

Tom Verbelen
Department of Cardiac Surgery, KU Leuven-University of Leuven and University Hospitals Leuven, Leuven, Belgium

Xinyu Zhao, Delang Liu, Chaowen Yu, Yong Sun and Shiyuan Chen
Department of Vascular Surgery, First Affiliated Hospital of Bengbu Medical College, Bengbu, Anhui Province, China

Thomas Kotsis and Panagitsa Christoforou
Vascular Division, 2nd Department of Surgery, National & Kapodistrian University of Athens Medical School, "Aretaieion" Hospital, Athens, Greece

Constantinos Nastos
2nd Department of Surgery, National & Kapodistrian University of Athens Medical School, "Aretaieion" Hospital, Athens, Greece

Fotios Eforakopoulos, Nikolaos Charoulis and Efstratios Koletsis
Department of Cardiothoracic Surgery, University of Patras, Patras, Greece

Maria Giovani
Department of Pediatric Surgery, Mitera Children's Hospital, Marousi, Athens, Greece

Petros Zampakis and Christina Kalogeropoulou
Department of Radiology, University of Patras, Patras, Greece

Fotini Fligou
Department of Anesthesiology and Intensive Care Medicine, University of Patras, Patras, Greece

Dimitrios Dougenis
Department of Cardiac Surgery, School of Medicine, National and Kapodistrian University of Athens, Attikon University Hospital, Athens, Greece

Jose Maria Pereira de Godoy
Cardiology and Cardiovascular Surgery Department of the Medicine School in São José do Rio Preto (FAMERP), CNPq (National Council for Research and Development), Brazil

Henrique Jose Pereira de Godoy
Medicine School of Universidade Federal do Mato Grosso-Cuiabã-UFMT and Research Group in the Clínica Godoy, Sao Jose do Rio Preto, Brazil

Ana Carolina Pereira de Godoy
Pediatrics Unit Intensive Therapy of Santa Casa de São Paulo, Brazil and Research Group of Clínica Godoy, São Jose do Rio Preto, Brazil

Maria de Fátima Guerreiro Godoy
Medicine School in São José do Rio Preto (FAMERP) and Research Group in the Clínica Godoy, Sao Jose do Rio Preto, Brazil

Nikolaos S. Ioakeimidis and Dimitrios Valasiadis
Department of Cardiology, General Hospital of Florina "Eleni Th. Dimitriou", Egnatias 9, Florina 53100, Greece

Andreas Markou
Department of Radiology, General Hospital of Florina "Eleni Th. Dimitriou", Egnatias 9, Florina 53100, Greece

Theodora Zaglavara
Department of Cardiovascular Imaging, Interbalkan Medical Centre of Thessaloniki, Asklipiou 10, Thessaloniki 57001, Greece

Javad Salimi
Trauma and Surgery Research Center, Sina Hospital, Tehran University of Medical Science, Tehran, Iran

Sayed Alimohammad Sadat and Mohammad Javad Yavari Barhaghtalab
Department of General Surgery, Shahid Beheshti Hospital, Yasuj University of Medical Science, Yasuj, Iran

Hormat Rahimzadeh
Department of Internal Medicine, Sina Hospital, Tehran University of Medical Sciences, Tehran, Iran

Ammar Mohammad and Wael Sahyouni
Department of Vascular Surgery, Al-Assad University Hospital, Damascus, Syria

Taisser Almeree
Department of Radiology, Al-Assad University Hospital, Damascus, Syria

Bayan Alsaid
Department of General Surgery, Al-Assad University Hospital, Damascus, Syria
Laboratory of Anatomy, Faculty of Medicine, University of Damascus, Damascus, Syria

Graham T. Endler, Karleigh R. Curfman, Jason H. Hwang and John L. Gray
Duke LifePoint Conemaugh Memorial Medical Center, Johnstown PA 15905, USA

Duncan Muir
University of Bristol Medical School, UK

Sachin R. Kulkarni
Gloucestershire Hospitals NHS Foundation Trust, Cheltenham, UK

Index

www.ingramcontent.com/pod-product-compliance
Lightning Source LLC
LaVergne TN
LVHW082231200926
848484LV00008B/2335